Human Rights and Wrongs in Psychology and Psychiatry

Human Rights and Wrongs in Psychology and Psychiatry

Edited by

Malcolm MacLachlan

*Professor of Psychology & Social Inclusion, Department of Psychology
Maynooth University, Ireland*

Ikenna D. Ebuenyi

*Assistant Professor, Department of Rehabilitation Science and Technology,
University of Pittsburgh, PA, USA*

Brendan D. Kelly

*Professor of Psychiatry and Consultant Psychiatrist, Department of Psychiatry,
Trinity College Dublin, Ireland*

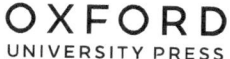
OXFORD
UNIVERSITY PRESS

OXFORD
UNIVERSITY PRESS

Great Clarendon Street, Oxford, OX2 6DP,
United Kingdom

Oxford University Press is a department of the University of Oxford.
It furthers the University's objective of excellence in research, scholarship,
and education by publishing worldwide. Oxford is a registered trade mark of
Oxford University Press in the UK and in certain other countries.

Published in the United States of America by Oxford University Press
198 Madison Avenue, New York, NY 10016, United States of America.

British Library Cataloguing in Publication Data
Data available

Library of Congress Control Number: 2025949510

ISBN 978–0–19–889157–4

DOI: 10.1093/med/9780198891574.001.0001

Printed and bound by
CPI Group (UK) Ltd., Croydon, CR0 4YY

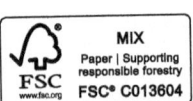

The manufacturer's authorised representative in the EU for product safety is
Oxford University Press España S.A. of Parque Empresarial San Fernando de Henares,
Avenida de Castilla, 2 – 28830 Madrid (www.oup.es/en or product.safety@oup.com).
OUP España S.A. also acts as importer into Spain of products made by the manufacturer.

Contents

Contributors

Cian Aherne
Clinical Psychologist, Jigsaw, The National Centre for Youth Mental Health, Limerick, Ireland

Naima Ali
Independent Researcher, Melbourne, Australia

Patrick Bracken
Independent Psychiatrist and WHO Consultant, Cork, Ireland

Rachel Brown
Department of Psychology, Maynooth University, Ireland

Anastasia Campbell
School of Law and Criminology, Maynooth University, Ireland

Cornelia Carey
Senior Registrar in Psychiatry, Discipline of Psychiatry, Trinity Centre for Health Sciences, Tallaght University Hospital, Trinity College Dublin, Ireland

Shemana Cassim
Senior Lecturer, School of Psychology, Massey University, Auckland, New Zealand

Kenneth Chambaere
Professor of Public Health, Sociology and Ethics, End-of-Life Care Research Group, Ghent University, Belgium

Finbarr Colfer
Health Information and Quality Authority, Galway, Ireland

Paul D'Alton
Associate Professor, School of Psychology, Department of Psychology, St Vincent's University Hospital, University College Dublin, Ireland

Ikenna D. Ebuenyi
Assistant Professor, Department of Rehabilitation Science and Technology, School of Health and Rehabilitation Sciences, University of Pittsburgh, PA, USA; Department of Behavioral and Community Health Sciences, School of Public Health, University of Pittsburgh, PA, USA

Priscille Geiser
Independent Consultant in Disability Rights and Inclusive Development, Lyon, France

Caoimhe Gleeson
National Office for Human Rights and Equality Policy, Health Service Executive, Donegal, Ireland

Kristijan Grđan
Mental Health Europe, Brussels, Belgium

Emma Hickey
Clinical Psychologist, Jigsaw, The National Centre for Youth Mental Health, Limerick, Ireland

Darrin Hodgetts
Professor of Societal Psychology, School of Psychology, Massey University, Auckland, New Zealand

Veronica Hopner
Senior Lecturer, School of Psychology, Massey University, Auckland, New Zealand

Edmund G. Howe III
Professor of Psychiatry, Uniformed Services University of the Health Sciences, Bethesda, USA

Julian C. Hughes
Honorary Professor, Bristol Medical School, University of Bristol, UK (Formerly consultant and professor of old age psychiatry)

Baher Ibrahim
Honorary Clinical Lecturer in Psychiatry,
Affiliate Researcher in History, University of
Glasgow, UK

Brendan D. Kelly
Professor of Psychiatry and Consultant
Psychiatrist, Department of Psychiatry,
Trinity College Dublin, Ireland

Jennifer Khan-Janif
Independent Researcher, Auckland, New
Zealand

Chapal Khasnabis
Head Office, World Health Organization,
Geneva, Switzerland

Thilo Kroll
Professor of Health Systems Management,
School of Nursing, Midwifery and Health
Systems, University College Dublin,
Ireland

Malcolm MacLachlan
Professor of Psychology and Social Inclusion,
Department of Psychology, and Assisting
Living and Learning Institute, Maynooth
University, Ireland
Visiting Professor, Department of Psychiatry
and Mental Health, University of Cape Town,
South Africa
Visiting Professor, Olomouc University
Social Health Institute, Palacky
University Olomouc, Czechia
Clinical Psychologist Advisor, Irish Health
Service (HSE)

Hasheem Mannan
School of Nursing, Midwifery and Health
Systems, University College Dublin, Ireland

Sílvia Marina
Faculty of Medicine, University of Porto,
Portugal
CINTESIS@RISE—Center for Health
Technology and Services Research, Porto,
Portugal

Claudia Marinetti
Mental Health Europe, Brussels, Belgium

Roy McConkey
Emeritus Professor of Developmental
Disabilities, Ulster University,
UK

J. McVeigh
Lecturer, ALL Institute and Dept of
Psychology, Maynooth University, Ireland

R. McVeigh
The Bar of Ireland, The Law Library,
Dublin, Ireland

Trudy Meehan
Lecturer, Centre for Positive Health Sciences,
RCSI, University of Medicine and Health
Sciences, Dublin, Ireland

Satish Mishra
European Office, World Health
Organization*, Copenhagen, Denmark

Cathal Morgan
European Office, World Health Organization,
Copenhagen, Denmark

Shaun T. O'Keeffe
Department of Geriatric Medicine, Galway
University Hospitals, Ireland

Derek Richards
School of Psychology, Trinity College Dublin,
Ireland
RED Digital Health Consulting, Dublin,
Ireland

Miguel Ricou
Faculty of Medicine, University of Porto,
Portugal
CINTESIS@RISE—Center for Health
Technology and Services Research, Porto,
Portugal

Sarah Robinson
Lecturer, School of Applied Social Studies,
University College Cork, Ireland

Matthé Scholten
Institute for Medical Ethics and History of Medicine, Ruhr University Bochum, Germany
Institute of Psychiatry, Psychology and Neuroscience, King's College London, UK

George Szmukler
Institute for Medical Ethics and History of Medicine, Ruhr University Bochum, Germany
Institute of Psychiatry, Psychology and Neuroscience, King's College London, UK

Rosalyn Tamming
National Disability Authority, Dublin, Ireland

Koen Titeca
Psychiatrist at AZ Groeninge Hospital, Courtrai, Belgium

Monica Verhofstadt
Expert with Lived Experience, Brussels, Belgium

Tony Wainwright
College of Life and Environmental Sciences, University of Exeter, UK

Michael Walsh
National Clinical Programme for People with Disability* (NCPPD), Ireland

Holly Wescott
Department of Psychology and Assisting Living and Learning Institute, Maynooth University, Ireland

---

*Affiliations are given for when authors were part of the Ireland/WHO Working Group on Rights Based Leadership and Governance

1

Rights and Wrongs in the Psych Professions

Malcolm MacLachlan, Ikenna D. Ebuenyi, and Brendan D. Kelly

Introduction

The practice of psychiatry and of several disciplines within psychology (e.g. clinical, counselling, educational, health and forensic psychology) presents a plethora of ethical issues, which also overlap with many concerns in other branches of medicine, as well as in nursing, social work, speech and language therapy and occupational therapy. Within this complex field of intersections between psychology, psychiatry, mental health, disability and human rights, different ideologies, social and power structures, and the role of patients or service users, compete for legitimacy, resources and authority. These varying perspectives 'read' ethical challenges and dilemmas in very different ways. This book addresses some of the most fascinating, uncomfortable, complex and pressing dilemmas experienced by both service users and service providers across mental health, disability, aging, rehabilitation and related services.

Our aim in this book is to help people *think through* ethics, by considering rights and wrongs, in: (1) a problem-based learning format, (2) the personal morality of 'right or wrong', (3) the professional ethics of clinical practice relating to 'right or wrong' and (4) through actions that promote 'human rights or wrongs' in terms of international conventions or national laws.

Professional bodies provide a set of ethical principles by which their practitioners should abide. However, these are rarely addressed in a problem-focused manner and the 'thinking through'—perhaps of competing ethical principles—is sometimes left to isolated individuals in pressing and difficult circumstances.

Most of the chapters in this book present no easy answers. The spirit of their dilemmas is not embraced by existing theories around morality, ethics, laws or rights; and indeed, these elements may contradict each other in some case studies. The practitioner is left with an uneasiness, an acute awareness of uncertainty, perhaps between their own morality, their professions' ethics, the State's laws and international human rights. We do not seek to provide 'fixes' for each of the difficult situations described, but rather to acknowledge that uncertainty and unease are common experiences to many clinical dilemmas. As Bekas (2013) acknowledges, 'uncertainty is the rule, and the individual and their context are as important as the syndrome in planning care'.

Morality, ethics and human rights are 'good things'. It is hard to find support for immoral or unethical acts, or for undermining human rights. But it's also hard to find explicit acknowledgement that all these 'good things' do not always go together, and indeed sometimes they may contradict each other. This volume explores the contradictions and difficulties that all practitioners in the psych fields experience, at least some of the time, when it comes down to deciding *what is the right thing to do*. We are interested in exploring those situations where rights and wrongs interplay; where personal morality, cultural diversity, professional ethics, national laws and international human rights treaties do not necessarily align; where practitioners may not feel comfortable airing private dilemmas in public, including with managers or other practitioners. We aim not to tell you how you should think about dilemmas, but to highlight things that should be considered, systematically thought through, influencing your conclusion and action. Sometimes this process may take weeks, at other times you only have minutes.

The applied sciences of psychology and psychiatry encompass both practitioners in those disciplines and those of other disciplines who use and contribute to the psych field—occupational therapists, general practitioners, occupational health physicians, social workers, speech and language therapists, nurses, and others. While there are certainly distinct challenges for each of these professions, there are also many common challenges across all of them. While we focus mostly on common challenges, we also consider some challenges distinct to some types of practitioners.

Morality, Ethics, Laws and Rights

Morality, rights and ethics are to do with values, and values are about what you feel is right and what is wrong, desirable or important, but it also refers to the 'worth, usefulness, or importance attached to something' (APA, 2018). Values are not just abstract, they are actual—they influence what you do. And values differ across groups, contexts and cultures (MacLachlan, 2006). In this volume we consider individual values to define a person's sense of morality, while the values of professional groups define ethical principles, that is, values to which members of a group feel an obligation to uphold. This obligation may be to each other, to the public or to both. Individual and professional values are of course embedded in broader cultural and subgroup identities. At the national level, one of the ways in which values are expressed is in laws which may well differ considerably across jurisdictions. At the international level, values are represented in human rights—a series of United Nations' declarations and conventions—that purport to describe values that apply to all people, everywhere.

Table 1.1 summarizes the relationship between values and how they play out at different levels of identity. They are not neatly stacked upon one another as the table might suggest, but rather may coexist uneasily, sometimes non-commensurate and sometimes simply contradictory. Indeed, as we move from the values of individuals to so-called universal values, there is great scope for difference. And so, sometimes, if

Table 1.1 The relationship between unit of identity, types of values and their associated meaning

Unit of identity	How values are expressed	Meaning
Individual	Morality	Personal values, an individuals' sense of right or wrong, of what is acceptable or unacceptable.
Group/ professional body	Ethics	Group value principles (or reasoned beliefs) established by distinct groups, including different professions, which develop ethical principles to guide both personal and collective behaviour, to promote positive outcomes and discourage negative outcomes, both for health service users and service providers.
National	Laws	Laws are societal rules that apply to all individuals and have a stated punitive or protective consequence if not followed.
International/ global	Human rights	Rights are entitlements, a service, opportunity or condition that a person should experience.

we want to act morally, be ethical, obey laws and uphold human rights, it is difficult to know what is the right thing to do. From the point of view of the psych disciplines, we now turn to look at these issues more closely.

Before we do that let us, as editors, acknowledge that while we all share a fundamental commitment to doing what it right for people, we do not necessarily always agree on what that is. We consider this to be one of the strengths of this volume—we take our differences as a useful starting point to navigate the challenges around morality, ethics, laws and human rights. To just take one example, between the three of us we may use different terms to refer to what we take to be the same experiences. One of the areas of interest in this volume is mental health. The terms 'mental illness' and 'mental health problems' are used by different members of the editorial team to refer to experiences of anxiety, depression, schizophrenia, and so on. The former term—'mental illness'—may be taken by some to imply a biological causal or at least a biologically mediated process, while the latter term—'mental health problems'—may be taken to imply that such problems are rooted in everyday living, psychological and/or social issues. In this volume we use the term 'mental health conditions' as something which is perhaps somewhere between the two, whilst also being the terminology used by the World Health Organization's QualityRights programme.

Its noteworthy that prominent diagnostic systems (such as Diagnostic and Statistical Manual of Mental Disorders 5th edition (DSM) or International Classification of Diseases, 11th revision (ICD11) do not use any of these terms (American Psychiatric Association, 2013; World Health Organization, 2022) rather they refer to 'mental disorders'. The names we give things influence how we think about them—that's why we name them the way we do! So, in using the term 'mental health conditions' we are not implying or privileging one causal pathway over another, one diagnostic tradition, or a categorical vs a dimensional approach. In the context of continued debate and contestation of causes, understandings and approaches to helping, we recognize that using words that seek to impose one understanding over others is not helpful, and indeed it is disrespectful to those with different views, whether they be service users or other service providers. Words that seek to disempower others have moral, ethical, legal and rights implications and illustrate just one of the ways in which many of us can unintentionally undermine others. As well as such subtle issues, this volume will also address very obvious and very difficult dilemmas—from involuntary confinement to the allocations of scarce resources, to how digital development may change services and offer new dilemmas and challenges.

Against this background, this volume presents a range of views on a wide diversity of themes. Clinical topics include euthanasia, assisted suicide, advance directives, treatment without consent, psychologists as community scribes and the use of antipsychotic medication in delirium and dementia. Other contributions focus on professions, politics and social change, the institutionalization of people with intellectual disability, the politics of diagnosis, constitutional law, and rights-based leadership and governance in health and social care services.

All these discussions present various ethical and moral dimensions, but ethics are brought into particular focus in chapters exploring ethical issues in different mental health conditions (including dementia) and developing theories of change to address human rights and wrongs. In terms of other initiatives and proposed solutions, various chapters examine mental health e-technologies, assisted decision-making, the WHO QualityRights programme, mental health advocacy, public and patient involvement in services, and task-shifting or task-sharing as a response to the dearth of human resources for mental health.

Self-Reflection in Psychiatry and Psychology

Before looking more into morality, ethics, laws and rights, we want to briefly stand back and acknowledge first that the history of the psych disciplines is one where at least some people feel that very significant harms and wrongs have been done. Furthermore, some contend that harms continue to be done, that we continue to undermine rights (Rubin & Flores, 2020). Part of the process of developing a self-conscious and critical-reflective approach is to be able to hear those criticisms and to understand the basis on which we react to them, our positionality and how that plays out in our personal behaviour and in the professional stances that we adopt. We must be open to the possibility of being wrong and needing to improve, without fearing that the edifice of the psych professions will crumble. Can they be that fragile in the view of some people and at the same time be as useful to humanity as many of us believe them to be, or to be as useful as they could be?

Wrongs in Psychology and Psychiatry

Both psychology and psychiatry attempt to understand and address human distress and to improve well-being across a broad range of areas including mental health, disability, neurodiversity, ageing, child development, reproduction and rehabilitation. It is important to remember that, as well as seeking to do good and doing good, individual practitioners and these professions have also, on occasion, done harm and increased distress. In retrospect, sometimes the methods they have used may—by today's standards—be considered naïve and harmful, and motivated more by a concern for professional power than for the well-being of those who should have received help. Perhaps in future some of what we do today will be viewed in a similar light. The only way we can guard against such harms is to seek out, acknowledge and reflect on the situations that we as practitioners, service users or others consider difficult, conflicting or wrong. Let's briefly consider some of the more notable historical wrongs associated with the psych professions.

The history of psychology is punctuated with changing practices and values. This includes Galton embracing eugenics, the Nazi party engaging *Völkerpsychologie* ('folk psychology') the utilization of psychology to justify apartheid (Hendrik Verwoerd the President of South Africa who introduced apartheid was previously a professor of psychology at Stellenbosch University), and the role of psychologists in the extra-judicial capture and containment of people in Guantanamo Bay, and their subsequent torture in a context designed to eschew national laws and international human rights (Hoffman et al., 2015). Such wrongs are not just a thing of the past: with aversion therapy, applied behavioural analysis, the industry of psychometric diagnosis and the 'industrialization' of therapy continue to draw strong contemporary critiques. Fundamentally the science of psychology has also been challenged by confirmation bias, underreporting of experiments that did not 'work', the difficulty in replicating some key studies, the misuse of statistics and the gap between theory and practice that is often observed, particularly in the field of psychotherapy. Equally concerning is the focus on WEIRD psychology. WEIRD stand for Western, Educated, Industrialized, Rich and Democratic (Henrich et al., 2010), and the critique is that the vast majority of participants in published studies in the leading journals are drawn from this very narrow selection of the world's population.

The history of psychiatry is also characterized by changing values and practices. These range from bizarre historic treatments such as hanging people up-side-down from ceilings, to ill-conceived and now abandoned lobotomies, to insulin-induced shock. Psychiatry is also of course linked with experimentation in World War II concentration camps and being complicit in the unwarranted confinement of 'enemies of the state'. Controversy continues around involuntary confinement, and the use of electric shocks and drugs to influence mental states and behaviours. Institutionalization and transinstitutionalization of individuals with disabilities or mental health conditions and those with dissenting voices by state actors continues (Schildbach &

Schildbach, 2018; Steinerte et al., 2012). Some of these topics are explored throughout this book.

Morality

Kohlberg's cognitive moral development (CMD) theory describes moral decision making from an individual perspective (Kohlberg, 1971). It identifies three levels of human moral development. At the pre-conventional level, individuals are motivated by self-interest, obedience, rewards and punishment. At the conventional stage, individuals do what is expected by others: they are concerned with social and interpersonal accord and conformity. The post-conventional stage (the most developed stage according to the theory) is where more autonomous decision making is demonstrated, including concerns with social contracts, universal principles and individual rights. Kohlberg's interest was in how decisions were made—the principles used—rather than if the decisions were right or wrong.

The theory is over 50 years old now and may be criticized in terms of its focus on social justice, as opposed to, or in combination with, other important values, such as caring; for being androcentric or culturally encapsulated; or simply because people demonstrate inconsistency in moral judgements (Krebs & Denton, 2005). Nonetheless, the theory does contain elements that may resonate with some of the challenges described in this volume. For instance, an individual's wish to avoid sanction, feelings of conformity and loyalty to an in-group, a concern with the social contract and individual's rights.

Like so many other areas of research in the psych disciplines there has been an exponential increase in interest and research on moral development and moral psychology in general, with some 21 different psychometric instruments now available to measure them (Martí-Vilar, et al., 2023). But let us consider one avenue of research on moral psychology which we believe is particularly relevant to our context. Building on research in cognitive psychology, Haidt (2007) argues that people respond to moral dilemmas in two separate but interconnected ways. Firstly, they use *moral intuition* to make judgements which are fast, automatic and usually emotional: so-called 'hot' affective responses. These tend to be simplistic evaluations—someone is good or bad, or I like or dislike someone. The second type of judgement is *moral reasoning*, which is a much slower, more deliberative and more rational process where the person is cognitively searching for and weighing up evidence. This process is therefore more complex and allows for more nuanced judgment. Moral intuition happens first, which may then be followed up by moral reasoning. Haidt uses the example of incest between two adult siblings who are both consenting, who enjoy a sexual experience, but do not repeat it. 'I don't know, I can't explain it, I just know it's wrong' is one response. The intuitive reaction frames the person's response, even though a more considered reflection might conclude that there is nothing fundamentally 'wrong', but it is emotionally unacceptable and evokes in many a response of disgust. Thus, it is an automatic response with emotional intensity that embodies moral judgement here. Does this happen in other contexts?

Moral foundations theory seeks to understand the origins and the variation in moral reasoning. It hypothesizes the existence of innate 'foundations' which are considered universal, but which may play out in different ways. These moral foundations are concerned with care, fairness, loyalty, authority and sanctity (Kesebir & Haidt, 2010).

The Harm/Care foundation is concerned for the suffering of others, with the primary moral emotion of compassion and its associated evolutionary benefit of more effective parenting. The Fairness/Reciprocity foundation is concerned with unfair treatment, cheating, justice and rights. The primary moral emotions associated with their presence or absence are anger/gratitude/guilt. This has the evolutionary value of encouraging cooperation and discouraging cheating.

The Ingroup/Loyalty foundation concerns obligations of group membership, such as loyalty, self-sacrifice and vigilance against betrayal. Here, the primary moral emotions are about the importance of ingroup loyalty and pride, belongingness and rage against traitors. From an evolutionary perspective, these emotions encourage more cohesive groups with better chances of survival in competitive or resource scarce environments.

The Authority/Respect foundation concerns social order, obligations to hierarchical relationships (obedience, respect) and fulfilment of role-based duties. The primary moral emotions are respect and fear. The idea here is that the ability to navigate complex social arrangements, including hierarchy, gave evolutionary advantage.

The Purity/Sanctity foundation concerns physical and spiritual contagion and virtues of chastity, wholesomeness and the control of desires. The primary moral emotion associated with failing to fulfil this foundation is disgust. Its evolutionary advantage is understood to be based on food-related evolutionary adaptations but also developed to encompass avoiding 'pollution' of the body.

Later versions of the theory incorporate other foundations and its five-factor structure does not necessarily hold up across different contexts (Kivikangas et al., 2021), where it may be argued that a two-factor structure ('Care/Fairness' and 'Loyalty/Authority/Purity'; Curry, 2019) provides a better model fit for the vast amounts of data that have been generated globally to empirically test the theory. Regardless of the distinctiveness of the five factors, their thematic relevance has been empirically demonstrated, and these themes resonate with health and social service contexts (Chan, 2021; Damsté & Kramer, 2023; Forkus & Weiss, 2021).

Ethics

According to the American Psychological Association (APA), evidence-based practice is about *integrating* the best research evidence available, with clinical expertise gained through experience and applied in relation to context of the person's/patient's characteristics, their cultural background and their personal preferences. However, Berg (2019) claims that while the APA extolls this tripartite model of evidence-based practice, in practice 'it is defined by science alone'. He also argues that clinical expertise and the person's/patient's preferences should be defined 'extra-scientifically' and not be 'perpetually controlled by scientific or propositional knowledge'. Berg sees the necessity of practitioner knowledge transcending scientific knowledge—which cannot reach into the peculiarities of everyday clinical practice contexts and clients. Furthermore, from a rights-based perspective if persons are to be able to influence their own treatment/actions then their preferences have to be meaningfully incorporated into practice, including treatment preferences which others may feel are unwise. Thus, acting on 'preferences' is an end in itself, and should not be seen simply as a means to other ends (such as, improved efficiency or efficacy, no matter how desirable these may be).

Berg (2019) also draws our attention to the fact that people's choices are culturally and contextually embedded. This is especially so where issues such as morality, ethics and rights are involved, especially in the context of different experiences, understanding and preferences about health and how to promote and achieve it, mental or physical. Berwick (2003) criticizes the approach of professional ethical codes as being counterproductive. Instead, he argues that to reduce the likelihood of errors and wrong-doing and to encourage and improve positive behaviours, a systematic approach to quality improvement is needed. Berwick fears that requiring adherence to professional ethics codes may in fact deter error reporting and limit the opportunity to learn from such errors. New approaches to error reporting could help address this matter.

In their paper 'Do Ethical Guidelines Give Guidance?', Eriksson et al. (2008) reviewed ethical guidelines, and particularly their stance on informed consent. They concluded that these guidelines do not really offer much guidance! They argued this was because of three problems which they identified as: the *interpretation* problem, the *multiplicity* problem and the *legalization* problem. The interpretation problem occurs where a practitioner must interpret generic rules in specific contexts and determine their applicability. To do this, they must have some ethical frame to make such an interpretation, and such theoretical frames may differ greatly between individuals. Furthermore, even within the same guidelines, there may be contradictory 'rules' regarding how a practitioner should respond in a given situation that may encompass several distinct ethical elements.

The multiplicity problem relates to the number of ethical codes, guidelines and values that practitioners and researchers encounter: 'there is a multiplicity of guidelines of both ethical and legal nature pulling in different directions [and] different guidelines may give different recommendations regarding how to handle a situation' (p. 2). The legalization problem refers to the increasing tendency for ethical issues to be pursued through legal recourse, while the role of legislation and its interaction with ethics, is rarely discussed in ethical guidelines. An example of the latter is where one of us (MM) was required to develop new clinical guidance because of a High Court decision (in Ireland), a decision which he disagreed with and felt that the approach required by the High Court was an inefficient and less effective use of the scarce resources available to serve people on lengthening waiting lists. Following the necessity to comply with the law and to implement revised clinical guidelines, within 2 years the number of people of waiting lists had increased five-fold. Thus, the clinical lead for the service was caught between the legal necessity of complying with a High Court decision and knowing that the consequence of doing so would disimprove the service. Whilst legally correct, it is hard to square this with professional ethics or a rights-based approach.

Eriksson et al. conclude that 'there simply are no quick fixes in the world of ethical decision making' (p. 14) and they argued that no number of new guidelines will address this. Rather 'Ethical competence is needed to deal with the problems as they arise' (p. 14). In this volume, our approach is very much aligned with Ericksson et al. as we seek to stimulate practitioners to critically reflect on the interplay between morality, ethics, rights and laws, and in so doing to enhance their competence in justly navigating clinical situations that often do not fit into neat boxes and often invite contradictory ethical interpretations. Sometimes, we need a compass, especially when there is no map.

Andersson et al. (2022) state that 'Healthcare professionals and students in clinical practice are confronted daily with difficult choices and must cope with questions of 'rightness' or 'wrongness' that influence their decision-making and the quality of the care provided' (p. 2). Developing the concept of ethical competence, Andersson et al. reviewed literature on education seeking to promote ethical competence among healthcare professionals and students. They identified three broad themes: firstly, creating the conditions and developing strategies that make learning ethical competence possible; secondly, being aware of your own thoughts and perceptions; thirdly, doing the right thing in terms of aligning with the person's/patient's interests. They also stress that 'An important aspect emphasised in the present study is the need to create a psychosocial climate that allows healthcare professionals and students to feel safe' (p. 22). And they go on to argue that 'To do the right and good thing, ... emphasises the healthcare professionals' and students' personal experiences, understanding, and views ... cultivated, for example, through reflection' (p. 23). This they stress is a skill, one which we aim to cultivate through this book.

Leach and Harbin (1997) analysing the percentage of the United States APA code found in other country codes. The overarching six 'Aspirational Principles' of the APA ethics code are Competence; Integrity; Professional and Scientific Responsibility; Respect for People's Rights and Dignity; Concern for Human Welfare; and Social Responsibility (with specific standards documented separately). While all the ethical principles were found to be mentioned in some form in the corresponding professional psychology ethical standards in Australia, Canada, Israel and South Africa, only half of them were found in Hong Kong, the Netherlands and Singapore; 17% in the Dominican Republic, and none in China. Overlapping ethical principles may reflect shared values with US ethical codes or cultural assumptions but do not support a universalist position for ethical principles. They may also reflect the different sort of work psychologists in different countries are involved in (e.g. a broad range of therapies in the US and primarily assessment in China). Reflecting on the complexity of human rights and ethical codes, Gauthier (2018) argues that 'it is unclear what source psychologists should use when interpreting references to human rights in codes of ethics'.

O'Donoghue (2020) articulates a number of criticisms of the APA ethics code including that it does not support ethical relativism, that is, the idea that principles may be contingent on contextual variable (e.g. time, place or demographic characteristics). Furthermore, he argues that some of the issues addressed in ethical codes are not ethical matters but rather issues of prudent practice, such as record keeping. He sees the codes as too broad in scope one the one hand and too narrow in their individualistic focus, seeing only individuals as making ethical decisions, rather than these also possibly being embedded in teams, institutions or cultures.

Holm's (2011) asks 'Who should decide the content of professional ethics?' and argues that while service users/patients have the strongest claim for influencing professional codes of ethics, as they are the most affected by them, they are rarely consulted or have any meaningful input to them. Furthermore, different categories of practitioners may well respond differently to the same ethical principles. For instance, Gilligan (2016) suggested that while females are more likely to reason with an 'ethics of care' and be concerned with relationships and interconnectedness, males are more likely to reason in relation to following rules. Clearly there are many other forms of intersectionality (age, experience, cultural identify, experience of difficulties, sexual orientation, etc.) that can influence how ethical codes or guidelines are interpreted or enacted (see later section in this chapter on positionality and reflection). We now briefly mention three dominant ethical frameworks, although we will not be recommending any particular one of them and will be noting how they can be in conflict.

Virtue ethics focus on the idea of being a 'good person'. According to Knapp et al. (2017), 'Virtues are character traits that have moral value' (p. 17): these traits are acquired over time, through practice, with the individual becoming a more virtuous person. This approach recognizes, correctly, that it is simply not realistic to have ethical rules for all circumstances; and so, it seeks to build character. The basic idea is that practicing virtues makes one more ethical. However, this approach does not lead to systematic ethical decision-making, but rather one that is more akin to being oriented by a moral compass.

Deontological ethics focus on fulfilling one's 'duty'. Kant believed that people should behave ethically to fulfil their duty as citizens towards society. In deontology, intention is key, while consequence is not. If people follow a series of rules then they can feel assured that they are fulfilling their duty to society. To this end, deontology sees a range of actions as being universally ethical and as people being obliged to uphold these written or unwritten 'rules'.

In *utilitarianism* the moral value of an act is determined by its consequences. It also refers to hedonism (maximizing good) and universalism, i.e. that this applies across all people, and is not just for the good of the individual.

Rest (1994) contended that we should go through a particular sequence of thoughts and actions to behave ethically. These were: *ethical sensitivity* (identifying the presence of an ethical issue); *ethical reasoning* (formulating an ideal course of action); *ethical motivation* (deciding what one is actually going to do) and *ethical implementation* (executing the action). These matters are considered in various ways, and in more applied ways, next.

The Trolley Problem

A classic ethics dilemma, which appears in a broad range of guises, is referred to as 'The Trolley Problem' (Thomson, 1984). In this hypothetical situation a train (or trolley) is heading down the tracks and is about to run over five people who have been tied to the tracks. An onlooker—you—could pull a lever and send the train down another track. However, on this alternative track there is one person tied to the track. So, what do you do? Do nothing (and act of omission) and five people die or pull the lever (an act of commission—you commit an act) and one person dies, but you save the other five who would have died if you did nothing. What would you do?

Let's change the scenario, rather than pulling a lever to change the direction of the train, imagine instead that you could push one very large older man off a bridge over the rail track and that this would bring the train to a halt before it reaches the five people tied to the track. Would you, do it?

Now change the large person to a young pregnant woman. Yes, that is very uncomfortable. Or imagine you are a surgeon with four patients on your in-patient ward who desperately need each of a heart, lung, liver and kidney, without which they will die within the next few weeks or months, unless they have these transplants. One of your patients has a visitor—she is strong, healthy and your guess has a perfectly good heart, lungs, liver and kidneys, and for a moment you wonder .... As you think through these scenarios did you apply virtue, deontological or utilitarian ethics? Did you think through the four stages described above? We imagine that most people do not do these things, and that they move from a utilitarian stance to one where this became increasingly uncomfortable, where you became more complicit and where your 'duty' may have felt unclear, and what might be considered virtuous also becomes opaque.

The Trolley Problem is a hypothetical thought experiment, and you will come across other thought experiments and reflective exercises throughout the chapters in this volume. But just how unrealistic are these sorts of 'Trolley Problems'—like dilemmas in the provision of services? Designing services often entails making deeply uncomfortable decisions capable of causing moral stress and injury. Virtually all health and social services are constrained by having fewer resources available than would be necessary to provide the services we want, and which people need and have a right to. For instance, with a given budget should a service support one individual with a very high level of support needs, being relocated from an institutional setting to live in a house in a community, as they have stated a wish to do? Or for the same budget should the service increase the number of personal assistance hours from 10 to 15 a week for 100 people who have a disability and live at home in the community, but do not have adequate opportunities to participant in their community, seek employment or access education?

Every year, budgets are allocated to some but not all needs. Should fewer but excellent services be provided to some, or should many people get an inadequate service that is better than no service at all? Do we continue to rely on specialized services provided by psych professionals, or should we adopt task sharing/shifting approaches to relieve the long waiting list for services? These decisions are being made all the time. People are being 'pushed off bridges' by inadequately addressing their needs, so that others can benefit from having the resources given to address their needs, but we are often too uncomfortable with these rationing decisions to make them clearly and openly. As a result, we disseminate decision-making about scarce resources across various systemic administrative functions, so that rationing occurs implicitly rather than explicitly. This means that, rather than deciding based on evidence and accountable moral choice, resource allocation is incremental and spread across multiple decision-makers, with few, if any, seeing the full picture the full consequences of making the big decisions. We often ration irrationally, in bursts and starts, often in the shadows.

Laws

As Dror (1957) stated, 'one of the more important repositories and expressions of the values of any society is its laws. … laws consist of a number of norms … closely related to various social values, being either a direct expression of them, or serving them in a more indirect way' (p. 440). Of course, some laws may be reflective of values from a previous age and are overturned by referendum or parliament to reflect the values of the current epoch. More emphatically, Maldonado (2019) states 'Law is culture, not its consequence' (p. 297). Temple University's Centre for Public Health Law (2024) research sees law as permeating culture, with legal rules becoming behavioural norms over time and thus law 'influences what people know or believe to be true, and shapes what people value' (p.1).

When it comes to national laws, different countries criminalize different sorts of discriminatory behaviour to different extents. Finland prohibits discrimination against persons with disability; Spain prohibits disability-based discrimination in employee recruitment; Luxembourg outlaws disability-based discrimination in the provision of goods and services. The breaking of disability laws can result in penalties of six months imprisonment in Australia or up to two years in Hong Kong. As Degener and Quinn (2021) conclude 'Our comparative survey found a wide diversity of legal approaches. To a degree, this is quite understandable given the diversity of the world's cultures and legal systems.'

Rains et al. (2019) found striking variations in the annual rate of involuntary hospital admissions in their comparison of 22 European countries, Australia and New Zealand; with Austria having the highest (282 per 100 000 individuals) and Italy the lowest (14·5 per 100 000 individuals). In the US, this varied from 29 per 100,000 to 966 per 100,000 across different states with a national average of 357 per 100 000

(Dunseith, 2020). From a values perspective different legal systems had different criteria for involuntary admission. For instance, 76% required that the individual poses a risk to themselves or others, and 24% did not. The exact opposite proportions related to a requirement that the individual does not have capacity—24% did have this requirement, 76% did not. Half of the countries (48%) required that the individual's condition should be treatable, and half did not (52%). Just over a third (38%) required that the next of kin or nearest relative be involved in the involuntary hospitalization process, whilst almost two thirds (62%) did not. Just under a third required that an individual be treated once hospitalized, whilst 71% did not. The criteria for admission (e.g. a diagnosis or not, or the type of diagnosis) and the rights of people confined involuntarily, also differed across countries.

Some of these differences no doubt reflect systematic and resource differences but also differences in values—what does the law require for those who are involuntarily admitted. Intriguingly, Rains et al. (2019) found that none of these differences in the legal frameworks across countries affected the rate of involuntary admission. Bed capacity which was related to admissions—the more beds in the system the more people were involuntarily admitted. Higher rates were also associated with higher GDP per capita purchasing power parity, healthcare spending per capita, the proportion of foreign-born individuals in the population and lower absolute poverty. Thus, values and cultural differences between countries may be 'trumped' by structural factors, but of course these structural factors (healthcare spending, proportion of foreign-born individuals and proportion living in absolute poverty) may also reflect national values enacted in relevant policies.

Rights

Human rights and wrongs are they core theme of this book. As the United Nations' Office of the High Commissioner for Human Rights (OHCHR) states: 'Human rights are rights we have simply because we exist as human beings—they are not granted by any state. These universal rights are **inherent** to us all, regardless of nationality, sex, national or ethnic origin, colour, religion, language, or any other status' (https://www.ohchr.org/en/what-are-human-rights, 2023).

Such rights have far reaching characteristics. They are *universal*, meaning they apply to all people, everywhere. This central right recurs in many international human rights conventions, declarations and resolutions. Human rights are also *inalienable*, meaning they cannot be removed, except where an established legal process has been followed (such as imprisonment for a crime removing the right to freedom, following an appropriate judicial process). Human rights are *indivisible and interdependent*, meaning it is the combination of a range of different rights that allows the full realization of single rights. So, the exercising or violating of civil and political rights affects economic, social and cultural rights, and vice versa.

Rights are also equal and non-discriminatory. Article 1 of the Universal Declaration of Human Rights (UDHR) asserts that 'All human beings are born free and equal in dignity and rights.' It is freedom from discrimination (Article 2) which ensures equality, and discrimination is one of the challenges which repeatedly presents itself across the broad range of situations described in this volume. Under international law, to ensure human rights are fulfilled, States have obligations and duties to all of us, as citizens. The three primary obligations are to *respect* (not interfere with or curtail) rights; to *protect* individuals and groups against human rights abuses; and to take positive action *fulfil* rights, not just hope they will be realized.

Morality, ethics, laws and rights express desired behaviours, but they are, of course, also themselves an expression of values, beliefs and practices that bind people together. However, values, beliefs and practices also differ, across cultures, contexts and social structures, especially within the context of health (MacLachlan, 2006). The scope and perception of rights are often shaped by national and cultural beliefs and practice which in turn limit a universal application of human rights (Ebuenyi et al., 2019). Also, national and political laws or boundaries may limit the realization of rights. For instance, although Article 13 of the UDHR declares that 'Everyone has the right to freedom of movement and residence within the borders of each state' in reality, this is individual and nation specific. Although it is understandable that individual choices may limit the exercise of this right when it concerns acts considered a deviation from set legal principles, which may or may not entail harm to another individual, there is evidence of limitation of these rights especially for individuals with mental health conditions. The institutionalization of individuals with intellectual and or psychosocial disabilities as documented in Chapter 7 curtails the freedom of movement.

Article 23 and 26 of the UDHR specifics that all have rights to Employment and Education. The extent to which this is feasible depends on several factors, and for people with various forms of disabilities, these rights are difficult to realize and, in some countries, non-existent. Individuals with psychosocial disabilities in low-resource settings are often consciously excluded from technical and vocational programmes which are means of education to prepare for work and or employment (Ebuenyi et al., 2018). Similarly, discriminatory employer practices continue to limit employment opportunities in both low- and high-income counties. In Africa, only about 1% of persons with psychosocial disabilities are employed (Ebuenyi, 2019) while in Europe and America this is between 20% and 40% (Harris et al., 2019). Hence, despite the elaborate recommendations of the UDHR and the Convention on the Rights of Persons with Disabilities on the inalienable rights to education, work and employment, realization of rights continues to elude the most vulnerable amongst us.

How Rights Are Structured within the United Nations

There are eight treaty bodies within the United Nations network of organizations:

a. The **Human Rights Committee** focuses on civil and political rights;
b. The **Committee on Economic, Social and Cultural Rights** (CESCR) monitors implementation of the International Covenant on Economic, Social and Cultural Rights;

c. The **Committee on the Elimination of Racial Discrimination** (CERD) addresses issues of racial discrimination;

d. The **Committee on the Elimination of Discrimination against Women** (CEDAW) addresses women's rights and discrimination against women;

e. The **Committee against Torture** (CAT) focuses on torture and ill treatment;

f. The **Committee on the Rights of the Child** (CRC) addresses child rights;

g. The **Committee on Migrant Workers** (CMW) focuses on the rights of migrant workers and members of their families; and

h. The **Committee on the Rights of Persons with Disabilities** is the newest body and addresses the rights of disabled people.

While these documents are meant to interact in complimentary ways, this does not always happen. The pronouncements of these bodies can contradict each other in fundamental ways, as is the case with admission and treatment without consent for severe mental health conditions, which is inconsistent with the UN Committee on the Rights of Persons with Disabilities' current interpretation of the Convention on the Rights of Persons with Disabilities, but accepted by the UN Human Rights Committee (2014) and UN Subcommittee on Prevention of Torture and Other Cruel, Inhuman or Degrading Treatment or Punishment (2016), under certain, limited circumstances (see Kelly, 2025, pp. 110–116, for more detailed discussion and sources).

Justice

There are some concepts that are related to morality, ethics, rights and laws, which are also worth highlighting in this Introduction to our volume. Haile et al. (2020) note that, while the APA's ethical principles have 'justice' as one of five core principles, it does not unpack the concept or think through its implications. The APA states: 'Psychologists recognize that fairness and justice entitle all persons access to and benefit from the contributions of psychology and to equal quality in the processes, procedures, and services being conducted by psychologists. Psychologists exercise reasonable judgment and take precautions to ensure that their potential biases, the boundaries of their competence, and the limitations of their expertise do not lead to or condone unjust practices' (APA, 2017, General Principles, Principle D)

Hailes et al. (2020) propose that three primary domains of justice—originating in social and organizational psychology—can be applied to flesh out the commitment to social justice: *Interactional* justice is about *how people treat each other*, that is, relational dynamics or the perceived fairness of interpersonal interaction, especially relating to power dynamics. *Distributive* justice is about the perceived fairness of *who gets what* outcomes (from remuneration, to prison sentences to promotion, etc.) and particularly so for the underprivileged. *Procedural* justice is about *how decisions are made*, that is, the perceived fairness of the process used to decide on the outcomes.

For at least some practitioners, it is insufficient to work only at the micro-level (e.g. providing psychotherapy or drugs for people) when an individuals' suffering is clearly also associated with oppressive social norms, policies or institutions (Goodman et al., 2004; Kinderman, 2021; MacLachlan & McVeigh, 2021). Increasingly there is recognition that practitioners also have a role in addressing meso-level (organizational) and macro-level (societal) injustices (Kelly, 2005)

Hailes et al. (2020) apply the three domains from organizational psychology to social justice through identification of seven issues to be addressed by practitioners: reflecting critically on relational power dynamics; mitigating relational power dynamics; focusing on empowerment and strengths-based approaches; focusing energy and resources on the priorities of marginalized communities; contributing time, funding and effort to preventive work; engaging with social systems; and raising awareness about system impacts on individual and community well-being.

Archer et al. (2020) also describe epistemic power: 'A person has epistemic power to the extent she is able to influence what people think, believe, and know, *and* to the extent she is able to enable and disable others from exerting epistemic influence' (p. 29). Clearly both psychiatry and psychology possess considerable epistemic power in terms of defining the existence or non-existence of problems/conditions/illnesses, legitimizing different interventions (such as different types of psychological or pharmacological treatments), and influencing research agenda and health services spending.

This can be problematic. Hutton and Cappellini (2022), in their article 'Epistemic in/justice: Towards "Other" ways of knowing' refer, in particular, to the role of knowledge hierarchies in this—that some 'ways of knowing' are credited as better than others. They talk about people being 'epistemically harmed' by having their knowledge dismissed or made less legitimate by others with more power and different types of knowledge, who do not give due credence to other types of knowledge. For instance, psychologists and psychiatrists may privilege diagnostic systems (such as DSM5 or ICD11) over other ways of understanding people's experience. When such arguments are anchored in professional standards or norms, they may be considered forms of 'identity-based social power' (Fricker, 2007).

The importance of 'lived experience' has been one response to the strength of professional power in health services. This is to counteract what Fricker describes as 'testimonial injustice', where in interpersonal communications, it is ' … the wrong that a speaker suffers in receiving deflated credibility from the hearer owing to identity prejudice on the hearer's part … ', leading to the speaker's knowledge not being accepted by the hearer (Fricker, 2007, p. 4). The term hermeneutical injustice is concerned with how power structures collective social understanding (Fricker, 2007). While there is a of course a very broad range of 'lived experience', acknowledging it does not necessarily imply difference to, or conflict with, professional knowledge or experience. Rather acknowledging lived experience is simply acknowledging that one person has not lived another person's experience, we have not 'walked in their shoes', even if we may travel in the same landscape. Acknowledging 'lived experience' is therefore about treating the person—and their perspective—with dignity, chiming with the UDHR's affirmation that all people should both have rights and be treated with dignity.

Trauma, Rights and National Laws

Those who seek to use health and social care services often come to those services because they have experienced difficult personal or social circumstances that may have had a traumatic effect on them. When these are experienced in childhood the term Adverse Childhood Experiences (ACEs) is often used to summarize them. The ACEs encompass a very broad range of experiences; from emotional, physical or sexual abuse, emotional or physical neglect, homelessness or incarceration; to witnessing domestic violence, maternal depression and withdrawal from the child, to divorce, substance misuse, and of course prior mental health or disability conditions. Such experiences are associated with a higher incidence of mental health conditions later in life (Ellis & Dietz, 2017). But there is also another type of ACE—Adverse Community Events. These include community violence or others forms of community disruption, poor quality housing, discrimination, poverty and a lack of opportunity, economic mobility and social capital. Where these factors interact—'double ACEs'—their effects may be greater and adverse community environments may predispose people to have fewer resources to manage the negative and potentially traumatizing effects of adverse childhood experiences.

The idea of trauma-informed services is not only that service providers should be aware of both personal and environmental factors that can precipitate mental health conditions, but also that practitioners should not adopt approaches to helping people which may in fact further traumatize them. While obvious examples of this may be forced treatments or involuntary admission to institutionalized care, other examples may include the person feeling disempowered by clinicians adopting paternalistic attitudes or hierarchical approaches to service delivery that may results in the person feeling they have little agency or decision-making power (Corrigan, 2016).

In many settings traumatizing behaviours or contexts are being reduced and staff are learning how to de-escalate difficult situations, but situations remain where staff believe that for a person's own good, or the good of others, they must take actions which may be traumatizing. So while national laws in many states require for those judged to be a danger, to themselves or others, to be detained, Article 1 (2) of the Convention on the Rights of Persons with Disabilities requires that 'Persons with disabilities include those who have long-term physical, mental, intellectual or sensory impairments which in interaction with various barriers may hinder their full and effective participation in society on an equal basis with others.' Furthermore, the Convention's Article 14—Liberty and security of the person requires that 'States Parties shall ensure that persons with disabilities, on an equal basis with others: (a) Enjoy the right to liberty and security of person; (b) Are not deprived of their liberty unlawfully or arbitrarily, and that any deprivation of liberty is in conformity with the law, and that the existence of a disability shall in no case justify a deprivation of liberty...'

This places practitioners in an invidious position where they might feel that they cannot uphold national law and international human rights at the same time; and where their professional ethics codes may not directly address this contradiction. The endorsement by some mental health service-users of the need for treatment without consent on the basis of impaired capacity adds a further layer of complexity to decision-making in this area (Gergel et al., 2021), along with the diametrically conflicting positions adopted by various UN bodies (see above, 'How Rights Are Structured within the United Nations'). We believe that the time is overdue for international human rights bodies, civil society, states representatives and professional bodies to acknowledge these difficulties and contradictions and to provide guidance that takes full account of the diversity of service-user views on this matter, and their families, This is certainly in the interests of service users, but also service providers who currently, in abiding by the law and executing their state-appointed, professional and ethical duties, may simultaneously be branded as 'human rights abusers' and experience moral injury, while also delivering effective care and support in accordance with the evidence bases of their professions (Kelly, 2025; Chapter 4).

Civil Society

Civil society organizations are key players in promoting and protecting human rights and preventing wrongdoing. Sometimes these organizations are comprised of a group with a single condition (e.g. the National Down Syndrome Society), or a group with diverse conditions but a common advocacy target (e.g. Psychiatric Survivors Movement), or they are more broadly representative in terms of umbrella bodies at national or international level (e.g. the International Disability Alliance, based in Geneva and New York, with a global mandate). The role of civil society is to push for what they see as improvements in services, informed by their range of experiences, and to hold government and other service providers to account in terms of its implementation of national laws or human rights treaties. For instance, the United Nations Disability Inclusion Strategy (UNDIS) was established to promote opportunities for civil society to influence both United Nations and state government laws and policies.

Many UN treaties are not 'justiciable', meaning they are not directly written into national laws but rather are meant to inform the application and sometimes the revision of those laws. States demonstrate their agreement with human rights instruments by *signing* them, and their commitment to abide by them by *ratifying* them. Such UN 'instruments' are thus often referred to as 'soft law'. They are attempting to influence social norms and what is considered acceptable by governments and citizens, but also what is considered acceptable by professions. Human rights are therefore often a process of persuasion, although sometimes they are also about litigation.

The representative bodies of professions seek to represent the interests of the members of their professions. They also wish to promote good services for those who use their profession. The balance between members' interests and the public interest is sometimes disputed. It is therefore also the role of civil society to hold professions to account and to advocate against what they consider to be practices which diminish the public's benefit—such as professions guarding their practice boundaries, charging high professional fees or engaging in coercive practices. Within the professions, practitioners may therefore feel 'attacked' by some civil society organizations, while supported by others. Sometimes this can result in professions 'othering' civil society, disregarding them or refusing to meet with them. We believe that all professional bodies should have a clear commitment to ways in which they can engage with civil society, to promote mutual learning and understanding, especially with those with whom we disagree most. Sometimes that understanding is simply understanding that there are many committed, passionate and expressive people, and that they are doing their jobs the best they can and/or living their reality as authentically as they can. The essence of the UN Convention on the Rights of Persons with Disabilities 'Nothing about us, without us'—calls for the participation of service users in all aspects of service development and provision.

Reflective Practice

Much of the research on the therapeutic relationship (between the person providing a service and the person receiving it) highlights its value in supporting beneficial outcomes (Duncan et al., 2010). The term 'transference' described how the person/client/patient may unknowingly transfer feelings about someone else onto the practitioner. The term 'countertransference' describes how the practitioner reacts to projections of the client/patient onto them, and it also includes the therapist's own transferring of feeling influencing some aspects of their encounters with other people. It is important for practitioners to be aware of what they bring with them and what they may symbolize to others, even if, and perhaps especially if, the practitioner does not embody what she may symbolize (MacLachlan, 2002). The term 'reflective practice' (Schon, 1983) describes the situation where practitioners seek to learn by reflecting on and are aware of how their prior experiences, their current circumstances or other factors may influence how they respond to others.

As stated by Andersson et al. (2022), 'Health-care professionals and students in clinical practice need a supportive learning environment in which they can experience a permissive climate for reflection on ethical challenges, conflicts, or dilemmas that influence everyday healthcare work.' (p. 24).

Practitioners are 'positioned' by many things—their professional identity, their social class, their experience of privilege, their colour, their gender identity, their experiences of mental health conditions or disabilities. Practitioners 'position' themselves and are 'positioned' by others. It is therefore important for us to think through morality, ethics, laws and rights by being aware of where we are thinking 'from'. As Nagel has demonstrated 'The View from Nowhere' (Nagel, 1989) does not exist, and it is actually being unscientific and biasing to ignore the experiences and views we bring to human encounters and how these may shape those encounters. Self-awareness adds rigor to what we can know from our interactions with others.

On this basis, we provide a selection of critical practice questions in Appendix 1.1. This list can be used in two ways. First, we suggest that it is useful to apply some of these questions to the case studies presented in various chapters within this volume. Second, we invite you to apply these questions to some of the moral,

Appendix 1.1

Rights & Wrongs—Critical Practice Questions

In relation to a case study in this book or a scenario in your own work use the questions below to help you critically reflect on it, including how you are positioned relevant to it.

1. **Emotional Response**

   What is your emotional reaction to it?

   Do you have a sense of liking/disliking any of the people in it?

   Have you experienced anything similar—either professionally or personally?

2. **Your own 'Social GRACES' which may influence your views***

   G: Gender, Gender Identity, Geography, Generation
   R: Race, Religion
   A: Age, Ability, Appearance
   C: Class, Culture, Caste
   E: Education, Ethnicity, Economics
   S: Spirituality, Sexuality, Sexual Orientation

3. **Structures**

   How does it relate to your own professional power, position or privilege?

   Do structural issues influence access or resources for some groups more than others, or the distribution of opportunities in relation to class, caste or location?

   Do cultural issues influence expectations or roles for people of different ages, different genders or regions?

4. **Re-telling**

   If you re-tell the story from the perspective of another person in the narrative, how does it change your view of it?

   Morals—what personal values does it trigger?

   Ethics—which professional ethical principles are most relevant?

   Laws—which national laws are most relevant?

   Rights—what Human Rights Conventions or Declarations or are most relevant to it?

   Conflict —do the above all align or is there some contradiction between them?

5. **Change**

   Would you do anything different in your own practice now?

   Has it changed your view of yourself in any way?

6. **Other**

   Are there other things that may influence how you feel, think or are likely to respond to it?

---

*See Burnham, J. (2018). Developments in Social GRRRAAACCEEESSS: visible–invisible and voiced–unvoiced 1. In *Culture and reflexivity in systemic psychotherapy* (pp. 139–160). Routledge.

ethical, legal, or rights difficulties or dilemmas you face in your daily life and your daily practice.

Ultimately, that is the fundamental purpose of this book: to bring moral and ethical reasoning more clearly into practice, for the benefit of all.

References

Adams, P. (2023a, 4 August). Blog post. https://www.routledge.com/blog/article/monster-metaphors-like-mental-illness-block-alternative-ways-of-tackling-big-issues

Adams, P. (2023b). *Monster metaphors: when rhetoric runs amok.* London: Routledge.

American Psychiatric Association. (2013). *Diagnostic and statistical manual of mental disorder* (5th ed.).

Andersson, H., Svensson, A., Frank, C. et al. (2022). Ethics education to support ethical competence learning in healthcare: an integrative systematic review. *BMC Medical Ethics 23*, Article 29 https://doi.org/10.1186/s12910-022-00766-z

APA. (2017). *Ethical Principles of Psychologists and Code of Conduct.* Washington: American Psychological Association.

APA. (2018). *Value: The American Psychological Association On-line Dictionary.* https://diction ary.apa.org/value

Archer, A., Cawston, A., Matheson, B., & Geuskens, M. (2020). Celebrity, democracy, and epistemic power. *Perspectives on Politics*, *18*(1), 27–42. doi:10.1017/S1537592719002615

Berg, H. (2019). Evidence-based practice in psychology fails to be tripartite: A conceptual critique of the scientocentrism in evidence-based practice in psychology. *Frontiers in Psychology: Theoretical and Philosophical Psychology*, *10.* https://doi.org/10.3389/fpsyg.2019.02253

Berwick, D. (2003). *Escape fire.* Jossey Bass.

Centre for Public Health Law. (2024). https://phlr.org/role-law-advancing-culture-health

Burnham, J. (2018). Developments in Social GRRRAAACCEEESSS: visible–invisible and voiced–unvoiced 1. In Inga-Britt Krause (Ed.), *Culture and reflexivity in systemic psychotherapy* (pp. 139–160). Routledge.

Chan, E. Y. (2021). Moral foundations underlying behavioral compliance during the COVID-19 pandemic. *Personality and Individual Differences*, *171*, 110463. doi: 10.1016/j.paid.2020.110463

Corrigan, P. W. (2016). Lessons learned from unintended consequences about erasing the stigma of mental illness. *World Psychiatry*, *15*(1), 67–73.

Curry, O. S. (2019). What's wrong with moral foundations theory, and how to get moral psychology right. *Behavioural Scientist*, 26 March. https://behavioralscientist.org/whats-wrong-with-moral-foundations-theory-and-how-to-get-moral-psychology-right/

Damsté, C., & Kramer, K. (2023). Moral intuitions about stigmatizing practices and *feeding* stigmatizing practices: how Haidt's moral foundations theory relates to infectious disease stigma. *Public Health Ethics*, *16*(1), 102–111. https://doi.org/10.1093/phe/phad002

Degener, T., & Quinn, G. (2021). *A Survey of International, Comparative and Regional Disability Law Reform.* In M. L. Breslin & S. Yee (Eds.), *Disability Rights Law and Policy: International and National Perspectives* (pp. 3–126). Brill. https://doi.org/10.1163/9789004478961_008

Duncan, B. L., Miller, S. D., Wampold, B. E., & Hubble, M. A. (2010). *The heart and soul of change: Delivering what works in therapy.* American Psychological Association.

Dunseith, L. (2020). Study finds involuntary psychiatric detentions on the rise. https://newsr oom.ucla.edu/releases/involuntary-psychiatric-detentions-on-the-rise

Dror, Y. (1957). Values and the Law. *The Antioch Review*, *17*(4), 440–454, https://doi.org/10.2307/4610000

Ebuenyi, I. D. (2019). *Inclusive employment: understanding the barriers to and facilitators of employment for persons with mental disability in East Africa* (Publication no: 9789402816877) [Doctoral dissertation, Vrije University, Amsterdam].

Ebuenyi, I. D., Regeer, B. J., Nthenge, M., Nardodkar. R., Waltz. M., & Bunders-Aelen, J. F. (2019). Legal and policy provisions for reasonable accommodation in employment of persons with mental disability in East Africa: A review. *International Journal of Law and Psychiatry, 64*, 99–105.

Ebuenyi, I. D., Rottenburg, E. S., Bunders-Aelen, J. F., & Regeer, B. J. (2018). Challenges of inclusion: a qualitative study exploring barriers and pathways to inclusion of persons with mental disabilities in technical and vocational education and training programmes in East Africa. *Disability and Rehabilitation, 42*(4), 536–544.

Ellis, W., & Dietz, W. (2017). A new framework for addressing adverse childhood and community experiences: the building community resilience (BCR) model. *Academic Pediatrics, 17*(7), S86–S93. https://doi.org/10.1016/j.acap.2016.12.011

Eriksson, S., Höglund, A. T., & Helgesson, G. (2008). Do ethical guidelines give guidance? A critical examination of eight ethics regulations. *Cambridge Quarterly of Healthcare Ethics, 17*, 15–29.

Fricker, M. (2007). *Epistemic injustice: Power and the ethics of knowing*. Oxford University Press.

Forkus, S. R., & Weiss, N. H. (2021). Examining the relations among moral foundations, potentially morally injurious events, and posttraumatic stress disorder symptoms. *Psychological Trauma: Theory, Research, Practice and Policy, 13*(4), 403–411. doi: 10.1037/tra0000968

Gauthier, J. (2018). References to human rights in codes of ethics for psychologists: critical issues and recommendations. Part II. *Bulletin of Peoples' Friendship University of Russia. Series: Psychology and Pedagogy, 15*(2), 131–146.

Gergel, T., Das, P., Owen, G., Stephenson, L., Rifkin, L., Hindley, G., Dawson, J., & Ruck Keene, A. (2021). Reasons for endorsing or rejecting self-binding directives in bipolar disorder: a qualitative study of survey responses from UK service users. *Lancet Psychiatry, 8*(7): 599–609. doi: 10.1016/S2215-0366(21)00115-2

Gilligan, C. (2016). *In a different voice*. Harvard University Press.

Goodman, L. A., Liang, B., Helms, J. E., Latta, R. E., Sparks, E., & Weintraub, S. R. (2004). Training counseling psychologists as social justice agents: Feminist and multicultural principles in action. *The Counseling Psychologist, 32*, 793–836. http://dx.doi.org/10.1177/0011000004268802

Hailes, H. P., Ceccolini, C. J., Gutowski, E., & Liang, B. (2020). Ethical guidelines for social justice in psychology. *Professional Psychology: Research and Practice*. Advance online publication. http://dx.doi.org/10.1037/pro0000291

Haidt, J. (2007). The new synthesis in moral psychology. *Science, 316*, 998–1002.

Harris, S. P., Gould, R., & Mullin, C. (2019). ADA research brief: Mental health, employment and the ADA. https://adata.org/research_brief/mental-health-employment-and-ada

Henrich, J., Heine, S. J., & Norenzayan, A. (2010). The weirdest people in the world? *Behavioral and Brain Sciences, 33*(2–3), 61–83. https://doi.org/10.1017/S0140525X0999152X

Hoffman, D., Carter, D., Lopez, C. et al. (2015). Report to the Special Committee of the Board of Directors of the American Psychological Association. https://www.apa.org/independent-review/APA-FINAL-Report-7.2.15.pdf

Holm, S. (2011). Who should decide the content of professional ethics. *Journal of Applied Ethics and Philosophy, 3*, 1–8.

Hutton, M., & Cappellini, B. (2022). Epistemic in/justice: Towards 'Other' ways of knowing. *Marketing Theory, 22*(2), 155–174. https://doi.org/10.1177/14705931221076563

Kelly, B. D. (2005). Structural violence and schizophrenia. *Social Science and Medicine, 61*(3), 721–730. https://doi.org/10.1016/j.socscimed.2004.12.020

Kelly, B. D. (2025). *The modern psychiatrist's guide to contemporary practice: discussion, dissent, and debate in mental health care*. Routledge. https://doi.org/10.4324/9781003378495 (Open Access: CC BY)

Kesebir, S., & Haidt, J. (2010). Morality. In S. Fiske, D. Gilbert, & G. Lindzey (Eds.), *Handbook of Social Psychology* (5th Ed.). Chichester: John Wiley & Sons.

Kinderman, P. (2021). From chemical imbalance to power imbalance: A macropsychology perspective on mental health. In M. MacLachlan & J. McVeigh (Eds.), *Macropsychology: A Population Science for Sustainable Development Goals*, 29–44. Springer. https://doi.org/10.1007/978-3-030-50176-1_2

Kivikangas, J. M., Fernández-Castilla, B., Järvelä, S., Ravaja, N., & Lönnqvist, J. E. (2021). Moral foundations and political orientation: Systematic review and meta-analysis. *Psychological Bulletin, 147*(1), 55–94. doi: 10.1037/bul0000308

Kohlberg, L. (1971). *From is to ought: how to commit the naturalistic fallacy and get away with it in the study of moral development*. Academic Press.

Krebs, D. L., & Denton, K. (2005). Toward a more pragmatic approach to morality: a critical evaluation of Kohlberg's Model. *Psychological Review, 112*(3), 629–649. doi:10.1037/0033-295X.112.3.629

Knapp, S. J., VandeCreek, L. D., & Fingerhut, R. (2017). *Practical ethics for psychology: A positive approach* (3rd ed.). APA.

Leach, M. M., & Harbin, J. J. (1997). Psychological ethics codes: A comparison of twenty-four countries, *International Journal of Psychology, 32*(3), 181–192. doi: 10.1080/002075997400854

MacLachlan, M. (2002). *Die Arbeit mit Psychotrauma. Persönliche, kulturelle und kontextuelle Probleme. [Working with psychotrauma: personal, cultural and contextual reflections]*. Überleben am Abgrund. Klagenfurt: Drava-Verlag, 231–244.

MacLachlan, M. (2006). *Culture & Health* (2nd ed.). Chichester: Wiley.

MacLachlan, M., & McVeigh, J. (2021). Macropsychology: Definition, scope, and conceptualization. In M. MacLachlan & J. McVeigh (Eds.), *Macropsychology: A population science for sustainable development goals*, 1–27. Springer. https://doi.org/10.1007/978-3-030-50176-1_2

Maldonado, D. B. (2019). The concept of culture and the cultural study of law. An essay. *Verfassung und Recht in Übersee / Law and Politics in Africa, Asia and Latin America, 52*(3), Special Issue: 'Law and Culture from a Comparative Perspective' 297–327.

Martí-Vilar, M., Escrig-Espuig, J. M., & Merino-Soto, C. (2023). A systematic review of moral reasoning measures. *Current Psychology, 42*, 1284–1298. https://doi.org/10.1007/s12144-021-01519-8

Nagel, T. (1989). *The view from nowhere*. Oxford University Press.

O'Donohue, W. (2020). Criticisms of the ethical principles of psychologists and code of conduct. *Ethics and Behaviour*, 30.

Rest, J. R. (1994). Background: Theory and research. In J. R. Rest & D. Narvaez (Eds.), *Moral development in the professions: Psychology and applied ethics* (pp. 1–25).

Rubin N. S., & Flores, R. L. (2020). *The Cambridge handbook of psychology and human rights*. Cambridge University Press.

Schon, D. A. (1983). *The reflective practitioner: How professionals think in action*. Sheridan.

Rains, L., Zenina, T., Dias, M. C., Jones, R., Jeffreys, S., Branthonne-Foster, S., Lloyd-Evans, B., & Johnson, S. (2019). Variations in patterns of involuntary hospitalisation and in legal frameworks: an international comparative study. *Lancet Psychiatry, 6*(5), 403–417. doi: 10.1016/S2215-0366(19)30090-2

Steinerte, E., Murray, R., & Laing, J. (2012). Monitoring those deprived of their liberty in psychiatric and social care institutions and national practice in the UK. *The International Journal of Human Rights, 16*(6), 865–882.

Schildbach, S., & Schildbach, C. (2018). Criminalization through transinstitutionalization: a critical review of the Penrose hypothesis in the context of compensation imprisonment. *Frontiers in Psychiatry*, *25*(9), 412622.

Thomson, J. J. (1984). The trolley problem. *Yale Law Journal*, *94*, 1395.

United Nations Human Rights Committee. (2014). General comment no. 35 (Article 9). United Nations.

United Nations Subcommittee on Prevention of Torture and Other Cruel, Inhuman or Degrading Treatment or Punishment. (2016). Approach of the Subcommittee on Prevention of Torture and Other Cruel, Inhuman or Degrading Treatment or Punishment regarding the rights of persons institutionalized and treated medically without informed consent. United Nations.

World Health Organization. (2022). ICD-11: International Classification of Diseases (11th revision). World Health Organization.

2

The World Health Organization's Programme on QualityRights

Ikenna D. Ebuenyi and Malcolm MacLachlan

Introduction

The World Health Organization's (WHO) QualityRights initiative was developed in 2012 with the aim 'to improve the quality of care and support in mental health and social services and to promote the human rights of people with psychosocial, intellectual or cognitive disabilities throughout the world' (WHO, 2012, 2019a). The development of this initiative was in response to the poor quality of care and human rights violations experienced by individuals with mental health conditions around the world (Funk & Drew, 2017; WHO, 2012). Much of the work of the QualityRights initiative has focused on mental health thus far, and so this will also be the primary focus of this chapter. Historically, the rights and mental health service experience of many individuals with mental health conditions have been associated with deprivation, discrimination, and limited access to care, associated with negative perceptions and misunderstandings about mental health (Thornicroft, 2006). According to the United Nations Report of the Special Rapporteur on the right of everyone to the enjoyment of the highest attainable standard of physical and mental health, there can be no mental health without rights (UN Human Rights Council, 2020). The report underscored the discrimination, disempowerment, coercion, social exclusion, and injustice experienced by individuals with mental health conditions, perpetuated by harmful sociopolitical systems, institutions, and practices. The special rapporteur recommended 'rights-based', holistic interventions that consider the lived experiences of affected individuals (UN Human Rights Council, 2020). This chapter reviews and reflects on the opportunities and challenges that the QualityRights initiative presents to the psych professions and to individual practitioners of these professions.

Across both low- and high-income countries, the treatment experience of individuals with mental health conditions and limitations of the personal liberty and human rights of some has led to the movement towards safeguarding the rights of individuals with mental health conditions through national and international human rights instruments. The United Nations Convention on the Rights of Persons with Disabilities (CRPD), which was adopted by the UN General Assembly in 2006, is one such international human rights instrument (United Nations, 2006). Presently, 187 countries have ratified the CRPD which requires individual countries to publish periodic reports on their progress towards the implementation of the CRPD recommendations. The CRPD advocates for a human rights approach to mental health and through its several articles provides a framework to advocate for the rights of persons with disabilities, including mental health. For instance, Article 12 of the CRPD affirms equal recognition before the law while Article 14 highlights the right to liberty and security of person (United Nations, 2006). Other relevant articles (Table 2.1) include Article 15 (Freedom from torture or cruel, inhuman or degrading treatment or punishment), Article 16 (Freedom from exploitation, violence and abuse), Article 19 (Living independently and being included in the community), Article 25 (Health) and Article 28 (Adequate standard of living and social protection). These articles and others in the CRPD advocate for an end to the rights violations experienced by individuals with mental health conditions in society, in the course of what is considered 'treatment' and after treatment. Mahdanian et al. (2023) highlight the bidirectional relationship between human rights and mental health. In their review, they suggest that while human rights violations can worsen mental health, human rights protections may improve mental health outcomes. These understandings and learnings from the recommendations of United Nations conventions on human rights informed the establishment of the QualityRights initiative (Mahdanian et al., 2023). The WHO QualityRights initiative is underpinned by the CRPD.

The QualityRights initiative objectives include to (1) build capacity to understand and promote human rights, recovery, and independent living in the community; (2) create community-based and recovery-oriented services that respect and promote rights; (3) improve quality of care and human rights in mental health and social

Table 2.1 WHO QualityRights Objectives and related CRPD article

QualityRights objectives	CRPD articles
Increase capacity to understand and promote human rights, recovery, and independent living in the community	Article 15 (Freedom from torture or cruel, inhuman, or degrading treatment or punishment)
Create community-based and recovery-oriented services that respect and promote human rights	Article 25 (Health) Article 27 (Work and employment)
Improve the quality of care and human rights conditions in mental health and related services	Article 12 (Equal recognition before the law)
Develop a civil society movement to influence policy-making and advocate for the integration of a human rights approach in mental health	Article 28 (Adequate standard of living and social protection)
Reform national policies and legislation in line with the CRPD and other international human rights standards.	Article 12 (Equal recognition before the law) Article 14 (Liberty and security of person)

services; (4) develop a civil society movement to conduct advocacy; and (5) influence decision-making in line with the CRPD and other international human rights standards (WHO, 2012, 2019a). The QualityRights utilizes several tools to further these objectives. They include the QualityRights toolkit (for assessing and improving quality and human rights in mental health and social care facilities) (WHO, 2012) and the other training packages (Table 2.2) developed with the objective 'to build capacity among mental health practitioners, people with psychosocial, intellectual, and cognitive disabilities, people using mental health services, families, care partners, and other supporters, nongovernmental organizations, organizations of persons with disabilities and others on how to implement a human rights and recovery approach in the

Table 2.2 WHO QualityRights trainings

Training type	Components
Core training	**Human rights.** WHO QualityRights Core training – for all services and all people **Mental health, disability and human rights.** WHO QualityRights Core training – for all services and all people **Legal capacity and the right to decide.** WHO QualityRights Core training: mental health and social services **Recovery and the right to health.** WHO QualityRights Core training: mental health and social services **Freedom from coercion, violence and abuse.** WHO QualityRights Core training: mental health and social services
Specialized training	**Recovery practices for mental health and well-being.** WHO QualityRights Specialized training **Strategies to end seclusion and restraint.** WHO QualityRights Specialized training **Supported decision-making and advance planning.** WHO QualityRights Specialized training
Training evaluation tools	WHO QualityRights training on mental health, human rights and recovery
Guidance	**Peer support groups by and for people with lived experience.** WHO QualityRights guidance module **One-to-one peer support by and for people with lived experience.** WHO QualityRights guidance module **Advocacy for mental health, disability and human rights.** WHO QualityRights guidance module **Civil society organizations to promote human rights in mental health and related areas.** WHO QualityRights guidance module
Service transformation	**QualityRights Assessment toolkit** **Transforming services and promoting human rights.** WHO QualityRights training and guidance: mental health and social services
Self-help	**Person-centred recovery planning for mental health and well-being self-help tool.** WHO QualityRights

area of mental health in line with the UN Convention on the Rights of Persons with Disabilities and other international human rights standards'(WHO, 2019b).

Achievements and Challenges of the QualityRights

Since its introduction, the QualityRights initiative has led to several positive achievements in the advocacy for a rights-based approach to mental health. Beyond being seen as an advocacy instrument for safeguarding the rights of persons with mental health, it has led to better understanding of the negative experience of individuals with mental health conditions across the world and a movement towards rights protection (Duffy & Kelly, 2023; Mahdanian et al., 2023; Moro et al., 2022a; Morrissey, 2020; Pathare et al., 2021). Across both low- and high-income countries, the QualityRights initiative has supported new legislation and changes in sociopolitical attitudes towards the rights or persons with mental health.

A 2015 survey on the quality of care and user's rights in Chilean psychiatric services using the WHO QualityRights reported reduced discrimination in health services, increased availability of psychotropic medications, but also less progress on community care and living, access to education and employment and respect for users' autonomy and freedom from maltreatment and cruelty (Minoletti et al., 2015). In 2019, a study in Iceland that evaluated attitudinal change towards CRPD rights among participants through delivery of the QualityRights training indicated relatively high levels of change in attitude (64% change in attitude of service providers) following completion of the training (Morrissey, 2020). In Ghana, the QualityRights assessment toolkit was used to assess mental health hospitals and quality of care and respect of human rights in the settings. The study findings indicated some shortcomings in the provision of care and recommended further aligning of mental health services to the human rights approach of the CRPD and the QualityRights initiative (Moro et al., 2022a). Moro et al. also highlighted that most mental health facilities were yet to initiate actions towards implementing the recommendations of the QualityRights initiative in relation to independent living in the community due to a lack of resources. In Kenya, a 2021 assessment of a large mental health hospital using the QualityRights toolkit indicated significant challenges in hospital infrastructure for care provision, inadequate human resources, lack of the right to legal capacity, abuse of patients, and lack of strategies towards community and independent living (Muhia et al., 2021).

In India, a 2021 study that evaluated the QualityRights programme in Gujarat reported improved attitudes towards service users, empowerment of service users and reduced 'burden of care' on caregivers. However, the study highlighted challenges with sustainability and advocated development of new community-based mental health services that are compliant with the human rights approach to increase access to care (Pathare et al., 2021). A 2022 evaluation of four West African countries (The Gambia, Ghana, Liberia, and Sierra Leone) using the QualityRights toolkit reported poor implementation of the rights in relation to an adequate standard of living and to enjoyment of the highest attainable standard of health, right to exercise legal capacity, the right to personal liberty and security, and promotion of the right to live independently and be included in the community. The study recommended improved human and financial resources for improved mental health services in line with the QualityRights initiative (Moro et al., 2022b). A 2023 editorial on the application of QualityRights in Ireland acknowledged the usefulness of the QualityRights training initiative following Ireland's ratification of the CRPD in 2018, but also stated the authors' position towards Articles 12, 14, and 27 (Duffy & Kelly, 2023). The authors suggested some challenges with the QualityRights and CRPD advocacy for an absolute implementation of Article 12 and the need for further funding of mental health services and implementation of the Assisted Decision-Making (Capacity) Act 2015 to help further legal capacity. As in many countries, in Ireland there are different constituencies advocating for different actions (or for resisting actions) to implement the CRPD. As authors of this chapter and editors of this book, it is important for us to openly acknowledge that we too have very different views to each other, each passionately and compassionately held, each respected, but not commensurate (see, for instance, MacLachlan, 2023; MacLachlan et al., 2021). It is these very tensions which are the workplace of the QualityRights initiative.

The foregoing has highlighted some of the applications of the WHO QualityRights programme across various settings, noting its achievements and challenges. A common feature of the settings is their ratification of the CRPD (United Nations, 2023). Despite ratification of the CRPD in these settings, implementation of the objectives of the QualityRights initiative has been problematic. If the QualityRights objectives are difficult to achieve in countries that have ratified the CRPD, what of countries that have yet to ratify it and hence may have no legal instrument to advocate for it? As authors of this chapter, our differing views on some of the objectives of the QualityRights arise from some of the practical implications of these rights for clinical practice. In the next sections, we use a case study to present such difficulties—some 'grey areas'—and we then analyse and reflect on them.

Case Study

AB was a senior civil servant who fled their country when the political problems degenerated to a civil war. AB escaped, leaving their partner and two children behind with plans to send for them. At the reception camp in AB's country of arrival the living conditions were difficult. Despite international aid and available support, life was difficult. The initial hopes of sending for the family faded as the civil war continued and AB's chances of making it to a safer and the higher-income country diminished. AB found no joy in daily activities, was unable to sleep, and was often observed talking to unseen persons. Friends at the camp were worried and brought AB to the camp clinic. At the camp clinic, AB was diagnosed with severe depression with psychosis by the community healthcare workers. Although AB had a family history of mental health conditions, AB had no prior diagnosed mental health issues.

It was only after a month that AB received antidepressants pills and was given a dose to last them a week. AB had no interest in taking the medication, believing that 'circumstances' were the problem rather than the diagnosis given. AB missed their family and their old job and was sad and frustrated that they could not legally work. AB soon joined others in the camp using cannabis, feeling that drugs and alcohol may efface their present difficulties. The impact of the drugs on AB was different. AB soon started neglecting self-care, seeing visions, and the voices in their head increased. In time, AB started to self-talk out loud and exhibited violent behaviours.

The reports from other residents led to AB being moved from the camp to the nearby 'mental rehabilitation hospital' in the same country. AB was chained to the bed and often sedated at the hospital. This was felt necessary due to the lack of personnel available to provide meaningful support to AB. In time AB hardly remembered who they were, and in time the memories of country and family faded, with just incoherent mutterings to the hospital nurses growing in extent and frequency.

Analysis

The objectives of the WHO QualityRights and CRPD are worthy, but we are concerned with the extent to which they can be realized where resources are scarce. AB's case is typical of many low- and middle-income countries and also, perhaps, resource poor health service settings in high-income countries. The nexus between social adversity and mental health and their bidirectional relationship has been extensively reported in literature (Lund et al., 2011).

The first paragraph of Article 25 of the CRPD states that 'States Parties recognize that persons with disabilities have the right to the enjoyment of the highest attainable standard of health without discrimination on the basis of disability.' The mental health condition that AB developed is a recognized form of disability under the CRPD, and AB's right to appropriate healthcare is also required by the CRPD. However, refugee status and the unmet need for mental health services meant that rather than receiving help from a psych professional, he was initially helped by less specialized community healthcare workers, who might not have been trained in the necessary skills to be of adequate help. It might be because of this, and a lack of effective alternative psycho-social interventions, that four weeks later AB received medication.

Studies in settings where the QualityRights initiative has been implemented or used for assessment highlight the need for more financial and human resources to achieve its objectives (Duffy & Kelly, 2023; Moro et al., 2022a). However, the review by Gastaldon et al. (2019) found that two-thirds of the studies used to create National Institute for Health and Care Excellence (NICE) guidelines did not use what they called 'pragmatic designs', meaning that they were not easily applicable to clinical practice, which often lacks the ideal conditions of well-resourced randomized controlled trials (Gastaldon et al., 2019). To implement rights requires both advocacy for resources allocated to appropriate types of staff rather than to traditionally orientated services, and research that evaluates the realities of their effectiveness.

Due to AB's personal choices and quality of treatment, their condition worsened. AB was not offered environmental, occupational or psychological services, or other interventions before medication. This outcome was largely shaped by social, political, and economic factors, rather than clinical ones. The case of AB begs many questions. It is possible that if AB had not had to leave their country, they might never have developed a mental health condition. If such a condition had developed in their own country, then family, community or other professional help might have been available. The circumstances that predisposed AB to, or were associated with, AB's mental health condition require as a much consideration as the consequences of their condition, if not more.

Socioenvironmental and political factors determine the landscape of risk for developing mental health conditions, predict access to treatment, often the types of treatment offered and influence the factors that shape recovery. High rates of mental health conditions in migrants and individuals in humanitarian crises have been previously documented (Ilozumba et al., 2022). The non-availability of purposeful training and employment were also relevant in AB's case. Although the CRPD supports inclusive employment of persons with disabilities, AB could not gain employment on account of refugee/immigrant status. The initial paragraph of Article 27 of the CRPD states that 'States Parties shall safeguard and promote the realization of the right to work, including for those who acquire a disability during the course of employment, by taking appropriate steps, including through legislation'. Work is relevant for social functioning and recovery (Ebuenyi, 2019). The lack of work/employment worsened AB's situation and strengthened the social distress associated with refugee status. Such a situation limits the relevance of any treatment or intervention, and constricts opportunity for recovery.

Intervention

The approach envisaged in rights documentation to supporting AB would require the availability of resources and actual implementation of legal and policy recommendations in the country where AB was a refugee. These conditions are necessary for the achievement of the objectives of the WHO QualityRights. The International Covenant on Civil and Political Rights (ICCPR) and the International Convention on the Protection of the Rights of All Migrant Workers and Members of Their Families (ICMW) recommend equal treatment of refugees and migrants, and meeting their basic needs for livelihood (United Nations, 1990, 2002). The enactment of these Conventions would have ensured that AB had access to work and employment which might have helped resolve their separation from family and community of origin.

Following AB's development of a mental health condition, the CRPD and WHO QualityRights ethos require that AB has access to the appropriate forms of help without restriction, based on the right to health (Article 25). Again, AB might have benefited from community mental health services, but this proved impossible in the refugee camp. It was only when AB's condition deteriorated that they were transferred to the hospital where some specialized services were available. There might have been no need to restrain and sedate AB. However, due to lack of financial and human resources for mental health in the country AB endured these interventions. AB could have been managed on an outpatient basis and followed up in the community, but again the social and political context made this impossible. Care at home requires a home. Care in the community requires a community. Neither of these was available to AB.

Theory

The rights-based ethos of the United Nations CRPD aspires to protect persons with disabilities across the world, especially in countries where it has been ratified. However, even after ratification, it can be difficult to realize the mandates of the Convention on certain issues, as seen in the case of AB. The right to health (Article 25) which is captured by the third objective of the WHO QualityRights ('Improve the quality of care and human rights conditions in mental health and related services') is dependent on the availability of mental health services and the contextual definition of quality care. The understanding of the concepts of care, services, and human rights is also contentious as, for some authors, certain rights perspectives can be seen as marginalizing or limiting the provision of care (Hoare & Duffy, 2021). The authors of that commentary suggest that characterizing involuntary treatment as inevitably abusing human rights closes the opportunity for debate on the issue and limits care for individuals with severe mental health conditions (Hoare & Duffy, 2021). In a rebuttal, McGovern argues that the WHO QualityRights is not antipsychiatry but an opportunity to offer person-centred care that is anchored in rights-based practice (McGovern, 2022).

The concept of rights and its application has always been dependent on duty holders (governments). The ethos of the WHO QualityRights is a lofty one and its helpfulness in promoting supported decision-making, recovery, and reduction of coercive practices are commendable. However, these objectives are dependent on the commitment of duty holders and system-level actors to safeguard these rights through provision of resources. The budgetary allocation for mental health around the world is still dismal and even in high-income countries, more financial resources are regarded as key towards achieving the objectives of the WHO QualityRights (Duffy & Kelly, 2023). For instance, achieving community mental health services or person-centred care would require having enough mental health service providers to ensure that individuals do not have to be sedated or chained as experienced by AB.

Rights Reflection

The rights-based ethos of the QualityRights is commendable. It has several advantages such as fostering supported decision-making, recovery, and reduction of coercive practices which are all in the interest of individuals with mental health problems. However, the absolute application of some of the tenets may also have implications for affected individuals.

First, ensuring legal capacity, human rights, recovery, and independent living is essential. However, these must also be individual- and context-driven. Insistence on independent living in the community, for example, might not be feasible in severe mental health conditions where there is no prior advance directive or insufficient resources to support the individual's ability to live independently.

Similarly, while community-based and recovery-oriented services that respect and promote human rights of individuals with mental health conditions are essential, it must be recognized that their realization is contingent on financial resources. At the same time, it is crucial that such additional resources are not used to reinforce oppressive models of practice but rather are allocated in ways that offer realistic service alternatives to the current inadequate services that dominate in most countries. Killaspy et al.'s review of the literature on community-based interventions for severe mental health conditions concluded that 'social interventions have considerable benefits but are arguably the most complex in the mental health field, and require multi-level stakeholder commitment and investment for successful implementation' (p. 960). Interventions should be designed and implemented with awareness of both the evidence base and the socioeconomic context of implementation (Killaspy et al., 2022).

The WHO QualityRights initiative advocates for improving the quality of care and human rights conditions in mental health and related services (WHO, 2012), while the WHO Mental Health Gap Action Programme Intervention Guide (mhGAP-IG) advocates for task-sharing approaches to reduce unmet need for mental services in low-income settings (WHO, 2016). We need to ensure that we are not bridging the gap at the cost of quality of care while still advocating for the right to quality care. The experience of AB highlights the ethical dilemma regarding task-sharing approaches as further elaborated in Chapter 16 of this book. However, we acknowledge here that modest training in mental healthcare for community workers may have significant benefits for service users (Deimling Johns et al., 2018). And so how much (training) is enough should not be a question answered by simply exporting traditions from or training from one country or context to a different country and different context.

The role of civil society movements in influencing policy-making and advocating for the integration of a human rights approach in mental health cannot be overemphasized. In Kenya, for instance, the 'users and survivors of psychiatry network' has been at the forefront of championing the rights of persons with mental health problems (Ebuenyi, 2019). It is essential that advocacy by civil society also respect the rights of the individual to choose the treatment that works for them.

Reforming national policies and legislation in line with the CRPD and other international human rights standards is perhaps the most important objective of the WHO QualityRights. However, we need to couple policy reformation with resourcing policy implementation through appropriate allocation of resources to mental health services. Mere endorsement of policies or ratification of the CRPD has been shown to be quite different from actual implementation of the recommendations of the Convention (Ebuenyi et al., 2019). Selective or convenient implementation of national policies is not sufficient to promote rights-based mental health services. In the case of AB, although the country had embraced the ethos of the WHO QualityRights, it was surprising that chains and sedation were also used in the same setting. It is essential that the advocacy and implementation of the WHO QualityRights is done in a reflective manner that promotes dialogue and understanding of the specific needs of individuals with mental health problems in diverse settings.

Questions and Thought Experiments

1. Do people with mental health conditions have the same rights as people without mental health conditions? If someone with a mental health condition needs additional support by public services, does that justify limiting the public services available to someone else?
2. When is it justifiable for a clinician to participate in limiting observance of a person's right to liberty? And, if there are occasions when it is justified, in what circumstances might it be considered to be torture?
3. If power and privilege are not equally distributed across the psych professions and an increased emphasis on rights challenges the status quo, how can change be encouraged?
4. Are the WHO QualityRights implementable in settings where legal and policy provisions do not reflect the ethos of the CRPD? If so, are 'rights' the most efficient way of achieving positive change?
5. What is the scope for safeguarding the rights of refugees and internally displaced persons with mental health problems towards enjoyment of the rights to health, employment and freedom from discrimination?

Further Reading

Ebuenyi, I. D., Guxens, M., Ombati, E., Bunders-Aelen, J. F., & Regeer, B.J. (2019). Employability of persons with mental disability: Understanding lived experiences in Kenya. *Frontiers in Psychiatry, 10, 539.*

Gill, N., Drew, N., Rodrigues, M., Muhsen, H., Morales Cano, G., Savage, M., Pathare, S., Allan, J., Galderisi, S., Javed. A., Herrman. H., & Funk. M. (2024). Bringing together the World Health Organization's QualityRights initiative and the World Psychiatric Association's programme on implementing alternatives to coercion in mental healthcare: a common goal for action. *British Journal of Psychiatry Open*, *10*(1), e23. doi: 10.1192/bjo.2023.622

Jenkins, R., Baingana, F., Ahmad, R., McDaid, D., & Atun, R. (2011). Social, economic, human rights and political challenges to global mental health. *Mental Health in Family Medicine*, *8*(2), 87–96.

Mahdanian, A. A., Laporta, M., Drew Bold, N., Funk, M., & Puras, D. (2023). Human rights in mental healthcare; A review of current global situation. *International Review of Psychiatry*, *35*(2), 150–162.

References

Deimling Johns, L., Power, J., & MacLachlan, M. (2018). Community-based mental health intervention skills: Task shifting in low-and middle-income settings. *International Perspectives in Psychology*, *7*(4), 205–230.

Duffy, R., & Kelly, B. (2023). Can the World Health Organisation's 'QualityRights' initiative help reduce coercive practices in psychiatry in Ireland? *Irish Journal of Psychological Medicine*, *40*(2), 114–117.

Ebuenyi, I. D. (2019). *Inclusive employment: understanding the barriers to and facilitators of employment for persons with mental disability in East Africa*. VU University Press, Amsterdam.

Ebuenyi, I. D., Regeer, B. J., Nthenge, M., Nardodkar, R., Waltz, M., & Bunders-Aelen, J. F. (2019). Legal and policy provisions for reasonable accommodation in employment of persons with mental disability in East Africa: A review. *International Journal of Law and Psychiatry*, *64*, 99–105.

Funk, M., & Drew, N. (2017). WHO QualityRights: transforming mental health services. *The Lancet Psychiatry*, *4*(11), 826–827.

Gastaldon, C., Mosler, F., Toner, S., Tedeschi, F., Bird, V. J., Barbui, C., & Priebe, S. (2019). Are trials of psychological and psychosocial interventions for schizophrenia and psychosis included in the NICE guidelines pragmatic? A systematic review. *PLoS ONE*, *14*(9), e0222891.

Hoare, F., & Duffy, R. M. (2021). The World Health Organization's QualityRights materials for training, guidance and transformation: preventing coercion but marginalising psychiatry. *The British Journal of Psychiatry*, *218*(5), 240–242.

Ilozumba, O., Koster, T. S., Syurina, E. V., & Ebuenyi, I. (2022). Ethnic minority experiences of mental health services in the Netherlands: an exploratory study. *BMC Research Notes*, *15*(1), 266.

Killaspy, H., Harvey, C., Brasier, C., Brophy, L., Ennals, P., Fletcher, J., & Hamilton, B. (2022). Community-based social interventions for people with severe mental illness: a systematic review and narrative synthesis of recent evidence. *World Psychiatry*, *21*(1), 96–123.

Lund, C., De Silva, M., Plagerson, S., Cooper, S., Chisholm, D., Das, J., Knapp, M., & Patel, V. (2011). Poverty and mental disorders: breaking the cycle in low-income and middle-income countries. *The Lancet*, *378*(9801), 1502–1514.

MacLachlan, M. (2023). Mental health services must be prised from grip of psychiatry. https://www.irishtimes.com/opinion/2023/05/22/mental-health-services-must-be-prised-from-grip-of-psychiatry/

MacLachlan, M., Murphy, R., Daly, M., & Hyland, P. (2021). Why it's time to stop saying 'mental illness': A commentary on the revision of the Irish Mental Health Act. *HRB Open Research*, *4*(28), 28.

Mahdanian, A. A., Laporta, M., Drew Bold, N., Funk, M., & Puras, D. (2023). Human rights in mental healthcare; A review of current global situation. *International Review of Psychiatry*, *35*(2), 150–162.

McGovern, P. (2022). The World Health Organization's QualityRights initiative: rights and recovery-oriented services should be at the centre not the margins of psychiatry. *British Journal of Psychiatry*, *221*(1), 428–430.

Minoletti, A., Toro, O., Alvarado, R., Carniglia, C., Guajardo, A., & Rayo, X. (2015). A survey about quality of care and user s' rights in Chilean psychiatric services. *Revista médica de Chile*, *143*(12), 1585–1592.

Moro, M. F., Carta, M. G., Gyimah, L., Orrell, M., Amissah, C., Baingana, F., Kofie, H., Taylor, D., Chimbar, N., & Coffie, M. (2022a). A nationwide evaluation study of the quality of care and respect of human rights in mental health facilities in Ghana: results from the World Health Organization QualityRights initiative. *BMC Public Health*, *22*(1), 1–14.

Moro, M. F., Kola, L., Fadahunsi, O., Jah, E. M., Kofie, H., Samba, D., Thomas, S., Drew, N., Nwefoh, E., Pathare, S., Eaton, J., Funk, M., & Gureje, O. (2022b). Quality of care and respect of human rights in mental health services in four West African countries: collaboration between the mental health leadership and advocacy programme and the World Health Organization QualityRights initiative. *British Journal of Psychiatry Open*, *8*(1), e31. https://doi.org/10.1192/bjo.2021.1080

Morrissey, F. (2020). An evaluation of attitudinal change towards CRPD rights following delivery of the WHO QualityRights training programme. *Ethics, Medicine and Public Health*, *13*, 100410.

Muhia, J., Jaguga, F., Wamukhoma, V., Aloo, J., & Njuguna, S. (2021). A human rights assessment of a large mental hospital in Kenya. *Pan African Medical Journal*, *40*(1), 199.

Pathare, S., Funk, M., Bold, N. D., Chauhan, A., Kalha, J., Krishnamoorthy, S., Sapag, J. C., Bobbili, S. J., Kawade, R., & Shah, S. (2021). Systematic evaluation of the QualityRights programme in public mental health facilities in Gujarat, India. *British Journal of Psychiatry*, *218*(4), 196–203.

Thornicroft, G. (2006). *Shunned: Discrimination against people with mental illness*. Oxford University Press.

UN Human Rights Council. (2020). *Report of the Special Rapporteur on the right of everyone to the enjoyment of the highest attainable standard of physical and mental health* (A/HRC/44/48). https://www.ohchr.org/en/documents/thematic-reports/ahrc4448-right-everyone-enjoyment-highest-attainable-standard-physical

United Nations. (1990). *International Convention on the Protection of the Rights of All Migrant Workers and Members of their Families*. https://www.ohchr.org/en/instruments-mechanisms/instruments/international-convention-protection-rights-all-migrant-workers

United Nations General Assembly. (1996). UN General Assembly. *International covenant on civil and political rights, 16 December 1966. United Nations, Treaty Series. 1996;999:171.*

United Nations. (2006). *Convention on the Rights of Persons with Disabilities (CRPD)*. https://www.un.org/development/desa/disabilities/convention-on-the-rights-of-persons-with-disabilities.html

United Nations. (2023). *Ratification Status for CRPD – Convention on the Rights of Persons with Disabilities*. https://tbinternet.ohchr.org/_layouts/15/TreatyBodyExternal/Treaty.aspx?CountryID=35&Lang=EN

WHO. (2012). WHO QualityRights tool kit to assess and improve quality and human rights in mental health and social care facilities. Geneva: World Health Organization.

WHO. (2016). mhGAP Intervention Guide-Version 2.0 for mental, neurological and substance use disorders in non-specialist health settings.

WHO. (2019a). Advocacy for mental health, disability and human rights: WHO QualityRights guidance module. Geneva: World Health Organization. https://apps.who.int/iris/handle/10665/329587

WHO. (2019b). QualityRights materials for training, guidance and transformation https://www.who.int/publications/i/item/who-qualityrights-guidance-and-training-tools

3
Professions, Politics, and Social Change

Paul D'Alton

> *Education is the point at which we decide whether we love the world enough to assume responsibility for it.*
>
> **Hanna Arendt**

Introduction: Professions, Politics, and Social Change

What do psychologists and psychiatrists and other health and social care professionals (HSCPs) have to do with ethics or human rights? Some might say the responsibility of HSCPs, when it comes to ethics, is with the service user sitting right in front of them or the research project they are responsible for that involves vulnerable participants, public finance, or sensitive data. Perhaps not uncommon among HSCP groups is the view that professional ethics are primarily circumscribed to issues of clinical care; such as the provision of treatments, involuntary admissions, issues of capacity and consent, the limits of confidentiality, and the assessment of risk. Human rights on the other hand are beyond the remit of HSCPs, and are the jurisdiction of civil society groups, and experts in national and international law experts.

Given such a circumscribed view concerning the separation of professional ethics and human rights, it is reasonable to question why practitioners should have anything to do with politics and social change. In the context of such a circumscribed model of professional ethics versus human rights, the domain of politics and social change are often understood as private and personal matters for HSCPs and have little or no bearing on their responsibilities as HSCP.

Overview

In this chapter I will be making the case for HSCPs to widen the lens from the individual to the collective: from the service user to the service provider; from pathology to policy; from the micro to the macro; from the consultation room to the constitution. I will briefly describe the evolution of professional codes of ethics over the 20th century and consider the antecedents such as the Holocaust and the resulting 1948 Universal Declaration of Human Rights to professional codes of ethics. In this context

I will make the case for the interdependent nature of professional codes of ethics and human rights.

Furthermore, I will make the case for why individual practitioners and their professional bodies, due to their codes of ethics and associated obligations as human rights-bearers, must occupy the policy and political arena because it is in the political arena that policies are formed that in turn shape the lives of the individuals they serve. My case will be based on the understanding that much, not all, of the human distress encountered by HSCPs is the result of inequity promoting policies.

Inequity and discrimination are not inevitable or a random outcome; inequity and discrimination are socially constructed, and the result of policy decisions. The absence of engagement in the political arena is itself a political act. However, the intersection of professional, politics, and social change is not straightforward; it is a layered and complex intersection of the personal, professional, and the political. It is an arena where personal and professional moralities can collide when we are forced to ask difficult questions when addressing difficult societal issues and when attempting to do the right thing.

In order to illustrate the role of professionals in the political arena and consequent social change, and the inherent complexity, I will describe the involvement of the Psychological Society of Ireland in the Marriage Equality referendum that took place in the Republic of Ireland in 2015 and the role that professional ethics and inherent human rights played in this process.

I will conclude this chapter with a summary and a reflection on the role of professionals, and politics and social change by briefly considering the emerging social issues where practitioners are called to grapple with difficult questions in their attempt to do the right thing.

Ethics and Human Rights for HSCPs

It is widely accepted and expected in contemporary society that HSCPs have an obligation to adhere to their professional codes of ethics. However, the concept of professional ethics is a relatively recent development (Scher & Kozlowska, 2018) and the development of professional ethics appears to have happened in tandem with, or at the very least been influenced by, the development of human rights after World War II (Marks, 2012).

The 1948 Universal Declaration of Human Rights

The Universal Declaration of Human Rights (UDHR) is considered to be the foundation of the wider human rights framework and a shared value system for human and societal well-being (Hagenaars & Thompson, 2020). Following the atrocities of World Wars I and II, the United Nations was established in 1945 and the UDHR was declared in 1948. The UDHR is considered to be the foundation of international human rights law; a declaration of fundamental values and agreed-upon standards, and represents a commitment by each State to its implementation (Patel, 2019).

However, it has also been argued that human rights pre-date the UDHR. Scholars have asserted that what we consider human rights are embedded in all religious, spiritual, and philosophical traditions, albeit selectively applied (Johnson & Symonides, 1998). Furthermore, the UDHR is not without criticism and controversy and on occasion is deeply contested. Human rights have drawn criticism as being neocolonial, eurocentric, male, and individualistic, as opposed to being collective in orientation (e.g. An-Na'im, 2016; Ignatieff, 2001; Panikkar & Panikkar, 1982; Shachar, 2001), and that as such our understanding of what it means to be human is mediated by these forces that underpin Western thought (Patel, 2019).

Patel (2019) argues that it is not surprising that human rights are Western in orientation and coloured by Western values give that they are a Western construct (Cerna, 1994; Mutua, 2002; Panikkar & Panikkar, 1982) since human rights were drawn up in the absence of equal and full participation of all nations, some countries were still under colonial rule at the time the UDHR was constructed.

However, it has also been argued that in an attempt to unify humanity, the UNDR and subsequent iterations may be as good as we can do (Tibi, 1994) and the search for an exhaustive, de-contextual, culturally neutral global guide is impossible, and many would argue undesirable since context is inescapable (Sørensen & Dalton, 2004; Tripathi, 2020).

Human Rights and Professional Codes of Ethics

Human rights are enshrined within the professional ethics of conduct of many different professional bodies including medicine, social work, psychology, and nursing (HIQA, 2019). Many professional HSCP groups have explicitly committed to issues of social justice and have grappled with these issues over the course of their respective professional development. Such a commitment is based on the recognition, to varying degrees by different HSCP groups, that social structures that promote inclusion or exclusion are a determinant of human well-being (Aldarondo, 2007; Burnes & Singh, 2010; Caldwell & Vera, 2010). This view does not advocate that all human suffering and distress be considered exclusively at a societal and policy level. It does, however, call for the consideration of the policy and political context and resulting inequity as potential determinants of human well-being. Critically this is the juncture of the intersection between HSCPs' professional ethics and human rights.

This is not a position where the rights of the individual are not considered or divorced from their own responsibilities. Furthermore, it is not a positioning that advocates particular political alliances or voting preferences. Rather, the contention is that professional ethics and their embedded regard for human rights inherently place an obligation on the practitioner to advance a more equal society by advocating for social change.

Such a widening of the professional ethics lens to include a broader human rights-based orientation in large part emerges from the antecedents to professional ethics, World Wars I and II, and the Holocaust, that emerged within the context of UDHR.

Human Rights Based-Approach for HSCPs

The Interdependent Nature of Professional Codes of Ethics and Human Rights

Health and social care practitioners do not operate in a political vacuum. They occupy professional roles that are not only influenced by social, economic and political factors but also shape these factors, passively or actively. The structural violence, the systemic and often invisible forms of harm and inequality perpetuated by social, economic, and political structures that disadvantage certain groups or individuals based on factors such as race, class, gender, or ethnicity and the resulting social inequalities, marginalization, discrimination, oppression, witnessed in society is, in my view, in large part the result of policy decisions.

Practitioners in psychology, psychiatry, and other specialisms are very often confronted with the pernicious impact of adversity, trauma, and inequality on the individual and discriminated groups of individuals. It is often, but not always, early life adversity, trauma or other human rights violations and structural inequality that act as the precipitant to an individual seeking help from a psychiatrist or a psychologist.

One could argue that it is the work of civil society groups to advocate for the victims of such structural inequalities and indeed to judge how governments are implementing international and constitutional obligations under the various human rights treaties. However, I am of the view that HSCPs have a similar obligation because their professional codes of ethics, for many professional groups, are embedded in human rights.

Furthermore, Patel (2019) asserts that it is the State and public authorities that are the duty-bearers who have the responsibility to uphold, protect, and fulfil human rights of individuals in society. According to Patel (2019), the duty-bearers include the policy-makers, regulatory bodies, hospital managers, bodies commissioned by the State to carry out work on behalf of the State, and HSCPs. For example, in many jurisdictions HSCPs have an explicit legal obligation to report infringements of human rights as they present in situations where vulnerable people are at risk of abuse or neglect.

In addition, given that many professional codes of ethics are influenced by human rights, a significant number explicitly reference human rights, there is, one could argue, an inherent added obligation as implicit duty-bearers, to promote human rights.

HSCPs and Social Justice

Health and social care practitioners are drawn to their roles in order to improve the lives of the people they serve and promote conditions that enhance human growth and flourishing. The concept of basic human needs is not new in health and social care (e.g. Maslow; 1943). It is widely accepted that basic human physiological needs such as shelter, food, and safety are prerequisite to human survival and to achieving subsequent well-being.

However, it appears that very often there is a cognitive disconnection between such basic human physiological needs and human rights. It seems that often basic human needs are disconnected from basic human rights in practice and in many of the theories underpinning our understanding of human development. It is also argued that if we do not approach our work as practitioners from a human rights-based perspective, we are at risk of neglecting the structural, discursive, economic, structural determinants of health, and State policies that maintain inequalities (Petel, 2020).

The apparent cognitive disconnection between basic human needs and basic human rights is not a natural relationship: the disconnection may result in practitioners inadvertently colluding in individualizing distress to a particular individual, family, or community or ethnic group which is often, however, the result in large part of the policy-driven determinants mentioned above. For many practitioners, perhaps for mental health practitioners in particular, inequalities and injustices happen outside the clinic walls and soundproofed therapy rooms. As a result, the adverse consequences that often present in practice are addressed as individual symptoms and the root causes such as the structural, political, and economic inequalities are left outside the consultation room.

There are, on the other hand, pockets within various disciplines that have a long history of such social justice and human rights based-approaches (HRBA: see *Advancing social justice through clinical practice*, edited by Etiony Aldarondo, 2007), where potential biological determinants of mental health conditions, such as genetics and physical health conditions, for example, are not disregarded but rather seen in the context of social contexts in which individuals and groups live.

It is interesting to note that in the psychology and psychotherapy field, historically at least, the arena of social justice has been championed by feminist therapists and community psychologists who have continually called for the recognition of the social factors that contribute to the distress people experience and have called for an activist stance for service providers and scholars (e.g. Emms, 2004, Nelson & Prilleltensky, 2005).

The social determinants of distress, often synonymous with a violation of human rights, must be considered as part of the approach practitioners adopt when faced with human suffering in my view. It has been suggested, however, that the social reformist, the activist, the human rights informed practitioner have had their tenacity and reach restricted by the needs of their respective professions, (Aldarondo, 2007, p.12).

A human rights based approach provides the ground from which practitioners can understand human suffering in a radically different way. From such a positioning, the causes of human suffering can be interrogated and provide a potentially potent antidote to the individualization of human distress. The human rights perspective for the practitioner allows for a radical reconsideration of human suffering, a brave challenge to often uncontested and established 'facts' and diagnostic categories, 'evidence based interventions', and decontextualized and de-politicized formulations of human distress.

Distress and Inequity: Social Structural Determinants of Physical and Mental Health

The structural, political, and economic conditions that create distress are often airbrushed away, or worse, located in the individual as some variant of personal failing—a view that seems prevalent in many neoliberal ideologies. When HSCPs obscure the social and economic inequalities, discrimination, and 'othering' that contribute to human distress, they are making a political statement. It is asserted that no act is politically neutral. This is demonstrated by the empirically supported research concerning the social determinants of health outcomes (Commission on Social Determinants of Health, 2008; Marmot & Commission on Social Determinants of Health, 2007) and evidence that there are sub-groups at greater risk of mental health problems due to adverse social, environmental, and economic conditions (Allen et al., 2014; Marmot et al., 2008).

The (WHO) Commission on Social Determinants of Health (2008) asserts that the unequal distribution of power, goods, income, and services and the resulting unequal distribution of negative health impacts, is not a naturally occurring phenomenon but rather the result of social and economic policies (Irwin et al., 2006). More recently the WHO (2024) has issued new guidance and a call for governments to rebuild societies in the context of climate change, Covid19, and conflicts across the world that are exacerbating health inequalities. If practitioners are consciously or unconsciously colluding with policies that undermine equity, it is perhaps fair to say the practitioners are complicit in creating the conditions for human suffering.

It is this interaction between professional ethics, human rights duty-bearing, politics, and policy that demands HSCPs enter the policy and political arena. The failure to do so is to support discriminatory social norms and in turn worsen the suffering of those HSCPs serve.

HSCP and the FREDA Principles

The application of human rights in the contexts in which practitioners work can sometimes be hard to grapple with. Indeed, this is often the criticism levied at the UDHR by many: it can appear somewhat abstract and to some extent illusive.

A HRBA is grounded in the core principles of the UDHR: dignity, freedom, inclusion, and the equal and inalienable worth of human beings. The FREDA principles (Fairness, Respect, Equality, Dignity and Autonomy) are an attempt to address the challenge practitioners encounter in the application of human rights to their work. FREDA is an internationally recognized framework through which a HRBA to health and social care can be approached (Curtice & Exworthy, 2010).

A HRBA for practitioners can be understood as the application of the FREDA principles to all aspects of health and social care, including direct service-user care, provision of supervision, research and audit, service development: an approach which places fairness, respect, equality, dignity, and autonomy at the heart of practice.

Maladjusted HSCPs and their Professional Bodies

Almost 20 years after the UDHR Martin Luther King stated:

> there are some things in our society, some things in our world, to which we … must always be maladjusted if we are to be people of good will … There comes a time when one must take a stand that is neither safe, nor politic, nor popular. But one must take it because it is right." (as cited in Newnes & Golding, 2017).

The absence of engagement in the political arena is itself a political act. However, the resulting interaction of the professional, personal, political, and moralities can challenge the individual HSCP and their respective professional bodies when we have to ask difficult questions to address difficult societal issues that cause human distress when attempting to do the right thing.

It is my firm contention that professional codes of ethics, grounded in human rights, and supporting policies will provide a framework in which professional bodies can approach difficult issues and be guided in how to do the right thing. Professional codes of ethics can also provide a relatively independent moral compass when tackling issues that may conflict with the personal morality of HSCPs.

LGBTI+ Death Penalty Discrimination and HSCPs

It is well recognized that individuals that make up members of the lesbian, gay, bisexual, transgender, and intersex community (LGBTI+) are marginalized, discriminated against, and victims of hate crimes (Gerber & Gory, 2014). In parts of the world homosexuality is still criminalized: 62 countries continue to criminalize homosexuality in their legal codes, several of which also outlaw forms of gender expression; several of these countries enforce the death penalty; many of these countries have sharia-based judicial systems (Bandera, 2023). In some parts of the world 'conversion therapy' is practised; for example, most states in the USA are still practising conversion therapy (Ducharme, 2023).

Professionals, most notably in psychiatry and psychology, historically contributed significantly to this discrimination and, I would argue, have vicariously contributed to the hate crimes inflicted on LGBTI+ people, and provided legitimacy to a range of discriminatory policies and laws internationally.

In the first edition of the *Diagnostic and Statistical Manual of Mental Disorders* (DSM), published in 1952, homosexuality was classified under 'sociopathic personality disturbance' (American Psychiatric Association, 1952). McHenry (2022) comments that 'the last 70 years have brought psychiatry a long way, but it is only in the most recent version of the DSM (fifth edition) that the last pieces of evidence of pathologizing homosexuality were removed' (American Psychiatric Association, 2013).

According to Drescher (2015) this change in focus highlights the impact of cultural context on the classification of diagnosis, whereby cultural norms impact what is considered pathological and the gay rights movement in the USA played a significant role in this regard. The work of gay activists, a number of brave psychiatrists and psychologists, and civil and legal reform groups brought about this change over decades of advocacy work.

The degree of functional impairment attributed to sexuality decreased as society became more accepting of sexual minority groups which Drescher (2015) asserts is mirrored in the depathologizing of homosexuality in the DSM. It is considered that one of the legacy issues resulting from this professional pathologizing of homosexuality is the influence it has on policy and legal discrimination: the restriction of civil marriage, and all the rights and privileges it provides to heterosexual couples is one concrete example.

The Psychological Society of Ireland and the Marriage Equality Referendum

In order to illustrate the role of professionals in the political arena and social change, and the inherent complexity, I will briefly describe the involvement of the Psychological Society of Ireland (PSI: the professional body for psychology in Ireland) in the Marriage Equality referendum that took place in the Republic of Ireland in 2015.

In May 2015 the citizens of the Republic of Ireland were asked to vote on changing the country's constitution to allow for same-sex marriage. In the months that preceded voting day, there was intense debate across print, radio, television, and social media concerning this proposed change.

Changing a country's constitution is no small matter—particularly the constitution of a country that was once considered the most Catholic country in the world. The Catholic Church remains vehemently opposed to same-sex marriage. The intense debate in the months leading up to the referendum was heated and many of the issues debated were psychological in nature; chief among them was the welfare of children.

If the constitution was amended to provide for same-sex marriage it would extend adoption rights to same-sex couples. There were several examples of inaccurate research being used to discriminate against gay and lesbian people, including citing dubious research from the 1960s that asserted gay men were more likely to sexually abuse children. It has been asserted that psychological research has been used as a threat to the welfare of those belonging to marginalized groups or even used as a destructive tool when conflict arises between groups (Wainwright & Leone, 2020).

Professional Bodies and Social Change

However, in May 2015, Ireland became the first country in the world to make same-sex marriage legal through popular vote. The professional bodies played a key role in this development: the PSI entered the public debate and in so doing, became one of the first professional associations to do so.

This was the first time in the history of PSI that it entered a debate on a matter concerning an amendment to the constitution. What was crucial in deciding PSI to depart from its usual position was the inaccurate use of psychological research in the public debate concerning marriage equality.

The PSI drew on its Code of Ethics where it states:

> Psychologists shall honour and promote the fundamental rights, dignity and worth of all people. They shall respect the rights of individuals to privacy, confidentiality, self-determination and autonomy, consistent with the psychologist's other professional obligations and with the law. (1.0)
>
> Make every reasonable effort to ensure the psychological knowledge is not misused, intentionally or unintentionally to harm others or infringe human rights. (3.3.5)

Following lengthy debate, the mandate to publicly support the amendment to the constitution in favour of same-sex marriage was based on the Code of Ethics and the PSI's policy on Equality and Inclusive Practice (EQuIP) (2008). The EQuIP policy states: 'The PSI supports legislation and social policies advancing equality and social inclusion for all people.' The PSI issued a position statement on marriage equality which concluded: 'In this context, and on the basis of existing evidence, the PSI is supportive of the proposed constitutional change to provide for full marriage equality for same-sex couples.'

This is an example of a psychology professional body getting involved in an issue concerning discrimination and inequality at national constitutional and policy level. It demonstrates the applicability of professional codes of ethics and associated policies in helping guide psychologists in a course of action in order to advance a more equal society. At some level, it represents a professional body being maladjusted to societal norms, to supporting a campaign to end discriminatory social norms and committing a political act—a different kind of political act—in advocating for the end of discrimination and injustice (Fox et al., 2009).

The process described above was one with personal relevance for the author. I was president of PSI during this time and I am a gay man. It served as an uncanny confluence of the profession, personal and political, with implications that have prompted reflection over the intervening years. I have contemplated whether the engagement of the professional body in the national debate preceding the referendum would have occurred if I had they not held the presidency at the time. This reflection raises a nuanced inquiry: to what extent do the personal backgrounds and experiences of leadership influence the stance of professional bodies on political and social issues? I am concerned that if such engagement is contingent upon the individual perspectives of leaders rather than being rooted in a broader commitment to human rights and social progress, it risks being arbitrary and insufficiently systematic in effecting meaningful societal change that positively impacts human well-being

Summary and Conclusions/Reflections

In adopting an HRBA to our work as practitioners we adopt a practitioner–activist position; we seek to understand and address the connection and intersection of discrimination, structural inequality, and ill health in all its various presentations. I contend that the commitment to a HRBA is based on our professional codes of ethics. Our codes of ethics are, in turn, influenced by human rights. Such a positioning penetrates our direct clinical care, our research, pedagogy, and service design and delivery, and has implications for how we train HSCPs and for the state regulatory bodies.

HSCP work with humans who are in need, these people come to us seeking alleviation of their suffering. Our ethics and inherent obligation as human rights duty-bearers involves more than alleviating or attempting to cure the distress after it has occurred. We are, in my view, duty-bound to not just alleviate distress but to address the source of the distress.

Reflective Questions

How does this chapter challenge your understanding of the role of HSCPs in promoting social justice and human rights? Reflect on any shifts in perspective regarding the intersection of professional ethics, human rights, and social change.

Reflect on the tensions and moral dilemmas highlighted in the chapter, particularly in relation to the intersection of personal, professional, and political values. How do these tensions influence your own decision-making processes and ethical reasoning within your professional practice?

Consider the implications of the case study involving the PSI's involvement in the marriage equality referendum. How does this example illustrate the potential impact of individual and collective action by HSCPs on policy and societal norms?

In what ways does the chapter challenge you to critically examine the structural determinants of health and well-being in your professional domain? Consider how you can contribute to addressing inequities and promoting social justice within your sphere of influence as an HSCP.

Reflect on the complexities inherent in navigating the intersection of personal, professional, and political spheres within the context of promoting social change as an HSCP. How does this intersection challenge traditional notions of professional neutrality and objectivity?

References

Aldarondo, E. (Ed.). (2007). *Advancing social justice through clinical practice* (pp. xxiv, 496). Lawrence Erlbaum Associates Publishers.

Allen, J., Balfour, R., Bell, R., & Marmot, M. (2014). Social determinants of mental health. *International Review of Psychiatry (Abingdon, England), 26*(4), 392–407. https://doi.org/10.3109/09540261.2014.928270

American Psychiatric Association. (1952). *Diagnostic and statistical manual of mental disorders* (1st ed.). American Psychiatric Publishing, Inc.

American Psychiatric Association. (2013). *Diagnostic and statistical manual of mental disorders: DSM-5TM* (5th ed.) (pp. xliv, 947). American Psychiatric Publishing, Inc. https://doi.org/10.1176/appi.books.9780890425596

An-Na'im, A. A. (2016). The spirit of laws is not universal: alternatives to the enforcement paradigm for human rights. *Emory Legal Studies Research Paper 17-428, Tilburg Law Review, 21*, 255–274. Available at SSRN: https://papers.ssrn.com/abstract=2891347

Bandera, G. (2023). Where is homosexuality illegal and punishable by death? https://www.fairplanet.org/story/death-penalty-homosexualty-illegal/

Burnes, T. R., & Singh, A. A. (2010). Integrating social justice training into the practicum experience for psychology trainees: Starting earlier. *Training and Education in Professional Psychology, 4*(3), 153–162. https://doi.org/10.1037/a0019385

Caldwell, J. C., & Vera, E. M. (2010). Critical incidents in counseling psychology professionals' and trainees' social justice orientation development. *Training and Education in Professional Psychology, 4*(3), 163–176. https://doi.org/10.1037/a0019093

Cerna, C. M. (1994). Universality of human rights and cultural diversity: implementation of human rights in different socio-cultural contexts. *Human Rights Quarterly, 16*(4), 740–752. https://doi.org/10.2307/762567

Commission on Social Determinants of Health. (2008). *Closing the gap in a generation: Health equity through action on the social determinants of health – Final report of the commission on social determinants of health*. World Health Organization. https://www.who.int/publications-detail-redirect/WHO-IER-CSDH-08.1

Curtice, M. J., & Exworthy, T. (2010). FREDA: A human rights-based approach to healthcare. *The Psychiatrist, 34*(4), 150–156. https://doi.org/10.1192/pb.bp.108.024083

Drescher, J. (2015). Out of DSM: depathologizing homosexuality. *Behavioral Sciences, 5*(4), 565–575. https://doi.org/10.3390/bs5040565

Ducharme, J. (2023, December 12). Conversion therapy is still happening. *Time*. https://time.com/6344824/how-common-is-conversion-therapy-united-states/

Fox, D., Prilleltensky, I., & Austin, S. (2009). *Critical psychology: an introduction*. SAGE Publications.

Gerber, P., & Gory, J. (2014). The UN Human Rights Committee and LGBT rights: What is it doing? What could it be doing? *Human Rights Law Review, 14*(3), 403–439. https://doi.org/10.1093/hrlr/ngu019

Hagenaars, P., & Thompson, A. D. (2020). The Universal Declaration of Human Rights: Foundations for a human rights based-and-oriented psychology. In *Human Rights Education for Psychologists*. Routledge.

Ignatieff, M. (2001). The attack on human rights. *Foreign Affairs, 80*(6), 102–116. https://doi.org/10.2307/20050331

Irwin, A., Valentine, N., Brown, C., Loewenson, R., Solar, O., Brown, H., Koller, T., & Vega, J. (2006). The Commission on Social Determinants of Health: tackling the social roots of health inequities. *PLoS Medicine, 3*(6), e106. https://doi.org/10.1371/journal.pmed.0030106

Johnson, M. G., & Symonides, J. (1998). *The Universal Declaration of Human Rights: a history of its creation and implementation, 1948–1998*. UNESCO Pub.

Kameny, F. (2009). How it all started. *Journal of Gay & Lesbian Mental Health, 13*(2), 76–81. https://doi.org/10.1080/19359700902735671

Marks, J. H. (2012). Toward a unified theory of professional ethics and human rights, *Michigan Journal of International Law, 33*(2), 1.

Marmot, M., & Commission on Social Determinants of Health. (2007). Achieving health equity: From root causes to fair outcomes. *Lancet, 370*(9593), 1153–1163. https://doi.org/10.1016/S0140-6736(07)61385-3

Marmot, M., Friel, S., Bell, R., Houweling, T. A. J., Taylor, S., & Commission on Social Determinants of Health. (2008). Closing the gap in a generation: Health equity through action on the social determinants of health. *Lancet, 372*(9650), 1661–1669. https://doi.org/10.1016/S0140-6736(08)61690-6

Maslow, A. H. (1943). A theory of human motivation. *Psychological Review, 50*(4), 370–396. https://doi.org/10.1037/h0054346

McHenry, S. E. (2022). 'Gay is good': history of homosexuality in the DSM and modern psychiatry. *American Journal of Psychiatry Residents' Journal, 18*(1), 4–5. https://doi.org/10.1176/appi.ajp-rj.2022.180103

Mutua, M. (2002). *Human rights: a political and cultural critique*. University of Pennsylvania Press.

Nelson, G., & Prilleltensky, I. (2005). *Community psychology: in pursuit of liberation and well-being*.

Newnes, L., & Golding, C. (Eds.). (2017). *Teaching critical psychology: international perspectives*. Routledge. https://doi.org/10.4324/9781315209319

Panikkar, R., & Panikkar, R. (1982). Is the notion of human rights a Western concept? *Diogenes, 30*(120), 75–102. https://doi.org/10.1177/039219218203012005

Patel, N. (2019). Human rights-based approach to applied psychology. *European Psychologist, 24*(2), 113–124. https://doi.org/10.1027/1016-9040/a000371

Petel, M. (2020). *Analyse de l'usage* stratégique des droits humains au sein du contentieux climatique contre les États (Analysis of the *strategic use of human rights in climate litigation against states*). Max Planck Institute for Comparative Public Law & International Law (MPIL) Research Paper No. 2020-33, Available at SSRN: https://ssrn.com/abstract=3692955 or http://dx.doi.org/10.2139/ssrn.3692955

Shachar, A. (2001). *Multicultural jurisdictions: cultural differences and women's rights*. Cambridge University Press.

Scher, S., & Kozlowska, K. (2018). The rise of bioethics: a historical overview. In *Rethinking health care ethics*. Palgrave Pivot. https://doi.org/10.1007/978-981-13-0830-7_3 -

Sørensen, B., & Dalton, P. (2004). The Convention against Torture and Other Cruel, Inhumane or Degrading Treatment or Punishment—limitations, restrictions and reservations. In *Reservations to Human Rights Treaties and the Vienna Convention Regime* (pp. 79–93). Brill Nijhoff. https://doi.org/10.1163/9789047413967_011

Tibi, B. (1994). Islamic law/Shari'a, human rights, universal morality and international relations. *Human Rights Quarterly, 16*(2), 277–299. https://doi.org/10.2307/762448

Tripathi, S. (2020). Companies, COVID-19 and respect for human rights. *Business and Human Rights Journal, 5*(2), 252–260. https://doi.org/10.1017/bhj.2020.16

Wainwright, T., & Leone, G. (2020). Use and misuse of psychological science, knowledge and research. In *Human Rights Education for Psychologists*. Routledge.

4
Psychosocial Perspectives on Euthanasia

Tony Wainwright, Miguel Ricou, and Sílvia Marina

Introduction and Overview

The discourse surrounding human rights, suicide, and voluntary euthanasia is a complex tapestry woven with threads of ethical, legal, and psychological considerations (Emanuel, 1994). This chapter aims to explore the intersection of these topics, focusing on the overlap between suicide behaviour and voluntary euthanasia within the context of human rights.

The right to life, a cornerstone of the Universal Declaration of Human Rights (United Nations General Assembly, 1948), is a fundamental human entitlement. However, the interpretation and application of this right becomes multifaceted when considering issues such as suicide and euthanasia. The right to life often extends beyond mere existence, encompassing the right to a life of dignity. This perspective inevitably raises questions about the quality of life and the right to die with dignity (Beauchamp & Childress, 2002).

Suicide, a global public health concern, is frequently associated with mental health disorders and psychosocial distress (World Health Organization, 2014). The World Health Organization's report on suicide prevention underscores the need for comprehensive strategies, emphasizing the importance of mental health care and support. However, the discourse becomes more intricate when considering euthanasia, an act of intentionally ending a life to alleviate pain and suffering.

Voluntary euthanasia, often referred to as 'assisted dying', is a contentious issue with diverse global legal perspectives (Emanuel et al., 2016). Some countries permit euthanasia under stringent conditions, while others have a mixed legal landscape allowing physician-assisted suicide. The debate around euthanasia often pivots on the ethical implications of 'right to die' versus 'sanctity of life' arguments (Ricou & Wainwright, 2018).

The Lancet Commission's reports concerning the Value of Death introduces a fresh perspective to this discourse (Knaul et al., 2018; Sallnow et al., 2022). They discuss the paradox of death in the 21st century, where some individuals receive excessive treatment in hospitals, while others succumb to preventable conditions without access to basic pain relief. The reports advocate for a rebalancing of death and dying, emphasizing the value of death and the importance of quality of life at the end of life.

The Convention on the Rights of Persons with Disabilities (CRPD) adds another layer of complexity to this discourse (United Nations, 2006). The CRPD underscores the inherent dignity of all persons with disabilities, including those with mental health conditions or terminal illnesses. This raises questions about the application of voluntary euthanasia in these contexts and the potential for coercion or undue influence. The same can be said about children and people with lack of competence (United Nations, 2006).

In this intricate narrative, the role of psychologists is becoming increasingly prominent, particularly in the context of hastened death (Marina et al., 2020). Psychologists are now recognized as key players in assessing patients, providing psychological support to patients and their families, exploring patient decision-making, and reorienting patients (Marina et al., 2020). However, these roles may vary depending on whether the patient has a terminal or non-terminal illness. The primary rationale for hastened death is unrelenting suffering, a profoundly personal experience of an actual or perceived impending threat to the integrity or life of the person, which has significant duration and a central place in the person's mind (Dees et al., 2011). This can be argued to be part of palliative care as the main goal should be the relief of suffering and improvement in the quality of life (Galushko et al., 2012).

In this chapter, the authors are concerned both to suggest there are specific roles for psychologists in end-of-life care as well as the more general point of the role of psychological expertise and psychological processes, where other professions, and indeed relatives and friends may be the key players. Our view is that psychologists, particularly clinical psychologists, through the nature of their training can have a useful role here as this will include areas such understanding the mental health issues involved as well as decision-making capacity and wider systemic questions.

Different legislatures have arrived at different conclusions concerning the involvement of professionals in voluntary euthanasia. It is generally a given that physicians are central to the process, but others are also often mentioned, for example psychiatrists, psychologists, social workers, and lawyers. We are not aware of any literature that explores how decisions about the identified role of different professions are reached in legal terms. In practice, we can speculate that it can be the specific training, power relationships, and institutional factors in play in particular countries. Nevertheless, the legislation in Portugal references the role of certain professionals in the process. It stipulates the involvement of a medical specialist in the disease of the person requesting euthanasia or assisted suicide. The law also highlights the need for a psychiatrist's consultation when there are doubts about the presence of a mental illness that could affect the individual's decision-making capacity. Furthermore, it advocates for the engagement of a clinical psychologist to accompany the person throughout the entire process, starting from the moment they request hastening of death.

However, it is clear that whether clinical psychologists are involved or not, psychological processes are critical in end of life decision-making, and in particular in considerations of voluntary euthanasia.

This chapter will delve into the heart of the decision-making process in hastened death, using two brief case studies, to illustrate the difficulties in the context where it is illegal and another where it is legalized. It will illuminate the shared decision-making (SDM) model, a critical tool in understanding the complex dynamics at play (Elwyn et al., 2012). The influence of psychological, social, and emotional factors on this process will be examined, providing a comprehensive view of the decision-making landscape. The three steps of SDM: choice talk, option talk, and decision talk, will be detailed, offering a step-by-step breakdown of this crucial process (Elwyn et al., 2012). In addition, it will show how the principles of ethical reasoning can be combined with a human rights-based approach (Plavšić et al., 2020).

The paper will emphasize the importance of monitoring and providing detailed information to patients and their families. It will advocate for further research in this area, underscoring the need for continued exploration and understanding. This conclusion will serve as a call to action, urging for more research to contribute to the role of psychologists in the global discourse on the right to life and to the importance of dignity as central to end-of-life care.

How Do We Decide What Is Right and Wrong: Lessons from Moral Psychology

The debate about what is the right thing to do when someone requests that their life be ended will not be settled in this chapter. We do not take a position on whether it is right or wrong to take one's own life, or indeed to help someone take their own life if it is lawful. All three authors have their own views about this, but for the purposes of this chapter, our aim is to explore what the 'right way' looks like from a psychological perspective to help someone who wishes to die and has full capacity, whether they are in a country where it is lawful or a country where it is not. For ease of understanding, we will provide separate commentary on the two situations, drawing on the situation in the UK, where it is not lawful, and in Portugal where it has recently become lawful. The same questions will arise, and the same principles apply.

Ethical Reflection on Euthanasia

Euthanasia, a term laden with emotion, ethics, and complexity, consistently invites intense debate. At its core, this debate is fuelled by its intersection with human rights and personal values, with contemporary discussions increasingly shifting towards the latter.

Modern societies are dynamic entities, always in a state of flux and evolution. With time, societal attitudes adjust, leading to a reconsideration of previously held beliefs and norms. As societies grow more diverse and interconnected, the balance between established norms and evolving individual beliefs becomes paramount. Notably, the global discourse around euthanasia is experiencing a significant paradigm shift. Once a topic primarily approached from moral and religious angles, it now finds itself enmeshed in a human rights framework (Pegram, 2015).

The European Association for Palliative Care (EAPC) has expressed concerns regarding the potential implications of legalizing euthanasia and physician-assisted suicide (Radbruch et al., 2016). They emphasize the importance of palliative care and its role in addressing the needs of patients facing life-threatening illnesses. The EAPC believes that the focus should be on ensuring access to high-quality end-of-life care rather than legalizing euthanasia.

A cornerstone of this new dialogue is the principle of dignity. Historically, the right to life was the most vehemently defended aspect of the euthanasia debate. However, the growing importance of individual dignity is reshaping perspectives. Dignity underscores the belief that every person's experience and agency is unique. Therefore, it becomes imperative that individuals should have a significant say in deciding their destinies, even when confronting the end of life (Pinker, 2011).

But the emphasis on dignity extends beyond individual agency. Recognizing and upholding a person's autonomy is fundamentally an act of conferring dignity upon them. To truly respect and validate an individual's choices, especially regarding something as personal and profound as their life's end, we must understand that decision-making is a complex process, based in rationality and emotions (Ricou et al., 2019).

Parallel to the value of autonomy runs the sanctity and intrinsic value of human life. This forms the bedrock of most ethical and societal structures. Within the myriad perspectives on euthanasia, two dominant values emerge: the respect for personal autonomy and the reverence for the sanctity of life.

The world of ethics often grapples with the challenge of defining and categorizing values. Are these values universal, or do they change based on context? Neumann and Olive (2003) noted that the perception of these values could significantly shape ethical choices. Professionals, when faced with scenarios where their core beliefs might clash with those of others, find themselves on difficult terrain (Page, 2012).

Beauchamp and Childress (2002) provided a pragmatic approach, introducing principles that are generally unyielding, except when they are in direct conflict. In such scenarios, healthcare professionals must often navigate a maze of ethical considerations to determine which principle should be prioritized.

One of the most pressing conflicts, especially in the euthanasia debate, is between autonomy and nonmaleficence. Both principles are crucial, but their interpretation and prioritization can differ based on the situation. It's a challenging conundrum: should the emphasis be on an individual's autonomy, potentially at the risk of causing harm? Or should the principle of nonmaleficence be paramount, even if it might be seen as paternalistic?

If society moves away from strictly absolute principles, the onus largely falls on healthcare professionals to make decisions on a case-by-case basis. However, such an approach comes with its set of challenges. Modern Western societies value both personal autonomy and life, making it a balancing act for professionals.

Legal structures, while essential, cannot capture the nuances and complexities of every individual case. Laws can provide broad guidelines and protections, but professionals must strike a balance between these rules and individualized care, which often demands deep ethical engagement.

For health-care professionals, the ultimate goal revolves around the patient's best interests. However, the term 'best' is inherently subjective. Is it about prolonging life, or is it about respecting the patient's wishes and autonomy? Adaptability, often seen as a marker of well-being, sometimes means supporting an individual's perception of their best path forward, even when it may be hard for others to understand or accept.

Complex factors, such as emotional fluctuations, cognitive capacities, and external pressures, further complicate these decisions. Such complexities are evident in the diverse decision-making processes observed in suicidal individuals (Damasio, 2010; Haidt, 2001; Mather & Lighthall, 2012).

Euthanasia and assisted suicide, although distinct, share thematic overlaps. Historical views on suicide have often been negative, but its potential decriminalization poses pressing questions about individual rights to determine one's life course.

In conclusion, the landscape of euthanasia is multifaceted and continues to evolve. Legal guidelines and ethical principles provide direction, but the heart of the matter lies in understanding and respecting individual choices, values, and rights. That is why psychologists have a major role to play. As society grapples with these challenges, it must strive for a balance that ensures compassion, dignity, and the highest ethical standards.

The Psychologists' Role

Voluntary euthanasia is usually discussed from either a medical or legal perspective, or both. However, the process of dying, while clearly having a physical dimension, can be seen as essentially a psychological one and so psychology is always relevant. Hastening death is a deeply personal decision that intersects with a person's emotional, psychological, and spiritual beliefs. This is where psychologists as professionals come into play.

It becomes evident that psychologists have a multifaceted role in the process of voluntary euthanasia. They are not just passive observers but active participants who can provide valuable insights into a patient's mental state, ensuring that the decision to hasten death is well informed and free from undue influences.

Psychologists can offer a unique perspective on the emotional and psychological turmoil associated with end-of-life decisions. They can help patients make decisions with a clear mind, free from external pressures, and with a full understanding of the implications. Furthermore, they can provide support to families, helping them navigate the emotional complexities of such a profound decision.

They can offer capacity assessment, education about communication, psychological counselling, research, and training. Additionally, psychologists can play a pivotal role in shaping public policy on voluntary euthanasia. They can advocate for more inclusive policies that recognize the psychological dimensions of hastened death and ensure that patients receive the psychological support they need.

Marina et al. (2020, 2021) systematized the potential roles for psychologists in voluntary euthanasia and assisted suicides:

a) *Psychological assessment.* We can split psychological assessment into two different perspectives: (1) the person's capacity to make decisions and cognitive stability, and (2) the motivators associated with the wish to die. The assessment of the person's capacity to make decisions typically assesses the rational understanding of information related to the decision, the ability to communicate, and an appreciation of the current condition and possible outcomes. On the other hand, many people with progressive and end-stage diseases have shown depressive symptoms (Wilson, et al., 2005) or other conditions that can influence their decision. Nevertheless, they can have the capacity to make decisions. Because depression and other psychological problems can have a negative impact on the quality of life and judgement of individuals, careful assessment is important in these cases. The characterization of suicidal ideation should also be considered. It is also of great importance to consider the wider context in which the person is requesting assisted dying, for example socioeconomic or cultural, among many others. A possible model for this is formulation, based on the Power Threat Meaning Framework[1].

b) *Need for assessment.* Given the complexity of this distinction, a thorough assessment is essential to determine whether death ideation stems from psychological issues like depression, which are treatable, or from a wish to relieve suffering due to an incurable illness. Regardless, it is impossible to make an absolute distinction and to make decisions free from errors. In fact, opting for legislation that allows for the possibility of assisted death acknowledges the potential for misjudgment in assessment. We must always be aware that in a society where this is not possible, there will be individuals who cannot adapt to their illness and will continue to suffer without the option of hastened death. Conversely, in societies that permit this, despite numerous safety measures, there will always be the risk of error, potentially leading to assisting the death of someone who might have been able to adapt to their illness and later appreciate having lived longer. This is why the involvement of clinical psychology is so crucial in this process.

c) *Psychological support to the patient and family.* This includes supporting the patient to manage psychological adjustment, well-being and distress, and communicating with families and other professionals. Psychologists can contribute

---

[1] https://www.bps.org.uk/member-networks/division-clinical-psychology/power-threat-meaning-framework

to more effective communication between the patient and their family and act as an advocate on behalf of the patient to ensure that his or her needs are met. The psychologist can also support families during the decision-making and later in bereavement, if necessary. Psychological support to patients and their families was the role most valued by psychologists for people with terminal illnesses.

d) *Explore patient's decision-making.* A patient with a severe prognostic likely faces an intense emotional condition that can influence their decision-making. Psychological counselling can be a very important tool for people who are facing difficult decisions in life. It is important to counsel the patient about all possibilities regarding the desire to die and how it can evolve over time. Discuss all possible consequences and alternatives, minimizing the possibility of external influence on the individual's decision. In that way, we can ensure that the patient is dealing with all the necessary information, starting from a neutral position by the psychologist. From the psychologists' view, for patients with non-terminal illnesses, the first line of intervention should be to explore decision-making.

e) *Reorientation of patients.* In some situations, patients need help to find meaning in their lives to adapt to their new situation, which initially led to the request to hasten death. Psychological techniques can be useful to encourage patients to maintain social roles, even in different ways, but emphasizing all the reasons for living. The importance of minimizing suffering with intervention techniques is also indicated. Reorientation of the patient was strongly emphasized in cases of patients without any kind of physical illness.

f) *Research and training.* Psychology has helped to develop knowledge across several fields, but in matters of the end of life, this knowledge should be deepened. Hastened death processes pose great challenges to healthcare professionals, both ethical and emotional. Professionals need to be trained and acquire skills in this area to respond to and understand a life-threatening choice. Psychologists can develop and provide training on the psychological aspects involved in the wish to hasten death and play a role in supporting other healthcare professionals with direct participation in these procedures.

g) *Help for healthcare professionals.* It has long been clear that healthcare professionals benefit from interventions, which can range from self-help initiatives—such as Balint groups—to psychological support, especially when dealing with emotionally demanding topics. Certainly, experiencing processes that may lead to the decision to assist in someone's death can be very challenging emotionally. In this regard, professionals directly involved in these processes should be identified as belonging to a risk group that could benefit from psychological support. Consequently, in addition to organizing peer intervision groups among these professionals, it is crucial to have readily accessible mental health professionals available for them.

h) Public policy. In most of the countries with voluntary euthanasia or assisted suicide legislation, no roles for psychologists are provided. However, this does not mean that psychologists can not be involved. In fact, it has been argued that interdisciplinary collaborative practice is important for increasing skills in this matter. Psychologists should advocate for changes to public policies to ensure adequate support for people with a request to die and for their families.

In conclusion, as the world grapples with the ethical implications of voluntary euthanasia, the role of psychologists becomes increasingly crucial. They offer a unique lens through which we can understand the psychological dimensions of such profound decisions. Their involvement ensures that the decision to hasten death is not just a medical one but also a well-informed psychological choice. As we move forward, it is imperative to recognize and amplify the voice of psychologists in this discourse, ensuring that the psychological well-being of patients is always at the forefront.

The Portuguese Law

In May 2023, Portugal approved a new law, named law No23/2023, that regulates the conditions under which hastened death is not punishable. Although the law is still awaiting regulation and is not yet in force, it has already been approved and no major changes are expected (Law No. 22/2023, Regulates the conditions under which medically assisted death is not punishable and amends the Penal Code).

In Portugal, medically assisted death is not considered a crime if it is the result of a decision made by an adult. This decision must be current, consistently expressed, serious, made freely, and with full understanding, in cases of intense suffering due to a severe, irreversible injury or a serious and incurable illness[2]. The procedure must be carried out or assisted by qualified health professionals (medical doctors or nurses). Voluntary euthanasia is only an option when the patient is physically unable to undergo medically assisted suicide. Additionally, the request for hastened death can be withdrawn freely at any time.

The patient directs their request to a doctor they have selected, known as the 'guiding doctor'. This guiding doctor reviews the patient's clinical history, considering it vital for their assessment.

Once the guiding doctor gives a favourable opinion, they seek the expertise of another doctor, a specialist in the patient's specific medical condition. This specialist's

---

[2] The law includes some definitions:

Serious and incurable disease: A life-threatening disease that is advanced, progressive, incurable, and causes intense suffering.

Definitive injury of extreme severity: A severe, definitive, and highly incapacitating injury that makes a person dependent on third parties or technological support for basic daily activities.

Intense suffering: Suffering resulting from a serious and incurable disease or a definitive injury of extreme severity, which is persistent, continuous, or permanent and considered intolerable by the person.

opinion either confirms or refutes the conditions outlined in the prior stipulations. If there is any uncertainty regarding the patient's ability to make an informed decision about hastened death, a psychiatrist's assessment becomes essential to ensure the patient's will is genuine, free, and informed. A clinical psychologist can be involved in the assessment at the request of the psychiatrist.

The role of mental health professionals in this context is not to act as gatekeepers, determining who can or cannot be permitted to hasten their own death. However, given the public's natural concern about individuals' capacity to make such a decision, the intent is to provide a safeguard. The aim is to conduct an assessment as objectively as possible of the person's capacity to make this decision, rather than evaluating the decision itself. Therefore, the focus is on identifying any mental illness diagnosis that might indicate incapacity to make such a decision. This is why recourse to psychiatry is necessary, as it is the field responsible for diagnosing psychiatric pathology.

Medically assisted death can only be carried out two months after the procedure's initiation request has been made. Throughout this process, the patient is assured access to palliative care and continuous support from a clinical psychology specialist.

Follow-up by a clinical psychologist is mandatory, except in situations where the patient expressly rejects it. This accompaniment is not intended to approve or reject the request for hastened death. The aim is to guarantee a space for free reflection between the patient and a specialist in clinical psychology, which is totally confidential and intends to increase the safety of the decisions made by the person.

The patient's family and the health professionals involved may also have access to psychological support by a clinical psychologist.

If both the guiding doctor and the specialist provide favourable opinions, the guiding doctor forwards a copy of the Special Clinical Record to the Verification and Evaluation Commission of Clinical Procedures for Hastened Death (VEC). This is to request a review of the procedure's adherence to the established requirements and its previous stages.

With approval from the VEC, the guiding doctor coordinates with the patient to schedule the date, time, location, and method for the hastened death procedure. While the guiding doctor and another health professional are required to be present during the administration of lethal drugs, other health professionals can also attend if deemed necessary by the guiding doctor. Additionally, individuals specified by the patient may be present. The patient has the final say in choosing the location for the procedure, as long as the appropriate clinical and comfort conditions exist for this purpose.

Case Study I: Hastened Death Discussed under the Portuguese Law

Background: Maria is a retired schoolteacher, with 70 years old, living in Lisbon, Portugal. She has been diagnosed with an advanced, incurable form of pancreatic cancer that causes her extreme suffering. Despite the best efforts of her oncology team, her condition is progressively worsening, and there is no hope of relief or recovery. Maria lives alone, her husband passed away five years ago, and her two children live abroad.

Request: Maria, in full use of her mental faculties, has expressed her wish to undergo medically assisted death. She has communicated this desire seriously, freely, and repeatedly over time, without any external pressure.

Initial consultation: Maria first discusses her wish with her primary care physician, Dr Silva. Dr Silva ensures that Maria understands her medical condition, the prognosis, and all available options for palliative care. Maria reaffirms her decision. Dr Silva records Maria's request in her medical file, noting her clear, consistent expression of her wish.

Second opinion: As per the law, a second doctor, Dr Costa, a specialist in oncology, is consulted. Dr Costa independently assesses Maria's condition and her request. He confirms the diagnosis and prognosis and agrees that Maria's request is serious and voluntary. Dr Costa writes a detailed report, confirming that Maria meets the criteria for hastened death. If there are any doubts about Maria's mental competence, a psychiatrist would be consulted to make that assessment. But, in this case, no request was made.

Psychologist: A psychologist, Dr Santos, is brought in to provide counselling to Maria. Dr Santos helps Maria explore her feelings about her decision, supports her in coping with the emotional aspects of her situation, and ensures that she has a safe space to discuss any fears or concerns. Dr Santos meets with Maria several times over a period of 3 months, providing ongoing emotional support and helping Maria process her decision, including exploring alternatives. Dr Santos also helps Maria prepare for the end of her life, discussing her wishes for her final days, and helping her communicate these wishes to her loved ones. In the end, one of Maria's sons asked the psychologist to draft a report that would express agreement with Maria's request. The psychologist, in a meeting with the son, clarified that the entire process was confidential and aimed at assisting Maria during this challenging period of her life. The objective was not to assess Maria's cognitive condition, something that had already been carried out by other healthcare professionals involved. Nevertheless, Dr Silva provided psychological support to the son, acknowledged their difficulties in navigating this phase of his mother's life, and assured him that Maria was receiving proper care, emphasizing that the decision she makes would undoubtedly be the best for her. In reality, it is not within the psychologist's role to pass judgment on whether to concur or disagree with the patient's request. Were this not the case, it would be more arduous for the interaction between the psychologist and the patient to cultivate the necessary trust and calmness, which is vital for the patient to articulate their doubts and anxieties during this particularly challenging moment in their life. Only if it were Maria, who requested, at the end of the process, a report from the psychologist, would the latter be able to do so. However, Dr Silva would need to discuss the potential consequences of this with Maria beforehand.

Health professionals involved in these cases may have doubts. This process is very personal, and they naturally experience a range of emotions during these assessments and support activities. They can try to put these feelings aside to do their job, but these emotions still affect them personally. That's why it's so important for them to have supervision, intervision, and psychological support. This not only helps in mitigating personal biases and influences in their decisions but also looks after their own mental health.

Verification and certification: The case is then referred to the Commission for Verification and Certification of Hastened Death. The Commission reviews the medical evaluations and verifies the legality of the procedures followed. The Commission takes into account all the details provided by the doctor's reports.

Final decision: Maria is given the opportunity to revoke her decision at any time. She chooses to proceed. The Commission certifies the case, and Maria's request for hastened death is granted. The procedure is scheduled for a date that Maria chooses, which was three months after the initial request. Nevertheless, Maria wanted to request voluntary euthanasia. However, as Maria possesses the physical capacity to undergo medically assisted suicide, this request was denied to her, leaving her with no choice but to accept the option for the latter.

Outcome: Maria's request is carried out in a dignified and humane manner, respecting her autonomy and her right to end her suffering. She is surrounded by her loved ones, and she passes away peacefully. Throughout the process, Dr Santos continues to provide psychological support to Maria, helping her navigate the emotional complexities of her decision and ensuring she feels heard and understood. It's important to note that Maria's family, despite their agreement at the time, may experience ongoing distress, uncertainty, and mixed emotions in retrospect. They might question the decision and the process for years to come. Therefore, ongoing psychological support should be made available to them, recognizing that the grieving process and the resolution of these complex feelings can take considerable time.

The United Kingdom Law

In the UK Assisted Dying is illegal[3]and so there are no conventional approaches. However, suicide itself has not been illegal in the UK since the 1961 Suicide Act, and for those who wish to hasten their death there are some choices. Some detail is provided here to indicate that every legislature will have somewhat different elements of permission and sanction. These permissions and sanctions in the UK are framed by the guidance published by the public prosecutors (in the UK known as the Crown Prosecution Service or CPS) and concern the action of those who help someone to die. These came about in 2015 because the then Director of Public Prosecution Sir

[3] https://www.cps.gov.uk/publication/assisted-suicide

Keir Starmer (the UK prime minister at the time of writing this chapter) told the House of Commons that his office had published guidelines because they had 'had to deal with a number of "right to die" cased including those of Debbie Purdy and Tony Nicklinson.' The guidelines explain who is likely to be prosecuted and who is unlikely to be if they are suspected of having helped someone to die. The criteria that make prosecution less likely include the person having full capacity, having a settled view that they wanted to die, and that the person helping them did not gain from their death. The criteria that make it more likely include that it was a young person, that there was no settled view that they wanted to die, and that the person helping them gained in some way. There is widespread acknowledgement that these guidelines are not satisfactory and the author of the guidelines himself said:

> We have arrived at a position where compassionate amateur assistance from nearest and dearest is accepted, but professional medical assistance is not unless you have the means of physical assistance to get to Dignitas. That, to my mind, is an injustice we have trapped within our current arrangements.[4]

To complicate matters further, the UK is, in fact, a federation of four nations, and some semi-autonomous legislatures. These include Scotland, Wales, Northern Ireland, Jersey, England, and the Isle of Man, each of which has somewhat different approaches to the Law. All are at various stages of considering a change to the Law.

Case Study II: Hastened Death Discussed under the UK Law

Meet Jane Emmerson, a 45-year-old schoolteacher who took early retirement from her job because she experienced high levels of stress and anxiety. She lives in a village in the south west of the UK. Jane has had a long history of mental health problems, which began during her childhood when she was sexually abused by her father. She has had a number of psychological treatments and is on a cocktail of psychiatric drugs but says none of it has been of much help. She reports repeated flashbacks to her childhood experiences and one of the many diagnoses she has is post traumatic stress disorder.

Jane used to be an active member of her community, known for her vibrant personality and zest for life, but even during these times Jane says she did not feel good.

For the past few years Jane has been supported by a community mental health team, following her leaving work as she was found to be failing as a teacher following an inspection by the education regulator.

She has approached the psychologist member of the team and said she has decided she wants to end her life but wants this to be assisted dying and as this is not possible

---

[4] https://www.bbc.co.uk/news/health-34208624

in the UK will go to Switzerland to the Dignitas organisation. She says that after years of contemplating her situation and discussing it with her close family, she has made the difficult decision to request assisted dying. She believes that this choice will allow her to end her suffering on her own terms, while still being able to say goodbye to her loved ones in a peaceful and controlled manner.

To do this, she wants to have an assessment of her mental capacity, to ensure that there is no debate about her ability to take this decision.

Analysis

For the purposes of this chapter, we have chosen to use the model presented Plavšić et al. (2020) which brings together the Four Component Model of Ethical Behaviour for psychologists (Rest, 1982) and the human rights-based approach developed by Urban Jonsson (Jonsson, 2003). James Rest's work has been developed over the years and has a formal assessment approach called the Defining Issues Test (Bebeau, 2002) that assesses someone's 'moral competence'.

The four components of the Four Component Model are ethical sensitivity, ethical reasoning, ethical motivation, and ethical action. Urban Jonsson's human right's model can be similarly divided into four components, human rights sensitivity, human rights reasoning, human rights motivation, and human rights action. These latter have two parties, those with human rights claims and those with human rights duties. These are shown in Table 4.1 taken with permission from Plavšić et al. (2020).

We will take Jane's situation and her request and view it through the components of the ethics and human rights models outlined in the Table 4.1.

Ethical and Human Rights Sensitivity

For there to be any reasoning, motivation, or action, there first needs to be recognition that there is an ethical or human rights issue involved. When Jane asks for an assessment, there are some general issues that would be considered as ethical whether it is about assisted dying or not. These include whether the assessment is necessary or not, whether the patient/client would be helped by the assessment, and so on. We will concentrate here on the specific purpose of the assessment as Jane wants to establish that she has the mental capacity to take decisions affecting her health and welfare. Jane has gone to the Dignitas website and found that they consider 'Any individual of legal age and full capacity of discernment may sign-up as a member of DIGNITAS'[5] which she says means she needs to demonstrate that she has full capacity.

---

[5] https://dignitas.ch/en/

Table 4.1 Comparison of the four-component model and the capability model

Rest four-component model		Jonsson capability/capability model	
	Ethical practitioner	Human rights claims holder	Human rights duty bearer
Sensitivity	Able to recognize an issue has an ethical dimension	Has the capability to assess a rights claim	Has the capability to assess a rights duty
Reasoning	Able to consider the pros and cons of different actions	Has the capability analyse the rights claim	Has the capability analyse the rights duty
Motivation	Has the motivation to take action on the ethical issues	Is motivated to communicate and take action about the rights claim	Is motivated to communicate and take action about the rights duty
Action	Has the competence to take effective ethical action	Has the capability to take action on the rights claim	Has the capability to take action on the rights duty

Ethical Issues Confronting Jane and the Team (Sensitivity and Reasoning)

Considering this context what are the ethical and human rights issues for Jane and the team? Beginning with the team, they would need to consider the legislative and professional context in which they worked. This team is working in England, and is part of the National Health Service, and the psychologist is a member of the British Psychological Society (BPS).

The BPS Code of Ethics and Conduct (British Psychological Society, 2021) has four principles to consider:

Respect: Members value the dignity and worth of all persons, with sensitivity to the dynamics of perceived authority or influence over persons and peoples and with particular regard to people's rights.

Competence: Members value the continuing development and maintenance of high standards of competence in their professional work and the importance of working within the recognised limits of their knowledge, skill, training, education and experience.

Responsibility: Members value their responsibilities to persons and peoples, to the general public, and to the profession and science of psychology, including the avoidance of harm and the prevention of misuse or abuse of their contribution to society.

Integrity: Members value honesty, probity, accuracy, clarity and fairness in their interactions with all persons and peoples, and seek to promote integrity in all facets of their scientific and professional endeavours.

The ethical questions that arise for the professional psychologist are:

1. Does it respect the patient and pay attention to the power relationships to carry out this assessment?
2. Does the psychologist have the competence to assess mental capacity in this context?
3. Is the assessment the responsible thing to do, in that it will avoid harm and not be an abuse of their knowledge and skills?
4. Will it be honest and fair to either carry out the assessment or decline?

A second series of ethical issues concerns the service.

1. Is it within the scope of a community mental health team to assess the mental capacity of someone who intends to seek assisted dying?
2. If it is considered ethical, is it lawful for the psychologist or other member of the team to undertake this assessment as it is unethical to break the law apart from limited circumstances where they are in conflict? The relevant legal frameworks might include the Mental Health Act (2007) and its counterpart, the Mental Capacity Act (2005), and the guidance from the UK Director of Public Prosecutions concerning those who assist someone in taking their own life (Director of Public Prosecutions, 2010 (updated 2014))
3. As Jane has hinted that if she is denied this assessment that she regards as a ticket to Dignitas, she might die by suicide instead, the service will need to consider the risks associated with withholding the assessment.

Human rights issues confronting the team: referring again to Table 2.1, does the team have the capability to assess what the human rights and duties are in this case? As Jane is an adult, there are no issues concerning the rights of the child. As she has had long-standing mental health conditions, the Convention on the Rights of People with Disabilities (CRPD) is relevant (Szmukler et al., 2014). From this perspective Jane would be entitled to access the same service as anyone else, so being discriminated because of her mental health condition would need to be considered carefully.

If Jane presented her request as a human rights issue, the team would need to be able to work out what the specific rights and duties involved would be in this situation.

Ethical issues confronting Jane and the team (motivation and action)

Following on from this, the team may not feel motivated to engage at all with Jane's request. They could take the view that it illegal to assist someone if you know they intend to take their own life. They may take legal advice that also reinforces this position. They would then be in a situation where they may be risking Jane taking her own life anyway, but not under the safe circumstances provided by Dignitas. On the other hand, they may be highly motivated to help Jane as she has been supported by the team for many years. They may feel that she is worthy of support and so ignoring the issue and dismissing it out of hand would not be favoured.

Integrating Decision-Making and Action

The considerations above cover a range of areas ranging from accurate analysis of the situation to what action is required, given the ethical and human rights issues involved. How does an individual practitioner or team integrate these various issues so that a coherent plan is undertaken?

Firstly, these sorts of considerations must be discussed with others through supervision or team meetings. Ideally Jane would be involved in the majority of these, but some, given the legal and ethical sensitivity, might need to be confidential to the team and/or practitioner. Here we just reiterate that in order to practice in any field where someone may ask for assisted dying, the team and or practitioners need to pay attention to all the areas outlined in Table 2.1. They need to be sensitive to the ethical and human rights questions, be able to reason about them, and be motivated to act in an ethical way consistent with human rights principles.

Where Could the Team and Jane Look for Guidance?

As noted earlier, each country will have its own specific rules about assisted dying. Jane's situation is not unlike one in Belgium from 2010, that of Tine Nys, a 38-year-old patient who said she was experiencing 'unbearable psychological suffering', and her death was hastened. This case was widely debated and resulted in a landmark ruling in Belgium that not only was Tine Nys entitled to assisted dying, but the law in Belgium was also incompatible with its constitution by being too restrictive (Watson, 2020). This could not be more different to the law in the UK or other countries where it is still illegal.

Conclusions

The discourse surrounding voluntary euthanasia and assisted dying is multifaceted, encompassing medical, legal, ethical, and psychological dimensions. The role of psychologists, as illustrated in the context of Portugal, is pivotal in ensuring that decisions about hastened death are deeply rooted in psychological understanding, safeguarding the mental and emotional well-being of the individuals involved.

The contrasting legal landscapes of Portugal and the UK underscore the complexities and challenges inherent in addressing this sensitive issue. While Portugal has delineated a clear framework for medically assisted death, the UK grapples with ambiguities and ethical dilemmas. The UK's stance on assisted dying, rooted in its historical and legal context, presents a myriad of challenges for individuals like Jane Emmerson, who seek a dignified end to their suffering. The guidelines provided by the Crown Prosecution Service offer some clarity but are widely acknowledged as unsatisfactory, leading to potential injustices.

The case of Jane Emmerson, juxtaposed with the Portuguese example, underscores the profound ethical and human rights considerations that professionals must navigate. The Four Component Model of Ethical Behaviour and the human rights-based approach provide a comprehensive framework for understanding and addressing these challenges. They emphasize the importance of ethical sensitivity, reasoning, motivation, and action, as well as the recognition and respect for human rights.

In the face of such complexities, it is imperative for professionals to engage in continuous dialogue, seek guidance from established guidelines, and prioritize the well-being of the individuals they serve. The contrasting approaches of Portugal and the UK highlight the need for ongoing discourse, research, and reflection on this pressing issue. As societies evolve and grapple with the ethical implications of voluntary euthanasia, it is crucial to ensure that decisions are informed, compassionate, and respect the dignity and rights of all individuals involved.

Questions to Consider

Psychological autonomy: How might the principles of cognitive psychology, particularly those related to decision-making, inform the discourse on the autonomy of individuals choosing euthanasia? To what extent does one's psychological state affect the ethical legitimacy of their choice?

Depression and voluntary euthanasia: Considering that depression can significantly impair judgment, should individuals diagnosed with depressive disorders be allowed to make decisions regarding voluntary euthanasia? What are the ethical and psychological implications?

Economics and voluntary euthanasia: Is it likely that economic considerations will play a part in lawmakers seeing an opportunity to save money on health care by making it easier for people to receive voluntary euthanasia. What are the ethical issues at play here? There is a general and profound ethical question concerning assisted dying in the context of inequality and limited resources. This has been extensively explored by Wolfensberger in his concept of 'Deathmaking' (see e.g. Wolfensberger, 1992) and the importance of effective safeguards to protect the most vulnerable.

Thought experiments: See Chapter 1 for more details of some of these examples.

The trolley problem reimagined: Imagine a variation of the trolley problem where the individual on one track is terminally ill and has expressed a wish for voluntary euthanasia. Would this change your decision on which track to divert the trolley? What does this reveal about your value judgments concerning the quality vs sanctity of life?

The ship of Theseus and identity[6]: If medical technology advances to the point where all of a person's consciousness and memories could be transferred to a machine, thus rendering their biological form redundant, would the act of terminating the biological life still be considered suicide or euthanasia? How do notions of identity and personhood factor into your ethical considerations?

Dual-Process Theory and Ethical Dilemmas: Drawing upon dual-process theories in psychology, imagine you are a healthcare provider faced with a patient requesting euthanasia. Your intuitive, fast-thinking System 1 tells you to preserve life at all costs, while your analytical, slow-thinking System 2 presents ethical arguments for honoring the patient's wish. How would you reconcile this internal conflict, and what does this reveal about your implicit theories regarding the role of psychology in ethical decision-making?

Cognitive Dissonance in Public Opinion: Suppose you encounter a society where public opinion strongly supports the right to life but also overwhelmingly endorses the legalization of euthanasia. How might cognitive dissonance theory explain this paradox? Would society benefit from interventions designed to resolve this cognitive dissonance, such as public health campaigns or educational programmes?

The Milgram experiment revisited: Imagine a modified version of the Milgram experiment, where participants believe they are administering life-ending medication to a willing patient, rather than electrical shocks to an unwilling subject. How might obedience to authority figures in a medical setting influence ethical considerations around euthanasia? What psychological mechanisms might be at play?

References

Beauchamp, T. L., & Childress, J. F. (2002). *Principles of biomedical ethics* (5th ed.). Oxford University Press.

Bebeau, M. (2002). The Defining Issues Test and the Four Component Model: Contributions to professional education. *Journal of Moral Education, 31*(3), 271–295. https://doi.org/10.1080/0305724022000008115

British Psychological Society. (2021). Code of ethics and conduct. https://cms.bps.org.uk/sites/default/files/2022-06/BPS%20Code%20of%20Ethics%20and%20Conduct.pdf

Damasio, A. (2010). *Self comes to mind: Constructing the conscious brain.* Pantheon/Random House.

Dees, M. K., Vernooij-Dassen, M. J., Dekkers, W. J., Vissers, K. C., & van Weel, C. (2011). 'Unbearable suffering': a qualitative study on the perspectives of patients who request

---

[6] https://open.library.okstate.edu/introphilosophy/chapter/ship-of-theseus/#:~:text=The%20ship%20of%20Theseus%2C%20also,from%20the%20late%20first%20century.

assistance in dying. *Journal of Medical Ethics*, *37*(12), 727–734. https://doi.org/10.1136/jme.2011.045492

Director of Public Prosecutions. (2010 (updated 2014)). *Policy for prosecutors in respect of cases of encouraging or assisting suicide*. https://www.cps.gov.uk/sites/default/files/documents/legal_guidance/assisted-suicide-policy.pdf

Elwyn, G., Frosch, D., Thomson, R., Joseph-Williams, N., Lloyd, A., Kinnersley, P., et al. (2012). Shared decision making: A model for clinical practice. *Journal of General Internal Medicine*, *27*(10), 1361–1367. https://doi.org/10.1007/s11606-012-2077-6

Emanuel, E. J. (1994). The history of euthanasia debates in the United States and Britain. *Annals of Internal Medicine*, *121*(10), 793–802. https://doi.org/10.7326/0003-4819-121-10-199411 50-00010

Emanuel, E. J., Onwuteaka-Philipsen, B. D., Urwin, J. W., & Cohen, J. (2016). Attitudes and practices of euthanasia and physician-assisted suicide in the United States, Canada, and Europe. *Journal of the American Medical Association*, *316*(1), 79–90. https://doi.org/10.1001/jama.2016.8499

Galushko, M., Romotzky, V., & Voltz, R. (2012). Challenges in end-of-life communication. *Current Opinion in Supportive and Palliative Care*, *6*(3), 355–364. https://doi.org/10.1097/SPC.0b013e328356ab72

Haidt, J. (2001). The emotional dog and its rational tail: A social intuitionist approach to moral judgment. *Psychological Review*, *108*(4), 814–834. https://doi.org/10.1037/0033-295X.108.4.814

Jonsson, U. (2003). *Human rights approach to development programming*. UNICEF.

Knaul, F. M., Farmer, P. E., Krakauer, E. L., De Lima, L., Bhadelia, A., Jiang Kwete, X., Arreola-Ornelas, H., Gomez-Dantes, O., Rodriguez, N. M., Alleyne, G. A. O., Connor, S. R., Hunter, D. J., Lohman, D., Radbruch, L., Del Rocio Saenz Madrigal, M., Atun, R., Foley, K. M., Frenk, J., Jamison, D. T., … Pain Relief Study, G. (2018). Alleviating the access abyss in palliative care and pain relief-an imperative of universal health coverage: the Lancet Commission report. *Lancet*, *391*(10128), 1391–1454. https://doi.org/10.1016/S0140-6736(17)32513-8

Marina, S., Wainwright, T., & Ricou, M. (2020). The role of psychologists in requests to hasten death: A literature and legislation review and an agenda for future research. *International Journal of Psychology*, *56*(1), 64–74. https://doi.org/https://doi.org/10.1002/ijop.12680

Marina, S., Wainwright, T., & Ricou, M. (2021). Views of psychologists about their role in hastened death. *OMEGA—Journal of Death and Dying*, *88*(1), 200–215. https://doi.org/10.1177/00302228211045166

Mather, M., & Lighthall, N. R. (2012). Risk and reward are processed differently in decisions made under stress. *Current Directions in Psychological Science*, *21*(1), 36–41. https://doi.org/10.1177/0963721411429452

Neumann, J. K., & Olive, K. E. (2003). Absolute versus relative values: Effects on family practitioners and psychiatrists. *Southern Medical Journal*, *96*(5), 452–457. doi: 10.1097/01.SMJ.0000054607.44960.49

Page, K. (2012). The four principles: Can they be measured and do they predict ethical decision making? *BMC Medical Ethics*, *13*(1), 10. https://doi.org/10.1186/1472-6939-13-10

Pegram, T. (2015). Governing relationships: the new architecture in global human rights governance. *Millennium-Journal of International Studies*, *43*(2), 618–639. https://doi.org/10.1177/0305829814562016

Pinker, S. (2011). *The better angels of our nature: why violence has declined*. Viking.

Plavšić, M., Wainwright, T., & Giotsa, A. (2020). Core competences for psychologists practising human rights-based approaches. In P. Hagenaars, M. Plavsic, N. Sveaass, U. Wagner, & T. Wainwright (Eds.), *Human rights education for psychologists* (pp. 235–247). Routledge.

Radbruch, L., Leget, C., Bahr, P., Muller-Busch, C., Ellershaw, J., de Conno, F., Vanden Berghe, P., & Board Members of EAPC. (2016). Euthanasia and physician-assisted suicide: A white paper from the European Association for Palliative Care. *Palliative Medicine, 30*(2), 104–116. https://doi.org/10.1177/0269216315616524

Rest, J. R. (1982). A psychologist looks at the teaching of ethics. *The Hastings Center Report, 12*(1), 29–36. http://www.jstor.org/stable/3560621 (The Hastings Center)

Ricou, M., Sa, E., & Nunes, R. (2019). The ethical principles of the Portuguese psychologists: an empirical approach. *Journal of Medical Philosophy, 44*(1), 109–131. https://doi.org/10.1093/jmp/jhy036

Ricou, M., & Wainwright, T. (2018). The psychology of euthanasia: Why there are no easy answers. *European Psychologist, 24*(3), 243–256. https://doi.org/10.1027/1016-9040/a000331

Sallnow, L., Smith, R., Ahmedzai, S. H., Bhadelia, A., Chamberlain, C., Cong, Y., Doble, B., Dullie, L., Durie, R., Finkelstein, E. A., Guglani, S., Hodson, M., Husebø, B. S., Kellehear, A., Kitzinger, C., Knaul, F. M., Murray, S. A., Neuberger, J., O'Mahony, S., ... Wyatt, K. (2022). Report of the Lancet Commission on the Value of Death: bringing death back into life. *The Lancet, 399*(10327), 837–884. https://doi.org/10.1016/S0140-6736(21)02314-X

Szmukler, G., Daw, R., & Callard, F. (2014). Mental health law and the UN Convention on the rights of persons with disabilities. *International Journal of Law and Psychiatry, 37*(3), 245–252. https://doi.org/https://doi.org/10.1016/j.ijlp.2013.11.024

United Nations. (2006). *Convention on the Rights of Persons with Disabilities.* https://www.un.org/development/desa/disabilities/convention-on-the-rights-of-persons-with-disabilities/convention-on-the-rights-of-persons-with-disabilities-2.html

United Nations General Assembly. (1948). *Universal Declaration of Human Rights.* https://docs.un.org/en/A/RES/217(III)

Watson, R. (2020). Assisted dying: Belgian doctors are acquitted of unlawful poisoning. *British Medical Journal, 368*, m425. https://doi.org/10.1136/bmj.m425

Wilson, K. G., Curran, D., & McPherson, C. J. (2005). A burden to others: a common source of distress for the terminally ill. *Cognition Behaviour Therapy, 34*(2), 115–123. https://doi.org/10.1080/16506070510008461

Wolfensberger, W. (1992). *A guideline on protecting the health and lives of patients in hospitals, especially if the patient is a member of a societally devalued class.* Training Institute for Human Service Planning, Leadership and Change Agentry, Syracuse University.

World Health Organization. (2014). *Preventing suicide: A global imperative.* WHO Press. https://iris.who.int/server/api/core/bitstreams/5bd12922-b362-458f-8025-f613da4922e7/content

5

The Institutionalization of People with Intellectual Disabilities

A Never-Ending Story

Roy McConkey

Our Inheritance

For centuries around the world, people who were different—whom today we recognize as intellectually disabled[1]—were ostracized within their tribes, clans, and communities. They were shunned as harbingers of misfortune who brought shame on their kin. Or as possessed by evil spirits that could not be exorcized. Many did not survive into adulthood as they succumbed to infanticide, childhood diseases, and malnutrition. The survivors though faced a pitiful future, often ending up as outcasts and beggars (Roth et al., 2019).

The industrial revolution across the Western world, and England in particular, sucked many people into the emerging cities and factories. Those unable to be productive workers often ended up in the 'workhouse'; the precursor of the institutions that were to follow. In those years, no distinctions were made about the different 'afflictions' besetting the unemployable, 'vagrants', and 'lunatics'. The priority, however, was to get them off the streets and reduce the threats they posed to responsible citizens. Prison provided only a short-term solution. The more enlightened medical doctors successfully argued for the opening of special hospitals—'lunatic asylums'—for those who were assessed as 'mentally disordered' through illness and/or disability (Bewley, undated).

Such institutions had a dual function. They provided a haven of safety for the persons where they might receive 'treatment' while at the same time protecting the wider public from any dangers the 'patients' might pose. Their location away from the cities reduced the risk of contact. In later years, the number of patients living their lives in institutions increased markedly as they became differentiated into those with mental health conditions and those who were deemed to be 'idiots' from birth. These institutions persisted for more than 100 years. They were copied in many other countries

---

[1] Other terms in past and present usage include: mental deficiency, mental retardation and learning disability.

throughout the British Empire, the USA, continental Europe, and Soviet Russia. This model of 'care' was guided by medical and nursing staff, local and national politicians, religious orders, and many other charities. For nearly 100 years it was the sole model of care for persons with intellectual disability provided by the State (Walmsley & Jarrett, 2021).

But the aspirations of institutions being a place of healing and asylum for people in need were subverted by inadequate funding, poor management, low morale, and ultimately squalid working and living conditions (Morris, 1969). One eminent visitor wrote in 1965 of people 'living in filth and dirt, their clothing in rags, in rooms less comfortable and cheerful than the cages in which we put animals in a zoo.' The person was Senator Robert Kennedy on a visit to Willowbrook, a state-run school for people with intellectual and developmental disabilities in Staten Island, New York.

In due course, whistleblowing by staff, media reports, and public inquiries revealed the extent of the deprivation and abuse perpetrated in such institutions. The move to close them and 'resettle' their inmates then became a policy objective of many countries, but it has been a slow and incomplete process and to this day, institutions and institutional thinking remain in many countries around the globe (Scoir et al., 2020). Furthermore, while their physical presence may have diminished, the forces that drove their creation and modes of working still live on, notably in the hierarchical model of medical care led primarily by psychiatrists and nurses, and which other professions have emulated.

In this chapter, we will explore why the closure of institutions is a never-ending story with no happy conclusion as yet. It is a reality to which psych professionals collude despite their rhetoric about human rights and evidence-based practice. And one that society tolerates because old fears and stigmas lie deep in our beliefs of what it means to be intellectually disabled (O'Hara & Bouras, 2007).

Present-Day Institutions

The old mental institutions and long-stay hospitals that housed many hundreds of thousands of people with intellectual disability in their heyday have long been emptied and the sites repurposed. But buildings do not define an institution, although their design and location did resemble a prison more so than a home. Rather the malign features of the institution were the crowding of people into communal dormitories, bathrooms and living areas, the rigid daily regimes, constant supervision, the lack of privacy, absence of choice, suppression of individuality, and often the threat or use of punishments, such as seclusion in locked rooms.

Of course, there were some positives. People's needs for food and shelter were broadly met, illnesses were treated, friendships were formed, and most staff were caring and loyal workers. But these positives could not outweigh the malign influences associated with congregating people with diverse needs and personalities into constrained spaces and limited opportunities for personal expression through recreation, education, or productive work. Hierarchical authoritarian management systems supervised the daily work of staff who were often lowly paid and undervalued.

Institutional practices have lived on in new guises and are not confined to people with intellectual disabilities. Residential and nursing homes, catering for upwards of 20 and more persons retain many institutional features (Cienkus, 2022; Hatton, 2017). These congregated living arrangements are favoured for those with higher dependency needs and persons with dementia but residents with intellectual disabilities enter younger and could spend many years in such homes due to the beneficial health and social care they receive. Once admitted they rarely leave.

Group homes became a preferred approach internationally to resettling residents from long-stay institutions and for people moving from family care (Braddock et al., 2001). Cost savings were gained by having larger establishments with up to 10 people living in the same house, albeit with their own bedroom but sharing all other facilities. Many residents had no choice over whom they lived with, nor could they easily move to another location. Paid staff came on a rota basis to support and supervise the residents but with insufficient time to focus on individuals while managing all the household tasks. Group homes also run the risk of becoming mini-institutions with fixed routines to maintain to keep everyone in order.

Latterly, 'assessment and treatment units' were created to meet the needs of persons identified as having behavioural and/or mental health issues. People were admitted from family homes or residential facilities when they could no longer be managed in those settings and especially when they posed a threat to themselves or to others—notably co-residents or staff. The units tended to function like a mini-hospital with 'treatments' provided by doctors, psychologists, therapists, and nurses. But even in the best-resourced units, the treatments often did not produce the intended outcomes in a timely manner, resulting in delayed discharges which were compounded when patients could not be returned to their previous abode. The units became a new form of long-stay hospital (MacDonald, 2017).

Alongside this specialist provision, a sizeable proportion of people with intellectual disability have been and are regularly detained in prisons (García-Largo et al., 2020; Murphy et al., 2017). Estimates of the numbers vary widely across jurisdictions but often their condition is not recognized or responded to within the prison and the wider criminal justice system. For most, prison will not be their long-term home but on release they often experience the same fate of the homeless; drifting between rough sleeping and hostels with increased risk of petty crimes and drug abuse.

Institutional practices can also live on in special schools—especially those which offer boarding arrangements—and in day centres and workshops catering for large groups of adult persons (McConkey et al., 2017). Nor are other care arrangements, such as respite breaks and domiciliary care, immune from institutional practices.

So, what explains the persistence of institutional care arrangements for persons with intellectual disability? The most common arguments stress economic considerations, such as shared costs across groups, the convenience for staff of having people in one location, and ease of supervision of both staff and residents. These justifications are further bolstered by comparison with how services are delivered to other client groups, such as care of the elderly and issues around prioritizing competing needs for scarce funds in health and social care. In sum, congregated care arrangements are seen to benefit the overall care system rather than the people who use them. But perhaps there are deeper reasons for a continuing reliance on institutional models, what we could call a mindset: 'a habitual or characteristic mental attitude that determines how you will interpret and respond to situations'[2] (Pelleboer-Gunnink et al., 2017).

The Institutional Mindset

When faced with decisions about the care of 'difficult' or 'complex children or adults with intellectual disabilities' especially but also more generally, it seems there is a bias towards institutional solutions. Psychiatrists and psychologists are not immune from these biases, despite their pledge to do no harm and to always act in the best interests of their often called 'patients'. Several influences come into play and although they are presented separately below, they interact, each influencing the other which makes it more difficult to appreciate and to reduce their possible malign effects on placement decisions and intervention strategies.

The Medical Model of Disability Lives On

Despite the international recognition of the social influences underpinning the functioning of persons with disabilities as manifest in the World Health Organization's (2009, updated 2018) International Classification of Functioning, Disability and Health, many service models are still predicated on assessing and reducing the person's impairments. This results in specialist assessment and treatments delivered in clinics, schools, and medical centres by discipline-specific experts. For their convenience, it is deemed better to gather them and their 'patients/clients' in one location with little attention paid to the wider social-environmental influences on the development and behaviours of their 'patients' and which may well have contributed to the extra support they may now require.

Implicit in this approach is that people with a common impairment will benefit equally from commonly delivered interventions such as pharmaceuticals or behaviour therapy. Admittedly an evidence base may exist on the effectiveness of the chosen treatments, but there is no guarantee these are equally effective across patients with differing life experiences. Moreover, if the treatments are delivered in specialized settings, the risk is that any gains may not transfer to the person's everyday life at home

---

[2] 'Mindset'. Vocabulary.com Dictionary, Vocabulary.com, https://www.vocabulary.com/dictionary/mindset. Accessed 14 Sep. 2023.

and in the community. Which begs the question why is the intervention not attuned to, and delivered in such naturally occurring settings?

Disabled People Do Not Enjoy the Same Rights as Their Non-Disabled Peers

The United Nations Convention on the Rights of Persons with Disabilities (2006) was the international response to a widespread conviction that a disability made a person less than human and that people who had disabilities did not deserve or were not capable of having the same rights as their non-disabled peers. The fact that their rights had to be specified by the United Nations was in itself recognition of a denial of their rights internationally. But UN Declarations or national policies and laws do not change the mindset and behaviours of long-established service systems, such as those which persist in modern education and health services. The rights to employment of people with intellectual disabilities (rather than attending day centres) or to have their own accommodation (rather than group living) are downplayed in favour of what has been traditionally provided and hence will continue to be available unless cultures and systems embrace a rights-basis to service delivery (Perlin, 2018).

Protecting Others Outweighs Protection of the Person

People with severely challenging behaviours of all ages pose a threat to the well-being of others around the individual, such as family members, paid caregivers, professional staff, and, albeit more rarely, the general public. A risk assessment will confirm the need to remove the person from their present setting as part of their duty of care to other persons to whom the person poses a threat. Were they not to do so and something untoward happens to the third party, then their managers, as well as the legal system, and even the media will accuse them of negligence and call for possible sanctions. In these instances, a speedy dispatch of the person to more institutional settings often occurs with the person legally detained under mental health orders if they do not go voluntarily. This decades old tradition places protection of others above protecting the individual from further harm.

But just reflect on the possible harm a person may face when removed to different settings. An abrupt change occurs in their living arrangements away from familiar caregivers and friends, disruption of their formal and informal supports, and familiar routines abandoned, all of which often results in increased stress and anxiety, especially for those on the autism spectrum (Quinn et al., 2022). Perhaps the biggest irony is that they may be placed in settings where there are others with challenging behaviour from whom they are at risk of harm or whom they may harm. In such settings, there is a greater risk, some may say *need,* to use seclusion, restraint, medication, and withdrawal of privileges. All of which seems more like punishment than therapy and their accommodation becomes more like prison than a place of healing.

Group-Based Services Are Cheaper

On the face of it, group-based services make sense, our school systems being a prime example. Pupils are organized into groups largely based on two considerations: what monies are available to spend on schools and a judgement as to the outcomes achieved. Would classes of 15 pupils produce better outcomes than those with 25 pupils? However, this balanced logic is largely absent in disability services mainly because attention has been focused solely on costs with scant attention given to the outcomes for users of services (Cronin & Bourke, 2017). Instead, service planners and providers have persisted in funding high-cost, group-based service models without assessing their value-for-money or seeking additional funds to ensure better outcomes for the users. More often they have done the opposite by reducing funds for services without considering that poorer outcomes may result. To use modern jargon, they offer poor value for money and diminishing returns on investment.

The Person Can't Object

Most people with intellectual disability are not verbally proficient and cannot marshal arguments against decisions made by those who are perceived to be cleverer than themselves. Family carers and junior staff in services may have similar feelings. But even when challenged, professionals may feel affronted that their advice is being questioned, especially when they have few or no alternatives to offer, compounded by a lack of time to listen or for negotiation.

More generally, the discrimination faced by persons with intellectual disability has not been matched by the vigour and consistency that challenged the discrimination experienced by women, people of colour, sexual orientation, and ethnic and religious minorities in our societies and services. The unconscious biases around discriminating practices remain even though the managers and professionals in health services espouse the language of equality for all (Shogren, 2022).

What Needs To Change?

To be clear, there are times when institutional care is indeed in the person's best interests. Rather my point is that this choice—indeed all professional choices—have to come after a process and that an institutional response should never be the first and only choice that is considered.

In more affluent countries, institutional care is fortunately on the decline. In poorer countries, the challenge is preventing its emergence. The shift from institutional care has been fuelled mainly by the advocacy of people with disabilities and their allies, notably parents of children who argued and fought for their sons and daughters to have a normal life. Changes in government policy and services were assisted by the scandals uncovered in large institutional settings which sadly continue to be repeated in more modern congregated settings, now called assessment and treatments centres, or nursing homes (Lodge, 2021). Regrettably, professionals such as medics, nurses, and psychologists were the most vocal for the retention of these options (Linker, 2013).

The insights gained from successful de-institutionalization can guide current efforts to avoid the tendency to fall back on institutional responses. In essence it involved a deep commitment to plan for each person individually.

Person-Centred Planning

Person-centred planning may have become a cliché but nevertheless the process for avoiding institutionalized responses is a simple but as complex as that. It's complex because existing systems have to be shut down and person-centred ones grown in their place. Experience tells us that the rhetoric from policy documents does not readily transform services nor will those gaining a livelihood from institutional provision willingly transfer their income to other forms of provision. Neither has the advocacy of and for persons with intellectual disability been sufficient to bring about the radical changes required. Caught in the middle have been well-qualified professionals—psychiatrists, psychologists, therapists, nurses, social workers, paediatricians—whose collective voices often have been muted with respect to reform possibly because they have been reluctant to challenge the managerial inertia around service reform (Perlin, 2018).

The challenge from professionals can take different forms but arguably the most effective is to promote tenaciously the welfare and best interests of the common people. In Victorian England, Florence Nightingale used it to transform hospitals, William Rathbone to instigate district nursing, and Octivia Hill to found what we today call social work. Similarly, the closure of institutions for people with intellectual disability had visionary leaders whose persistence and determination brought about the swift closure of many hospitals (Beadle-Brown et al., 2007).

So, what can professionals do to effect change? Here are the key strategies that have proved to be effective, especially when used in combination (Eklund et al., 2019; McGill et al., 2020).

Know the Individual

The core strategy is to plan what is best for the person. This means listening, observing, and discovering each individual's experiences, aspirations and needs, and doing this in the settings where they currently live. There are various tools available for obtaining and documenting the information gathered (National Development Team for Inclusion, 2020). Admittedly this process can take some time but in essence the goal is to find out what is important for the person, what they like and don't like and similarly who are the important people in their lives. More detailed gathering could be entrusted to persons who know the individual well and have done so for some time in order to complement the person's clinical assessments. Importantly the plan explicitly identifies the outcomes to be attained for the individual. These form the basis for evaluating the effectiveness of the planned actions.

Multidisciplinary and Cross-Sector Team Working

The lack of joined up working across the various professionals involved in the person's care is a long-standing complaint and which could be avoided if multidisciplinary—or better still transdisciplinary—working became the norm (Burrows et al., 2023). Small teams of core professionals are easier to manage and seem to work more efficiently and effectively but the membership should be determined by the person's aspirations and needs. Modern technology allows for meetings to happen virtually and for information to be shared quickly. One named person should be the co-ordinator for the individual. Decisions should be made through consensus as far as possible, but the most senior person—based largely on peer recognition or on rotating the chairing role at meeting—may have to take responsibility for a decision, documenting clear reasons for its choice.

Options and Choices

Exploration of the options that are currently available or could become available is a necessity. Engage with the person and their advocates as to their preferences. Facilitate visits to different options as well as scrutinising websites, videos and booklets. Undertake an option appraisal and if no existing service is available then engage with management in devising a new service tailored to the individual but likely one that will also address the unmet needs of others.

Range of pathways and gradations of services

Following on from the above, the team of professionals should develop a pathway through the various options that can or could be available across the relevant sectors, such as health, housing and day-time occupation (Royal College of Psychiatrists, 2014). Moreover, the pathway can also illustrate how differing needs will be met through having different tiers of service, from least to most intensive. Charting these pathways can illustrate the gaps in current services especially the preventative actions that can be taken to avoid triggering referrals to a 'higher tier' of service.

The pathway approach also enables costs to be determined for services across the tiers so that value-for-money analyses can be undertaken when costs are set against outcomes.

Mobilising informal supports

Professional services need to look beyond their own resources if they are to have an impact on a person's overall quality of life. Connecting with the community and voluntary sector will open up options around informal supports for the individual through leisure and sports activities, voluntary work and membership of social clubs with the potential for developing networks of acquaintances from which friendships might merge. Similar activities can also be enjoyed by groups of people with intellectual disability where friendships and romantic relationships have also developed (McConkey & Lorenzo, 2022).

New Professional Support Roles

Workforce planning in intellectual disability services is still dominated by outmoded service models with more investment going to highly trained and paid professionals whose engagement with service-users is typified by short consultations for a limited time. By contrast, support workers who have up to 24/7 contact with service users are the least qualified and lowest paid. It is long past the time for rebalancing the professional workforce away from the former to the latter (National Quality Board, 2018). This will mean new forms of training and accreditation opportunities to enable new cadres of support workers to take on greater responsibilities in meeting the needs of people with intellectual disability and their family carers through personalized provision and in community settings. Salary scales will then need to reflect their increased responsibilities and expertise but even then many more persons of this grade can be employed from current health budgets that are biased towards well-paid professionals and clinicians.

Self-Directed Support

A major innovation in social services that has also been trialled in health services, has been to allocate the funding of service supports to the person themselves so that they choose the supports and services best suited to them, for example, a personal assistant for daily living tasks rather than residential care (Morrow & Kettle, 2021). The principle is fine, but the administrative procedures associated with it have blunted its use and effectiveness, especially for people with intellectual disability most of whom will need a broker to manage the payments. Also, to maximize the effectiveness of self-directed support, ideally the fore-going strategies need to be in place, otherwise the range of supports available for purchase by individuals will not be available.

Making the Seemingly Impossible, Possible

The foregoing strategies can seem impossible to attain with many factors working against them. Worn-down family carers will take whatever option is available and have no energy to explore alternatives. In cash-strapped services, energies are directed at maintaining current service provision with little appetite to embark on their transformation. Visionary professionals are fearful of raising the expectations of people with disabilities that may not materialize. In poorer countries, these factors combine to ensure little changes and unmet needs continue to grow. Sadly there are no quick fixes other than one: change comes not in giant leaps but one step–one person at a time. Foot soldiers rather than generals can bring about change.

Changing the Singer and the Song

In this final section, I want to challenge you. I have outlined how the 'song' around institutionalization needs to change. But that cannot happen without changing the singers—that may include you! I will assume that you might be a lone voice singing 'the times they are a'changin' although I suspect that if you start to openly question existing practices you will find liked-minded people to join the choir. But again it has to start with one person—you.

Think about a person you have recently worked with for whom the decision was their admission to a congregated setting for either a time-limited placement or an extended stay. It might have been to an assessment and treatment unit (in area or out of area), a nursing or residential home, a special school (day or residential)—see section above on 'Present Day Institutions' for other examples. You might use the pro forma below to reflect on the factors that lead to that decision and ones that on reflection you might have neglected to consider.

	I did this	I could have done this
Assessment of the person's problems.		
Assessment of the person's social and environmental context.		
The risks the person posed at the time.		
The risks the person could be exposed to in the new setting.		

	I did this	I could have done this
The person was involved in making the decision.		
Who advocated for the person?		
I took account of the person's rights (e.g. informed consent, assisted decision making services).		
I investigated other options.		
Other colleagues were involved in the decision.		
I detailed the outcomes that the placement would/should provide.		
Systems are in place to ensure the outcomes are being monitored or achieved.		
I am hopeful that the person now has a better quality of life and I am seeking evidence of it.		
Any other comments and thoughts?		

If you can find a colleague with whom you can discuss your responses, it may give you further insights.

Also, if you repeat the exercise but this time for another patient/client for whom a congregated placement was avoided, that might also illuminate the influences on your decision-making.

The table below is an opportunity to highlight the key points you took from this exercise and how you might act differently.

Summary	Your response
In retrospect was this a good decision you and/or others made? Note the reasons for your answer.	
What would you like to have done or would do differently?	
What stopped you from doing the above?	
What have you learnt from this exercise?	

A Never-Ending Story?

Knowing what can be done to avoid institutional care is no guarantee that it will happen. Rather circumstances and events may make it unavoidable as the 'least-worst' option. Those particularly at risk are persons with the most complex needs for whom our best staff struggle to provide the interventions required to meet their needs. But it is not just a few persons who are affected but other pressures threaten many more. At present in the United Kingdom and other countries, the factors sustaining institutional care are a lack of trained staff, increasing numbers of people requiring services, and cost pressures within health, social and educational services. The business solution is a return to group-based options despite their known imperfections and poorer value of money in terms of outcomes for the service users with the clinching argument being that in a crisis, any type of support is better than none. Professionals and the organizations that represent them can collude in maintaining imperfect models of care through an unwillingness to opt for alternatives over which they will have less influence. Their power as decision-makers will be ceded to others, even though intellectually they can knowledge the force of arguments for moving away from institutional models of care.

Admittedly too, there are family carers and some people with disabilities who take comfort from institutional provision for the security and continuity that it offers whereas newer forms of service are perceived as involving too many risks while discounting the opportunities they could offer to the person.

And what of individual professionals, such as psychiatrists and psychologists? Do they accept the constraints imposed on them by their business managers and the preferences of family carers when they know it may not be in the best interest of their clients based on their clinical judgements and research evidence? But how best can they challenge the system? I suspect local solutions will be needed rather than national plans coupled with persistence and support from allies.

Alas for all these reasons I suspect that we will not see a speedy end to institutional care and may never do so, much as it pains me to say so. Yet I take hope, knowing that services have changed remarkably in the past decades and can do so again. I hope too a future generation—you included—will prove me wrong and that your advocacy, creativity, and ingenuity will confine to history the long shadow of institutional care practices.

References

Beadle-Brown, J., Mansell, J., & Kozma, A. (2007). Deinstitutionalization in intellectual disabilities. *Current Opinion in Psychiatry, 20*(5), 437–442. https://doi.org/10.1097/YCO.0b013e32827b14ab

Bewley, T. (undated). *Madness to mental illness. A history of the Royal College of Psychiatrists. Learning disability psychiatry*, Online archive 25b, (iii). https://www.rcpsych.ac.uk/docs/default-source/about-us/library-archives/archives/madness-to-mental-illness-online-arch ive/development-of-specialties/specialties-learning-disability.pdf?sfvrsn=b61ff72e_6

Braddock, D., Emerson, E., Felce, D., & Stancliffe, R. J. (2001). Living circumstances of children and adults with mental retardation or developmental disabilities in the United States, Canada, England and Wales, and Australia. *Mental Retardation and Developmental Disabilities Research Reviews, 7*(2), 115–121. https://doi.org/10.1002/mrdd.1016

Burrows, L., Page, G., Plugaru, E., Kent, B., Odiyoor, M., Jaydeokar, S., Williams, J., Elliot, K., Laugharne, R., & Shankar, R. (2023). Ideal models of good inpatient care for adults with intellectual disability: Lessons from England. *International Journal of Social Psychiatry, 69*(4), 814–822. https://doi.org/10.1177/00207640221140290

Castro-Kemp, S., & Samuels, A. (2022). Working together: A review of cross-sector collaborative practices in provision for children with special educational needs and disabilities. *Research in Developmental Disabilities, 120*, 104127. https://doi.org/10.1016/j.ridd.2021.104127

Cienkus, K. (2022). Deinstitutionalization or transinstitutionalization? Barriers to independent living for individuals with intellectual and developmental disabilities. *Notre Dame Journal of Law, Ethics and Public Policy, 36*, 315.

Cronin, J., & Bourke, J. (2017). Value for money? An examination of the relationship between need and cost in intellectual disability services. *Health & Social Care in the Community, 25*(3), 1227–1236. https://doi.org/10.1111/hsc.12425

Eklund, J. H., Holmström, I. K., Kumlin, T., Kaminsky, E., Skoglund, K., Höglander, J., Sundler, A. J., Condén, E., & Meranius, M. S. (2019). 'Same same or different?' A review of reviews of person-centered and patient-centered care. *Patient Education and Counseling, 102*(1), 3–11. https://doi.org/10.1016/j.pec.2018.08.029

García-Largo, L. M., Martí-Agustí, G., Martin-Fumadó, C., & Gómez-Durán, E. L. (2020). Intellectual disability rates among male prison inmates. *International Journal of Law and Psychiatry, 70*, 101566.

Hatton, C. (2017). Living arrangements of adults with learning disabilities across the UK. *Tizard Learning Disability Review, 22*(1), 43–50. https://doi.org/10.1108/TLDR-11-2016-0040

Linker, B. (2013). On the borderland of medical and disability history: A survey of the fields. *Bulletin of the History of Medicine, 87*(4), 499–535. https://www.jstor.org/stable/26305957

Lodge, M-K. (2021). Winterbourne 10 years on: how much has changed? *BMJ, 373*, Article 1389. https://blogs.bmj.com/bmj/2021/05/28/winterbourne-10-years-on-how-much-has-changed/

McConkey, R., Kelly, F., Craig, S., & Keogh, F. (2017). A longitudinal study of post-school provision for Irish school-leavers with intellectual disability. *British Journal of Learning Disabilities, 45*(3), 166–171. https://doi.org/10.1111/bld.12190

McConkey, R., & Lorenzo, T. (2022). Leisure and friendships. In H. L. Atherton & D. J. Crickmore (Eds.), *Learning disabilities: toward inclusion* (7th ed., pp. 428–445). Elsevier.

MacDonald, A. (2017). Variation in rates of inpatient admission and lengths of stay experienced by adults with learning disabilities in England. *Tizard Learning Disability Review, 22*(4), 218–221. https://doi.org/10.1108/TLDR-07-2017-0027

McGill, P., Bradshaw, J., Smyth, G., Hurman, M., & Roy, A. (2020). Capable environments. *Tizard Learning Disability Review, 25*(3), 109–116. https://doi.org/10.1108/TLDR-05-2020-0007

Morris, P. (1969, Reprinted, 2006). *Put away: institutions for the mentally retarded.* Taylor & Francis Inc.

Morrow, F., & Kettle, M. (2021). Self-directed support: ten years on. *IRSS Insights* no. 61. https://hub.careinspectorate.com/media/4549/sds-ten-years-on.pdf

Murphy, G. H., Gardner, J., & Freeman, M. J. (2017). Screening prisoners for intellectual disabilities in three English prisons. *Journal of Applied Research in Intellectual Disabilities, 30*(1), 198–204. https://doi.org/10.1111/jar.12224

National Development Team for Inclusion. (2020). Introduction to person-centred planning. https://www.ndti.org.uk/resources/publication/introduction-to-person-centred-planning-tools

National Quality Board. (2018). Safe, sustainable and productive staffing: An improvement resource for learning disability services. https://www.england.nhs.uk/wp-content/uploads/2021/04/learning-disability-services-safe-staffing.pdf

O'Hara, J., & Bouras, N. (2007). Intellectual disabilities across cultures. In D. Bhugra & K. Bhui (Eds.), *Textbook of cultural psychiatry* (pp. 461–470). Cambridge University Press. https://doi.org/10.1017/CBO9780511543609.037

Pelleboer-Gunnink, H. A., Van Oorsouw, W. M. W. J., Van Weeghel, J., & Embregts, P. C. M. (2017). Mainstream health professionals' stigmatising attitudes towards people with intellectual disabilities: a systematic review. *Journal of Intellectual Disability Research, 61*(5), 411–434.

Perlin, M. L. (2018). Your old road is/rapidly agin': International human rights standards and their impact on forensic psychologists, the practice of forensic psychology, and the conditions of institutionalization of persons with mental disabilities. *Washington University Global Studies, Literature Review, 17,* 79.

Quinn, S., Rhynas, S., Gowland, S., Cameron, L., Braid, N., & O' Connor, S. (2022). Risk for intellectual disability populations in inpatient forensic settings in the United Kingdom: A literature review. *Journal of Applied Research in Intellectual Disabilities, 35*(6), 1267–1280. https://doi.org/10.1111/jar.13030

Roth, E. A., Sarawgi, S. N., & Fodstad, J. C. (2019). History of intellectual disabilities. In J. L. Matson (Eds.), *Handbook of intellectual disabilities. Autism and child psychopathology series* (pp. 1–20). Springer, https://doi.org/10.1007/978-3-030-20843-1_1

Royal College of Psychiatrists. (2014). Care pathways for people with intellectual disability. *Faculty Report FR/ID/05.* https://www.rcpsych.ac.uk/docs/default-source/members/faculties/intellectual-disability/id-fr-id-05.pdf?sfvrsn=11e73693_4

Scior, K., Hamid, A., Hastings, R., Werner, S., Belton, C., Laniyan, A., Patel, M., & Kett, M. (2020). Intellectual disability stigma and initiatives to challenge it and promote inclusion around the globe. *Journal of Policy and Practice in Intellectual Disabilities, 17*(2), 165–175. https://doi.org/10.1111/jppi.12330

Shogren, K. A. (2022). Presidential Address, 2022—Dismantling Systemic Barriers: Re-Envisioning Equity and Inclusion. *Intellectual and Developmental Disabilities, 60*(6), 520–529. https://doi.org/10.1352/1934-9556-60.6.520

United Nations. (2006). Convention on the rights of persons with disabilities. https://www.un.org/development/desa/disabilities/convention-on-the-rights-of-persons-with-disabilities/convention-on-the-rights-of-persons-with-disabilities-2.html

Walmsley, J., & Jarrett, S. (2021). *Intellectual disability in the twentieth century: transnational perspectives on people, policy, and practice.* Policy Press. Bristol.

World Health Organization. (2009, updated 2018). *International Classification of Functioning, Disability and Health.* Geneva. https://www.who.int/standards/classifications/international-classification-of-functioning-disability-and-health

6
Assisted Suicide and Mental Health

Monica Verhofstadt, Koen Titeca, and Kenneth Chambaere

Introduction

In numerous countries worldwide, there is a growing momentum towards the legalization of euthanasia and/or physician-assisted suicide (E/PAS) (Mroz et al., 2021). Euthanasia involves an active intervention by a physician to end a patient's life at their own request, through the administration of a lethal dose of medication. In the case of physician-assisted suicide, the physician and/or nurse fulfil a more passive role by prescribing and/or supplying the lethal dose, that the patient self-administers.

The vast majority of jurisdictions limit E/PAS to patients suffering from conditions where death is expected in the foreseeable future. However, Belgium (2002), along with the Netherlands (2002), Luxembourg (2009), and Spain (2021), stands out as one of the few countries with a legal framework allowing adults primarily with severe mental health conditions[1] to qualify for E/PAS, if and only if all legal requirements are met. Furthermore, Switzerland has implemented a policy of legally *condoning* PAS in these conditions. In March 2023, Canada decided to expand its legislative framework to include adults with predominantly mental health conditions, but recently the government put this expansion on hold for one year to address critics' concerns adequately and allow expert panels sufficient time to incorporate additional safeguards for this specific patient group into the law (BBC News, 2022; Government of Canada 2023).

For the past two decades, Belgium has been at the forefront of legalizing and implementing euthanasia[2]. While the law is accessible to adults with mental health conditions, euthanasia for this patient group was initially rare. However, the number

---

[1] In striving for inclusive language, we use 'mental health' and 'mental health conditions' in this chapter. These terms best describe euthanasia's principle, allowing everyone, even those mainly experiencing psychological distress without severe psychiatric conditions, to request euthanasia. Although such requests are seen in practice and deserve to be taken seriously, it is crucial to note that the law requires suffering to stem from a severe and incurable condition or accident, excluding psychological suffering alone as grounds for euthanasia.

[2] There exist differences in the terminology and practices of E/PAS among these countries. While the legislation in the Netherlands, Luxembourg, and Canada distinguishes between the two, Belgian law explicitly mentions only the concept of 'euthanasia' but lacks specific guidelines on its implementation. This has resulted in an ethical distinction between euthanasia and PAS in clinical practice, with varying perspectives on whether or not PAS is also covered by the Euthanasia Law. Although efforts are underway to incorporate PAS into Belgian euthanasia law, this chapter consistently employs the term 'euthanasia' as this term is explicitly used by the Belgian legislator.

of reported cases has been increasing since 2008 (from 1 per year to approximately 10 per year between 2009 and 2010), with a fourfold increase between 2011 and 2014, and has stabilized at around 25 patients between 2019 and 2022 (Verhofstadt, 2022, p. 152). In 2022, a total of 2,966 people died through euthanasia in Belgium, accounting for 2.5% of all reported deaths in the country[3] (FCEE, 2022). While the majority of euthanasia cases were related to somatic conditions, 26 individuals (0.9%) died through euthanasia based on mental health conditions (FCEE, 2023).

Hence, Belgium stands at the forefront of navigating uncharted territories of ethical contemplation in the context of legislative progress and societal change. Originally conceived with non-mental health patient populations in mind[4], Belgium's euthanasia legislation aimed to provide solace and dignity to those enduring unbearable suffering from any grievous, incurable medical condition. Nevertheless, the changing circumstances have brought about intricate difficulties, specifically concerning adults with mental health conditions who are progressively recognizing their possible qualification under existing legislation. These individuals are thus making up a growing number of requests for euthanasia.

Consequently, various dilemmas have emerged in the realms of clinical practice, ethics, law, and society. Ongoing debate primarily revolves around 'factual issues', with ethical, clinical, and scientific discussions seeking to address the permissibility and implementation of euthanasia in mental health conditions from a practical–clinical standpoint. These discussions aim to establish appropriate legal requirements within mental health services, recommend additional safeguards, understand the prevalence and motivations behind patient requests for euthanasia, and evaluate physicians' readiness to participate in euthanasia assessment procedures[5]. Some issues have led to cases being brought before the European Court of Human Rights (ECHR), including two cases related to E/PAS in mental health contexts.[6] The court has recognized the potential for evolving obligations on member states to establish regulations ensuring

---

[3] To put this into perspective, in 2022, Belgium had 11 and half million inhabitants.

[4] In the electronic databases of the Belgian parliaments' debates preceding euthanasia legislation, (Belgian Chamber of Representatives (no date); Belgian Senate (no date)); there was only mentioning of physical and to a lesser extent psychological suffering, but there was no mentioning of the specific context of psychiatry. Hence, it can be deemed clear that the Belgian legislator did not have adults, predominantly suffering from mental health conditions in mind when stipulating the legal framework.

[5] Unlike the Canadian and Australian legislators, the Belgian legislator has *only* assigned a formal role in euthanasia assessment procedures to the professional group of physicians (i.e. not to the professional group of nurses). Note that the law had been extended to minor patients in 2014 but under more strict conditions. The law applies to these minors *only* in cases of, e.g. physical suffering due to a medically terminal condition. During the euthanasia assessment procedures, the professional group of psychologists can also be consulted for formal advice in this specific subpopulation. In the context of mental health, it is rare for minors to suffer from a terminal condition, except in the final stages of anorexia. Therefore, in this chapter, the main focus concerns the role of physicians.

[6] In the first 'Haas vs Switzerland' case (2011), it concerned an individual suffering from severe bipolar disorder, who argued for their supposed 'right to a dignified death'. Although the court did not explicitly recognize this right, it acknowledged the potential for member states to have evolving obligations in establishing regulations that ensure dignified deaths. The court ruled that granting or denying euthanasia for individuals with mental disorders should be accompanied by stringent safeguards to prevent abuse, particularly among vulnerable patients. The second 'Mortier vs Belgium' case involved a patient with chronic depression and a personality disorder who underwent euthanasia in 2012. The patient's son filed

dignified deaths but has emphasized the need for stringent safeguards to prevent abuse, particularly among vulnerable patients. In Belgium, even criminal proceedings have been initiated in some euthanasia cases.[7] The outcome of the latest legal proceeding seems to have made physicians' more reluctant to engage in euthanasia trajectories based on mental health reasons, due to potential legal issues raised by patients' relatives (Vande Casteele & Distelmans, 2022).

However, more extensive ethical dilemmas concerning the implications, effects, and repercussions of euthanasia laws continue to go unresolved. Specifically, clinical practice was confronted with certain ethical issues for which neither practice nor the legislature was prepared.

This chapter aims to shed light on some of the overlooked complexities and ethical dilemmas associated with procedural aspects of euthanasia, particularly in mental health practice. It explores the interplay between the ECHR's Article 2, which relates to 'the right to life', and in the context of mental health also the tension between suicide prevention and allowing euthanasia, and Article 8, which navigates the delicate balance between individual privacy and familial bonds. Through a thorough examination of these themes per the main stakeholders (the patient, the professional, and the close relatives, this chapter seeks to promote an informed and nuanced understanding of euthanasia in mental health practice.

The Patient

First and foremost, it is essential to fully comprehend the patient's intended meaning when expressing a request for euthanasia, with a particular focus on understanding

a complaint with the ECHR, alleging violations of the 'right to life' and the 'right to respect for private and family life'. The court determined that the Belgian euthanasia law met the requirements of the ECHR, except for the regulation of posteriori control by the Federal Control and Evaluation Commission, which failed to guarantee the independence of all members. As a result, amendments to the euthanasia law in Belgium are considered necessary to ensure the independence of commission members.

[7] In 2015, the first and only 'euthanasia case' was transferred by the Federal Control and Evaluation Committee on Euthanasia to the Belgian Prosecutor because not all legal requirements were deemed to have been met. However, the Public Prosecutor decided that the case did not fall under the Law on Euthanasia, because the patient drank the lethal dose herself and thus dismissed the physician from further legal proceedings. The most recent and most notable trial involved the euthanasia of a young woman with borderline personality disorder and autism, filed by some of the patient's relatives, where all three physicians involved were acquitted. However, the performing physician was required to provide further justification in an additional civil procedure, as the previous judgment was annulled due to insufficient reasoning for the acquittal. Recently, there was also an acquittal of the charges against the performing physician in that case. Note that by 'performing physician', we mean the physician responsible for administering (or supplying) the legal dose of medication. Also note that any physician can act as the 'performing physician' or 'advising physician', as the legislator does not attribute specific qualifications to this role, i.e. being a physician and having knowledge of the euthanasia law is sufficient to be deemed capable of handling euthanasia requests and procedures. According to the legislation, however, in cases involving non-terminally ill patients, formal advice from not just one, but two independent advising physicians is required. This includes the necessity of involving either a psychiatrist or a specialist in the patient's specific disorder as the second advising physician.

the underlying motive behind the request. The annual reports of an end-of-life consultation centre in Ghent reveal that approximately half of the patients withdraw from their euthanasia procedure after one or two consultations (Vonkel een luisterend huis, 2021, 2022). This suggests that not all euthanasia requests arise from a persistent desire for death. Scientific research conducted in Belgium (as well as in The Netherlands) further supports this finding, indicating that patients may have various reasons for making a euthanasia request (Pronk et al, 2021; Verhofstadt et al., 2021a). While some consider it a contingency plan in case their suffering becomes unbearable without any prospect of improvement, others seek acknowledgment of their intolerable suffering while still holding onto hope for a chance of recovery. It is important to note that in these cases, euthanasia is not necessarily sought as an end to their lives, but more reflecting a search for recognition of their relentless agony and for increased support to critically examine and reassess the current therapeutic trajectory and to find alternative ways to alleviate their perceived unbearable suffering.

However, ethical dilemmas arise when attempting to incorporate the ambiguity surrounding thoughts of death into the euthanasia assessment procedure. Moreover, striking a balance between suicide prevention on the one hand and allowing euthanasia on the other presents challenges. Can euthanasia be viewed as a therapeutic measure to prevent suicide? To shed light on this connection, a recent qualitative interview study was conducted with individuals who had requested euthanasia and explored their perspectives on euthanasia in relation to suicide (Verhofstadt et al., 2001). Most participants expressed that their euthanasia request stemmed from a well-considered desire for a hastened death, while acts of suicide or suicide attempts often arose from despair or a plea for attention. Participants regarded euthanasia as a more dignified and acceptable end-of-life option compared to unassisted suicide. However, some participants also considered suicide as an alternative if their euthanasia request were to be rejected or delayed. Additionally, the perception of euthanasia being more dignified disappeared for some participants when they realized they had little control over the procedure or its outcome. This led them to reconsider their euthanasia procedure and, in some cases, even revert to suicide (ideation). A recent interview study among health-care workers confirmed this double-edged nature of the euthanasia option (Verhofstadt et al., 2022a). While it may empower some patients to refocus on life and improve their well-being, it may discourage or further demoralize others, causing them to lose motivation to explore life's possibilities and become more inclined toward death.

To address these complexities, a two-track approach during the handling of euthanasia requests has been recommended in advisory texts, that were published in 2017--2019 (Verhofstadt et al., 2019). This two-track approach involves a 'death track' and a 'life track'. Whereas the death track entails creating space for serenely and openly discussing thoughts of death, the life track focuses on understanding the (underlying) meaning of the euthanasia request and exploring opportunities to continue living. Note that there is no clear division between the two tracks, and that the two-track policy recommends adhering to the legal procedural sequence and effectively communicating one's intentions. Note also that the law explicitly states that no one should be compelled to participate in euthanasia assessment procedures. Understanding that a portion of physicians view adherence to the 'death track' as conflicting with their personal and/or professional ethics or values (Verhofstadt et al., 2024a), the advisory texts clarify that physicians engaged in euthanasia procedures can participate in or prioritize either track to varying degrees. The primary principle is that each physician has the option to blend these two tracks or to concentrate solely on one. However, both tracks must always be concurrently considered. Consequently, other mental health caregivers may also actively engage in the euthanasia process (with patient consent) or focus on the life-oriented track.

However, the implementation of this two-track approach faces some obstacles. Some patients whose euthanasia requests are under review may experience distress and uncertainty due to the uncertain outcome, paradoxically also the possibility of being deemed eligible for euthanasia. As regards the latter, they fear that being labelled as 'having an incurable mental health condition' could negatively impact their remaining rehabilitation options, social relationships, and societal reintegration (Verhofstadt et al., 2021). Conversely, a portion of health-care workers seems significantly frustrated by the euthanasia law, due to e.g. conscientious objection, which leads them to disregard the euthanasia procedure, to respond aggressively, or to withhold treatment from individuals seeking euthanasia or already undergoing the procedure, ultimately compromising the principle of not abandoning patients within healthcare.

In addition, when a patient faces a physician who remains unresponsive to a euthanasia request—either refusing discussion or reacting aggressively—it might undermine the therapeutic relationship. Dismissing such a critical patient concern damages trust and places the patient at risk of abandoning the current clinical trajectory themselves, potentially driving them to seek another therapist or becoming excessively focused on the death track (Verhofstadt et al., 2022b). In addition, meaningful referral has been made legally enforceable in recent law adjustment. In the revised Law, it is stipulated that: 'the physician who refuses to examine/explore a euthanasia request, must provide the patient (or the person in confidence) the contact details of a centre or association, specialized in euthanasia legislation, as well as provide the patient's medical record to the physician, who is designated by the patient or the person taken in confidence, within 4 days of the explicit request' (Nationale Raad Orde der Artsen, 2003).

Neglecting the life track, which involves exploring alternatives to death, has also been identified as problematic. Some health-care providers appear to fall short in properly addressing all the legal and due care criteria, e.g. the exploration of all reasonable therapeutic options for a sufficient period of time (Verhofstadt et al., 2021b, 2022a, 2024b). In addition, although legally mandated to provide their formal advice to the attending physician—who subsequently informs the patient—the consulting physician is not legally obligated to directly communicate their findings to the patient (although they are allowed to do so). In practice, however, some physicians provide formal advice directly to the patients rather than to the attending physician, potentially undermining e.g. the trust and coordination necessary for effective patient care. Furthermore, concerning procedural aspects, there is evidence of health-care workers *initiating* discussions about euthanasia (Verhofstadt et al., 2024b). This is also contrary to the legal sequence—albeit implicitly—outlined in the Belgian euthanasia law, which suggests that the patient should initiate the request and the physician should then decide whether or not to engage in it. In contrast, the legal frameworks in e.g. New Zealand (End of Life Choice Bill, 2019) and some Australian states (Voluntary Assisted Dying Act, 2019, 2020) explicitly state they are *prohibited* from initiating discussions about euthanasia.

Furthermore, media coverage can have a substantial influence on shaping how euthanasia is perceived and discussed, and is sometimes not using the correct terminology, which can lead to confusion, especially in the context of mental health conditions.

Patients have stressed an urgent need to challenge the distorted portrayal of euthanasia and strive for a more intricate discourse, transcending the simplistic and polarizing pro-versus-contra arguments that often surround euthanasia, particularly within the context of mental health conditions. In certain instances, patients found themselves amidst fervent advocates and adversaries of euthanasia laws, entangled in the wider euthanasia debate on a personal level (Verhofstadt et al., 2021a). This prevailing situation was confirmed not only by healthcare workers but also by some patients' loves ones, who indicated that disclosing the personal narrative could be perilous for the patient as it tends to shift the focus predominantly towards the death track (Helinck et al., 2025; Verhofstadt et al., 2022a). Other patients feel intrinsically compelled to raise awareness and gain recognition for individuals suffering from mental anguish and euthanasia ideation and decide to make their story public themselves. However, sharing personal stories publicly can have detrimental consequences. Some members of patient's close relatives testified that, once these stories become public, patients are subjected to a barrage of opinions, judgments, inaccurate and misplaced media scrutiny, and public pressure, significantly worsening their mental well-being (Helinck et al., 2025).

The Physician

Ethical concerns surrounding physicians in the practice of euthanasia encompass various aspects that demand careful consideration. One concern pertains to the establishment of End-of-Life Consultation (EoLC) centres[8], which tend to attract a majority of euthanasia cases for mental health reasons to only a few physicians. In 2003, the Belgian National Board of Physicians issued a warning in this direction,

---

[8] These End-of-Life Care (EoLC) centers comprise multidisciplinary teams, where both general physicians and specialized physicians (e.g., psychiatrists) receive support in their operations from professionals like psychologists and psychiatric nurses.

deeming the creation of such teams or centres undesirable (Nationale Raad Orde der Artsen, 2003). In this regard, it is noteworthy to mention that there are multiple end-of-life information and end-of-life consultation centres in Belgium, whose role of expertise is embedded in the revised Law of 2020, stating that 'the physician who refuses to explore a euthanasia request, must provide the patient (or her person in confidence) the contact details of a centre or association, *specialized* in euthanasia legislation' (Belgisch Staatsblad (Moniteur Belge), 2020). These centres were founded from 2003 onwards with the aim of providing information about, education on, and/ or assistance in medically assisted dying and throughout the years, they have gained extensive experiences in the management of complex euthanasia cases. Former research revealed that these end-of-life consultation centres are both praised and criticized. They are considered a much needed addition to the 'individual professional' and more easily allow for in-depth assessment for patients with complex clinical features, such as psychiatric and/or somatic comorbid conditions that mutually reinforce or hinder each other, further complicating the clinical trajectory (Verhofstadt et al., 2022a). However, this 'lower threshold' for such discussions is currently threatened by waiting lists and understaffing. In addition, limited professional collaboration and even patients being victim of internal rivalries between these centres have been reported (Verhofstadt et al., 2022a). One recent study adds another critical consideration, namely, that too many euthanasia requests are evaluated by the same EoLC team: the main risks associated with a limited group of physicians acting as a 'circuit' poses concern lack of independence, desensitization, uniformity of perspectives, and potential biases in assessing euthanasia requests (Verhofstadt et al., 2024a). Moreover, these centres are not a preferred gateway for all health-care professionals, as some perceive these centres as having lenient attitudes toward euthanasia. They might prefer assistance from individuals or facilities that exercise more caution and stricter criteria in end-of-life care, differing from what they perceive these centres to offer.

Hence, a debate is needed on what should be the 'position' or generally accepted role of these centres. In the future, it may be helpful to discuss if their mission could be restricted to a more advisory role as third, independent partner for the attending physicians and a more supporting role for patients. In this way, these centres could serve and support euthanasia assessment procedures as much as possible, without the need to take over from treating psychiatrists who are generally expected to maintain a leading and coordinating role in the assessment procedure.

Another ethical concern revolves around the notion of 'expertise' for physicians engaging in euthanasia practice. Presently, physicians can engage in euthanasia procedures for people with mental health conditions even without extensive expertise or training. Knowing that half of the recently surveyed psychiatrists feel insufficiently competent to participate in euthanasia assessments, with less than 5% having received specific courses or training in end-of-life care (Verhofstadt et al. 2020), this contributes to the raised concerns about the thoroughness of the assessment and monitoring of euthanasia requests, highlighting the importance of ensuring that physicians possess the necessary expertise in this sensitive and complex area.

One barrier lies in the insufficient recognition of the need for enhanced expertise, both legally and in practical terms. A recent interview study highlighted e.g. that current training, which covers euthanasia and mental health, only lasts for 1.5 hours. This training lacks appeal due to its focus on rigid procedural aspects, resulting in the absence of ethical debates, practical-clinical implications, rehabilitation integration, and case studies. This underscores the insufficiency of the current training in offering a comprehensive understanding and practical examples within this specific field. The Flemish Psychiatric Association provided recommendations for the specific skills required for physicians, emphasizing that a single end-of-life education programme might not sufficiently address the inherent complexity of evaluating a euthanasia request presented by a psychiatrist. This evaluation necessitates diverse expertise, 'encompassing the evaluation of decision-making capacity, diagnostic and therapeutic proficiency in the relevant psychiatric condition, assessment of medical hopelessness, and psychotherapeutic acumen regarding the intricate layers, implicit meanings, and dynamics (transference and countertransference) associated with the desire for death and the euthanasia request' (Vlaamse Vereniging voor Psychiatrie VVP (Flemish Association for Psychiatry), 2017, p. 11). Hence, handling euthanasia requests and procedures presents physicians with a multifaceted and demanding task that surpasses usual medical expertise. In addition, it also implies that physicians can be tasked with addressing inherently societal problems beyond the purely medical. Negotiating these intricate layers requires physicians to delicately balance complex considerations while upholding ethical standards and legal requirements. Developing proficiency in these diverse areas demands extensive training, and ongoing professional development, potentially taking a high amount of time to achieve a comprehensive understanding and mastery in each aspect.

As regards the abovementioned, strongly recommended two-track approach, there are certain factors that can be considered as facilitators. Two important factors to consider are avoiding 'offloading' referrals to other physicians and instead engaging in open and calm discussions about the patient's thoughts on euthanasia. It is not intended for the physician to simply agree to the euthanasia request. If the patient is deemed not (yet) eligible for euthanasia, the physician can openly communicate this to the patient. A recent interview study with patients has shown that those who remain adherent to therapy as long as the treating physician can provide a well-founded explanation for the refusal of a request, allows the patient to continue discussing thoughts of death during therapy, and/or refers the patient to someone else to further clarify the euthanasia request (Verhofstadt et al., 2022b).

This seamlessly brings us to the second facilitator, i.e. 'effective referral'. It is crucial to allow meaningful referrals in situations where physicians have 'conscientious objections'. While physicians should have the discretion to decide whether or not to engage in euthanasia practice, it is important not to disregard the patient's euthanasia request. This approach aligns with the principles of non-maleficence and patient autonomy, to prioritize well-being. Also, the attending physician should refer the patient to advising physicians, including at least one specialist in the specific mental disorder.

However, in practice, this suggested sequence is often reversed, as in some cases, the search for the attending or performing physician begins *after* formal advice has already been given. This is to the patient's detriment, as it can lead to false expectations. For example, if the advice of the consulted physicians is positive, the patient may get the false impression that the search and consultation of the performing psychiatrist is a mere formality (which it is not).

A barrier is the time constraints within the referral process. A physician who refuses to examine or explore a euthanasia request must provide the patient with contact details of a specialized centre or association 'within four days'. This can be frustrating for the treating physician who needs (and deserves) more time to engage in meaningful conversations with the patient, e.g. to fully comprehend the (meaning behind the) euthanasia request, and to consider their own involvement in a potential euthanasia procedure. It may also lead to 'pass-the-buck scenarios'. These barriers emphasize the need to address time constraints, ensure adequate training, and establish a more streamlined and effective referral process in euthanasia practice.

Another barrier is that the position, role, and needs of certain other health and social care workers seem to be overlooked. To date, the Belgian Legislator stipulates that the attending physician must inform only the nursing team about the euthanasia request, if the nursing team is in close relation with the patient. However, in mental healthcare there are often many various health-care workers deeply involved in patients' clinical trajectory and consequently, they can be significantly affected by and can affect the euthanasia trajectory themselves. It can be important to provide them with specific protocols that cater to their unique role and needs.

Close Relatives

The Law provides minimal details concerning the patient's close relatives. It only specifies that physicians must meet the following two conditions regarding involving the close relatives. Firstly, the attending physician may engage in discussions about the euthanasia request with the patient's close relatives, chosen by the patient. Secondly, the attending physician ensures that the patient has the opportunity to discuss their euthanasia request with anyone they choose, enabling them to seek support and guidance from their social network.

It is important to acknowledge other health-care workers and the patient's close relatives in the euthanasia process. Involving other health-care workers through gathering information from others helps form a complete understanding of the patient's situation, providing valuable support for managing several issues they may face. Similarly, involving the close relatives can allow for a comprehensive understanding, additional support to the patient and mutual support within their circle. It also creates an opportunity for social healing and overall well-being (Verhofstadt et al., 2022b).

However, there are barriers to involving the patient's close relatives. Practical difficulties include a lack of guidance on when and how to inform specific individuals and determining responsibility in terms of e.g. which health-care provider is best positioned to inform the family. Emotional difficulties arise from managing mixed or extreme reactions within the inner circle, potentially leading to conflicts (Verhofstadt et al., 2022b). Legal difficulties also arise due to patient privacy rights and situations where family members oppose euthanasia (Verhofstadt et al., 2022b).[5] Clear guidelines, emotional support, and legal considerations are needed to manage the involvement of the close relatives effectively (Verhofstadt et al., 2022a, 2022b).

Close relatives involved in the euthanasia trajectory also embark on a profound journey that deepens their understanding and empathy for the patient's suffering (Helinck et al., 2025; Pronk et al., 2023). It is important to note that not all wish to be equally involved, as it depends on e.g. the unique bond and history between them and the patient, on the stage of the euthanasia process (exploratory phase versus formally advising stage) and the motivations behind the euthanasia request (tentative versus persistent). The inner circle generally desires to be involved in the euthanasia procedure during certain consultations with the physician and the patient, in which they seek recognition, the opportunity to express their perspectives without imposing their views, and a deeper understanding of the request. However, a recent study among loved ones showed that not all are (equally) involved in the euthanasia procedure, showed inconsistency in the information and support provided by the involved physicians, and a lack of aftercare for family members (Helinck et al., 2025).

Clear communication with(in) the patient's close circle was occasionally perceived as obstructed. This could be due to the patient and/or physicians not being forthcoming, or due to a lack of trust on the part of either the patient or the physicians. For instance, this lack of trust might arise when some of the inner circle expressed notably negative views about the euthanasia procedure or had even sought legal counsel. As a result, the physician and/or the patient refrained from sharing everything with even the supportive family members (Helinck et al., 2025).

Furthermore, the patient's close relatives faces diverse reactions from their own social circles, depending on their level of knowledge or previous confrontation with chronic mental health issues. Some close relatives were criticized for supporting euthanasia and felt the need to 'constantly justify' it.

In addition, it has been found that there is not only a significant gap in structured care for the inner circle being confronted with such euthanasia trajectories, but also in structured aftercare, particularly in the grieving process that they go through after the patient's death, but also after an intense farewell process where the patient ultimately put the euthanasia procedure on hold. The inner circle has emphasized that this support does not necessarily have to be provided by the involved physicians in order to avoid taking away too much precious consultation time from the patient. However, they pointed out that this potential assistance should be systematically embedded within euthanasia procedures so that they can be referred to health-care professionals who are adequately knowledgeable about euthanasia, and that financial barriers should also be eliminated.

Finally, the 'close relatives' concept is often used interchangeably with 'family' in advisory literature. This raises the question of automatic inclusion based solely on legal family status and biological ties. Or, to put it differently, it suggests that non-blood relatives might be part of this circle, potentially even as the most significant person in a social network. This involves understanding relationship dynamics, emotional bonds, and support levels.

Questions and Thought Experiments

Up to this point, we have illuminated the ethical complexities encountered in practical implementation. Below, we take a step further by delving into certain aspects and challenging the reader with some final reflections.

Redefining Expertise: Beyond Quantity to Comprehensive Competence in Euthanasia Practice

In the realm of euthanasia practice, expertise goes beyond the sheer quantity of cases a physician has encountered. Could redefining the role of these centres to prioritize providing additional support to patients, their close relatives, and colleague physicians, rather than assuming sole responsibility for managing the entire euthanasia trajectory from start to finish? Would this new model not better emphasize continued education, specialized training, and the development of reflective practices, ultimately enhancing the delivery of high-quality euthanasia practices? Should the assessment itself involve a standard multidisciplinary approach? Considering the wide scope of associated issues, is it peculiar that the medical field predominantly oversees the entire euthanasia trajectory, even though the underlying meaning of euthanasia requests often extends beyond medical problems? Consequently, can physicians be expected to handle all aspects of this complex terrain?

Beyond a Mere Checklist: Examining the Acceptability of Euthanasia in Mental Health Services from a Multifaceted Perspective

Assessing eligibility for euthanasia in the context of mental health requires more than a straightforward checklist evaluation based on meeting legal criteria. It involves delving into societal factors in death requests, such as stigmatization, marginalization, and insufficient access to adequate mental healthcare. Recent interview studies, for instance, shed light on the often restricted access to quality care for people considering euthanasia (with the abundant possibilities for the easy-to-treat at the detriment of the difficult-to-treat), the inadequacy of existing recovery-oriented and palliative care approaches within mental health, highlighting the urgent need for transformative change (Verhofstadt et al., 2021a, 2022a).

Euthanasia in mental health demands a nuanced perspective that acknowledges the broader societal landscape, which also delves into the underlying societal factors contributing to their distress and profoundly impacting their well-being and quality of life, which can leave them feeling trapped and devoid of hope, potentially shaping their inclination towards euthanasia. Resolving these issues necessitates a comprehensive approach that not only evaluates the patient's individual circumstances but also endeavours to enhance the mental healthcare and overall socioeconomic system, diminish stigma, and expand access to quality care options.

Reimagining Multidisciplinary Approaches in Euthanasia Trajectories: A Thought Experiment Challenging Medical Dominance and Advocating for Collaborative Ethical Care

The current landscape of euthanasia assessments in Belgium centres heavily on the role and responsibilities of physicians, potentially neglecting significant contributions from non-medics. This dominance appears logical given physicians' typical responsibility for medical decisions, as in medical end-of-life care. However, beyond physicians, psychiatric nurses, psychologists, and volunteers actively supporting patients during euthanasia procedures lack proper recognition and support. Recent interviews suggest non-physician health-care providers seek specific protocols tailored to their needs, similar to those in managing suicide cases, to navigate euthanasia laws effectively (Verhofstadt et al., 2022a). A recent study, however, highlighted concerns about involving too many caregivers, citing efficiency as well as privacy issues, e.g. the nature of the treatment relationship and the bond of trust with the patient may change if non-medics were to become more involved in euthanasia assessment procedures (Verhofstadt et al., 2024a).

In addition, surveys have revealed emotional and moral challenges faced by psychiatrists. Approximately half of the surveyed psychiatrists encountered difficulties in implementing euthanasia requests in their standard clinical therapeutic setting (Verhofstadt et al. 2020). Among those involved in carrying out euthanasia cases, half reported feeling pressured by patients to approve euthanasia, a quarter felt pressured by close relatives either to approve or disapprove of euthanasia, and a quarter struggled to assess patients' legal compliance due to the subjective nature of mental health (Verhofstadt et al., 2021b). The entire euthanasia trajectory significantly impacted psychiatrists emotionally, with up to 72% experiencing strain, and over half seeking emotional support (Verhofstadt et al., 2021b). However, surveys have not comprehensively gauged the broad spectrum of moral and emotional strain experienced by non-medical professionals.

Moreover, concerns may arise regarding increased involvement in clinical practice, potentially prompting expansions of euthanasia legislation, especially concerning individuals with dementia or those who express a 'feeling tired of life'. These concerns provoke significant moral challenges and ethical deliberations, urging thorough reflection on managing diverse viewpoints within the multidisciplinary health-care team and advocating strategies to alleviate their personal and moral distress.

Countries with similar legal frameworks or those considering it are therefore encouraged to contemplate situations where physicians, as well as other health-care workers, are provided comprehensive guidelines and protocols for managing euthanasia trajectories in a clinical setting. While these guidelines offer a structured framework for procedural aspects, they should also encompass guidance for scenarios where a physician faces significant ethical and moral dilemmas despite following these guidelines. For instance, when a patient's request for euthanasia conflicts with a colleague's conscientious objection or causes tensions due to conflicting viewpoints among the patient, their relatives, and/or medical colleagues. In such scenarios, it becomes evident that merely providing tick-box guidelines does not adequately equip physicians and other health-care workers to navigate the complex web of moral, ethical, and emotional challenges inherent in euthanasia decisions. This thought experiment emphasizes the necessity for a more comprehensive approach that addresses not only the procedural aspects but also the intricate moral, ethical, and emotional dimensions involved in euthanasia practice in general, particularly in the context of mental health.

Further Reading

Nicolini, M. E. (2021). *Euthanasia and assisted suicide for psychiatric disorders. Clinical and ethical perspectives*. [PhD Thesis, KU Leuven]. https://www.marienicolini.com/_files/ugd/bb0ea8_c6c0318080b94d9a969a982a2ae9accd.pdf

Pronk, R. (2021). *A dialogue on death: On mental illness and physician-assisted dying*. [PhD Thesis, Universiteit van Amsterdam]. https://pure.uva.nl/ws/files/65781146/Thesis_complete_.pdf

van Veen, S. M. P. (2022). *The art of letting go: A study on irremediable psychiatric suffering in the context of physician assisted death*. [PhD-Thesis, Vrije Universiteit Amsterdam]. https://books.gildeprint.nl/thesis/575842-vanveen/

Verhofstadt, M. (2022). *Euthanasia in the Context of Adult Psychiatry: Walking the Tightrope Between Life and Death*. [PhD-Thesis, Vrije Universiteit Brussel & Ghent University]. https://cris.vub.be/ws/portalfiles/portal/86844133/Verhofstadt_Monica_PhD_thesis_23.05.2022.pdf

References

BBC news. (2022, December 16). Canada looks to delay assisted dying for mentallyill. https://www.bbc.com/news/world-us-canada-63991452

Belgian Senate. (no date). Database of the Belgian Senate. https://www.senate.be/www/?MIval=/index_senate&MENUID=12000&LANG=nl

Belgian Chamber of Representatives. (no date). Database of The Belgian Chamber of Representatives. https://www.dekamer.be/kvvcr/index.cfm##

Belgisch Staatsblad (Moniteur Belge). (2020). *Wet Tot Wijziging van de Wetgeving Betreffende de Euthanasie (15 Maart 2020)*. 2020:16623. https://www.ejustice.just.fgov.be/cgi_loi/change_lg.pl?language=nl&la=N&table_name=wet&cn=2020031502

End of Life Choice Bill. (2019). *New Zealand Parliament*. https://www.legislation.govt.nz/act/public/2019/0067/latest/DLM7285905.html

FCEE (Federal Control and Evaluation Committee for Euthanasia. (2022). *Tenth Report to the Parliament (2020-2021)*. Brussels, Belgium. https://overlegorganen.gezondheid.belgie.be/nl/documenten/fcee-verslag-euthanasie-2022

FCECE (Federal Control- and Evaluation Committee on Euthanasia). (2023). Euthanasie—Cijfers van 2022. https://overlegorganen.gezondheid.belgie.be/nl/documenten/euthanasie-cijfers-van-2022

Government of Canada. (2021). Medical assistance in dying. Web Page modified on 18 March 2021. https://www.canada.ca/en/health-canada/services/medical-assistance-dying.html

Helinck, S., Pardon, K., Chambaere, K., & Verhofstadt, M. (2025). Understanding the experiences and support needs of loved ones in psychiatric euthanasia trajectories—a qualitative exploration. *Qualitative Health Research*, 35(1), 56–73. doi: 10.1177/10497323241237459.19

Mroz, S., Dierickx, S., Deliens, L., Cohen, J., & Chambaere, K. (2021). Assisted dying around the world: a status quaestionis. *Annals of Palliative Medicine*, 10(3), 3540–3553. doi:10.21037/apm-20-637

Nationale Raad Orde der Artsen. (2003). *Advies Betreffende Palliatieve Zorg, Euthanasie En Andere Medische Beslissingen Omtrent Het Levenseinde*. https://ordomedic.be/nl/adviezen/deontologie/consent-fully-informed/advies-betreffende-palliatieve-zorg-euthanasie-en-andere-medische-beslissingen-omtrent-het-levenseinde

Pronk, R., Willems, D. L., & van de Vathorst, S. (2023). What about us? Experiences of relatives regarding physician-assisted death for patients suffering from mental illness: a qualitative study. *Culture, Medicine and Psychiatry*, 47(1), 237–251. doi:10.1007/s11013-021-09762-1

Pronk, R., Willems, D. L., & van de Vathorst. S. (2021). Feeling seen, being heard: perspectives of patients suffering from mental illness on the possibility of physician-assisted death in the netherlands. *Culture, Medicine and Psychiatry*, 46(2), 475–489 doi:10.1007/s11013-021-09726-5

Vande Casteele, L., & Distelmans, W. (2022). Is de houding van LEIFartsen veranderd na het euthanasieproces? Bevraging van LEIFartsen in februari 2021 na het proces Tine Nys. [in Dutch]. *Huisarts Nu*, 51, 8–11.

Verhofstadt M. (2022a). *Euthanasia in the context of adult psychiatry: walking the tightrope between life and death. (Dissertation)*. [PhD Thesis, Vrije Universiteit Brussel, Ghent University].

Verhofstadt, M., Audenaert, K., Mortier, F., Deliens, L., Liégeois, A., Pardon, K., & Chambaere, K. (2022b). Concrete experiences and support needs regarding the euthanasia practice in adults with psychiatric conditions: a qualitative interview study among healthcare professionals and volunteers in Belgium. *Frontiers in Psychiatry*, 13, 859745. doi:10.3389/fpsyt.2022.859745

Verhofstadt, M., Audenaert, K., Van den Broeck, K., Deliens, L., Mortier, F., Titeca, K., Pardon, K., & Chambaere K. (2020). Belgian psychiatrists' attitudes towards, and readiness to engage in, euthanasia assessment procedures with adults with psychiatric conditions: a survey. *BMC Psychiatry*, 20, 374. doi:10.1186/s12888-020-02775-x

Verhofstadt, M., Audenaert, K., Van den Broeck, K., et al. (2021b). Euthanasia in adults with psychiatric conditions: A descriptive study of the experiences of Belgian psychiatrists. *Science Progress, 104*(3), 003685042110297. doi:10.1177/00368504211029775

Verhofstadt M, Chambaere K, Pardon K, et al. (2022c). The impact of the euthanasia assessment procedure: a qualitative interview study among adults with psychiatric conditions. *BMC Psychiatry, 22*(1), 435. doi:10.1186/s12888-022-04039-2

Verhofstadt, M., Moureau, A., Pardon, K., & Liégeois, A. (2024a). Ethical considerations regarding euthanasia in the context of adult psychiatry: a qualitative interview study among healthcare workers in Belgium. *BMC Medical Ethics, 25*(1), 60. doi: 10.1186/s12910-024-01063-7

Verhofstadt, M., Pardon, K., Audenaert, K., Deliens, L., Mortier, F., Liégeois, A., & Chambaere, K. (2021a). Why adults with psychiatric conditions request euthanasia: A qualitative interview study of life experiences, motives and preventive factors. *Journal of Psychiatric Research, 144*, 158–167. doi:10.1016/j.jpsychires.2021.09.032

Verhofstadt, M., Van Assche, K., Pardon, K., Gleydura, M., Titeca, K., & Chambaere, K. (2024b). Perspectives on the eligibility criteria for euthanasia for mental suffering caused by psychiatric disorder under the Belgian Euthanasia Law: a qualitative interview study among mental healthcare workers. *International Journal of Law and Psychiatry, 93*. https://doi.org/10.1016/j.ijlp.2024.101961

Verhofstadt, M., Van Assche, K., Sterckx, S., Audenaert, K., & Chambaere, K. (2019). Psychiatric patients requesting euthanasia: Guidelines for sound clinical and ethical decision making. *International Journal of Law and Psychiatry, 64*, 150–161. doi:10.1016/j.ijlp.2019.04.004

Vlaamse Vereniging voor Psychiatrie VVP (Flemish Association for Psychiatry). (2017). *Hoe Omgaan Met Een Euthanasieverzoek in Psychiatrie Binnen Het Huidig Wettelijk Kader? (How to Deal with Euthanasia Requests from Psychiatric Patients within the Legal Framework?).* Kortenberg, Leuven. https://vvponline.be/wp-content/uploads/2024/06/VVP_advies_euthanasie_2017_clear_NL.pdf

Voluntary Assisted Dying Act 2017, s. 61. Parliament of Victoria. https://content.legislation.vic.gov.au/sites/default/files/2023-08/17-61aa006-authorised.pdf

Voluntary Assisted Dying Act 2019 (Western Australia). https://www.legislation.wa.gov.au/legislation/prod/filestore.nsf/FileURL/mrdoc_42491.pdf/$FILE/Voluntary%20Assisted%20Dying%20Act%202019%20-%20%5B00-00-00%5D.pdf?OpenElement

Vonkel een luisterend huis. (2021). *Jaarverslag Vonkel 2020 [Annual Report of the End-of-Life Consultation Center Vonkel, 2020].* https://www.vonkeleenluisterendhuis.be/teksten/jaarverslag2020.pdf

Vonkel een luisterend huis. (2022). *JAARVERSLAG VONKEL 2021 [Annual Report of the End-of-Life Consultation Center Vonkel, 2021].* https://www.vonkeleenluisterendhuis.be/teksten/jaarverslag2021.pdf

7
Assisted Decision-Making, Moral Rights, and Changing Legislation

Cornelia Carey and Brendan D. Kelly

Introduction

Assisted decision-making policy and legislation have significant potential for both protection and violation of rights. Increasingly, states aim to move away from a 'best interests' decision-making framework to a 'will and preference' basis in policy and legislation (Curtis et al., 2022). This is in keeping with the United Nations (UN) Convention on the Rights of Persons with Disabilities (CRPD) which seeks to promote, protect, and ensure the full and equal enjoyment of all human rights and fundamental freedoms by all people with disabilities, including people with mental health conditions or neurological conditions (United Nations, 2006).

Assisted decision-making is relevant to many articles in the Convention, especially Articles 12 ('Equal recognition before the law'), 19 ('Living independently and being included in the community'), 21 ('Right to freedom of expression, opinion and access to information'), and 28 ('Adequate standard of living and social protection'). The Republic of Ireland signed the Convention in 2007, ratified it in 2018, and issued its initial State Report to the Committee on the Rights of Persons with Disabilities in 2021 (Department of Children, Equality, Disability, Integration and Youth, 2021).

In line with the Convention, Ireland introduced the Assisted Decision-Making (Capacity) Act 2015 and Assisted Decision-Making (Capacity) (Amendment) Act 2022 to overhaul legal provisions for people who have, or may shortly have, impaired ability to make decisions. The main aims of the new legislation are to ensure that the individual's rights to autonomy and self-determination are respected, to adopt a human rights-compliant legal framework for supported decision-making, and to provide legal clarity regarding who can assist formally with decision-making.

In this chapter, we will describe this change in approach to capacity assessment and assisted decision-making in Ireland, comparing this to England and Wales (a comparable neighbouring jurisdiction that ratified the CRPD in 2009 after the commencement of the current Mental Capacity Act 2005). Notably both jurisdictions have common law as opposed to civil law systems meaning that judicial rulings on individual cases guide new legislation. We will describe and analyse two relevant case studies, exploring the potential for conflict between new legislative frameworks,

Table 7.1 A comparison of capacity legislation between Ireland, England, and Wales and their adherence to CRPD guiding principles

Capacity legislation	Ireland	England and Wales
Former capacity legislation	Lunacy Regulation (Ireland) Act 1871.	Common law.
Former approach to decision-making capacity assessment	Binary, i.e. either an individual had the capacity to make their own decisions, or they did not. The High Court considered whether the person was of 'unsound mind' and 'incapable of managing their own affairs'. If not, they could be made a 'Ward of Court' and a 'Committee' was appointed to manage the person's property, money, and overall care.	The courts developed specific tests relating to particular forms of decision making e.g., entering into a contract ('Boughton v Knight' (1873).
Prompt for change to legislation	The Supreme Court acknowledged the 'over-broad' and 'disproportionate' impact of wardship (AM vs Health Service Executive, 2019).	English capacity law was criticized by the Law Commission as being 'unsystematic' and 'out of step' with disability rights (Law Commission, 1995).
Current capacity legislation	Assisted Decision-Making (Capacity) Act 2015	Mental Capacity Act 2005
Functional capacity assessment	Yes. See note (A) below for requirements under the functional assessment of capacity.	Yes. Quasi-diagnostic requirement for 'an impairment of, or a disturbance in the functioning of, the mind or brain' (Section 2(1)).
Provision for decision making assistance	Three levels of assisted decision-making. See note (B) below.	Legislation allows for the appointment and functions of an 'independent mental capacity advocate service' which can perform similar functions (Sections 35–41 of the Act) to Ireland's three tiers of decision-making assistance.
Future planning arrangements	'Advance healthcare directive' (Part 8 of the 2015 Act). 'Enduring power of attorney' (Part 7 of the 2015 Act).	'Advance Decision to Refuse Treatment' (Part 1, Section 24 of the 2005 Act). 'Lasting Power of Attorney' (Part 1, Section 9 of the 2005 Act).
Deprivation of Liberty Safeguards	No (but might be introduced separately in the future).	Yes.

(*continued*)

Table 7.1 Continued

Capacity legislation	Ireland	England and Wales
Respect for inherent dignity, individual autonomy including the freedom to make one's own choices, and independence of persons	The Assisted Decision-Making (Capacity) Act 2015 states that, wherever possible, people should be facilitated in making their own decisions and uses a 'will and preference' framework.	The Mental Capacity Act 2005 uses a best interests framework rather than 'will and preference'.
Non-discrimination	Functional capacity assessments are to be applied to all individuals in the same manner.	Quasi-diagnostic requirement for 'an impairment of, or a disturbance in the functioning of, the mind or brain' (Section 2(1)).
Full and effective participation and inclusion in society	As part of the transition to the new Act, all Wards of Court are scheduled to undergo a review process and be discharged from wardship, with some transitioning to the new system of supported decision-making under the 2015 Act and others leaving the system if capacity were demonstrated. Treatment and care provided to someone who lacks capacity should involve the least possible restriction on basic rights and freedoms.	Deprivation of Liberty Safeguarding is in place to prevent unlawful detention.
Respect for difference and acceptance of persons with disabilities as part of human diversity and humanity	A person should not be treated as lacking the capacity to decide just because they make an unwise decision (see Thought Experiment 4).	Quasi-diagnostic requirement for 'an impairment of, or a disturbance in the functioning of, the mind or brain' (Section 2(1)) remains an issue.
Equality of opportunity	As part of the transition to the new Act, all Wards of Court are scheduled to undergo a review process.	The Mental Capacity Act 2005 signalled a move away from specific tests created by the courts to a more standardised approach of assessing functional capacity.
Accessibility	Presence of a Decision Support Service.	Presence of independent mental capacity advocate service.
Equality between men and women	Binary gender pronouns, e.g. 'if he or she'.	Use of male pronouns only in the Mental Capacity Act 2005.

Table 7.1 Continued

Capacity legislation	Ireland	England and Wales
Respect for the evolving capacities of children with disabilities and respect for the right of children with disabilities to preserve their identities	Children are not referenced.	Children are not referenced.

Notes

(A) Functional capacity assessment criteria under the Assisted Decision-Making (Capacity) Act 2015:

(1) […] a person's capacity shall be assessed on the basis of his or her ability to understand, at the time that a decision is to be made, the nature and consequences of the decision to be made by him or her in the context of the available choices at that time.

(2) A person lacks the capacity to make a decision if he or she is unable (a) to understand the information relevant to the decision, (b) to retain that information long enough to make a voluntary choice, (c) to use or weigh that information as part of the process of making the decision, or (d) to communicate his or her decision (whether by talking, writing, using sign language, assistive technology, or any other means) […]

(3) A person is not to be regarded as unable to understand the information relevant to a decision if he or she is able to understand an explanation of it given to him or her in a way that is appropriate to his or her circumstances (whether using clear language, signing, visual aids or any other means).

(4) The fact that a person is able to retain the information relevant to a decision for a short period only does not prevent him or her from being regarded as having the capacity to make the decision.

(5) The fact that a person lacks capacity in respect of a decision on a particular matter at a particular time does not prevent him or her from being regarded as having capacity to make decisions on the same matter at another time.

(6) The fact that a person lacks capacity in respect of a decision on a particular matter does not prevent him or her from being regarded as having capacity to make decisions on other matters (Section 3).

(B) In Ireland, the Assisted Decision-Making (Capacity) Act 2015 provides for three levels of assisted decision-making:

(1) Decision-making assistant: Any individual can appoint a decision-making assistant, who is someone they trust to advise them about their decision. The decision-making assistant does not make the decision for the person, and therefore has no decision-making responsibility, but they provide information, advice, and opportunity for discussion. While many people already seek assistance in this way for certain decisions, the new legislation formally recognises such arrangements (Part 3 of the 2015 Act).

(2) Co-decision-maker: Subject to certain conditions, a person can appoint a co-decision-maker either at their own initiative or if the Circuit Court finds that appointing a co-decision-maker would mean the person no longer lacks capacity. The co-decision-maker is a joint decision-maker who can veto certain decisions in situations of sufficient risk. The creation of a co-decision-making agreement requires a statement by a healthcare professional (not necessarily a registered medical professional) and the appointer must have capacity to decide to enter into the co-decision-making agreement (among other matters) (Parts 4 and 5 of the 2015 Act).

(3) Decision-making representative: the Circuit Court can appoint a decision-making representative to make substitute decisions on behalf of a person in respect of certain areas of decision-making, if the Court feels that this is appropriate (Part 5 of the 2015 Act).

human rights, and moral theories related to assisted decision-making, and conclude by providing thought experiments for further reflection.

Case Study 1

An 86-year-old man is admitted to hospital following his third fall at home with subsequent head injury and broken ribs. He does not require surgery. The man has advancing dementia and lives alone. Two trials of a discharge home had already been made by the team in line with the patient's wishes. Following consultation with him, enhanced community supports had been provided, his bed was moved downstairs, a downstairs toilet was installed, and regular visits from health-care assistants were organized and funded. Despite this, the man continued to sleep upstairs on the floor and refused to allow health-care assistants to enter his home.

Following his most recent admission, the clinical team suggested supported residential care, but the man refused to consider this. He could not provide an explanation as to why this was the case and so the clinical team performed a functional assessment of his decision-making capacity about discharge home. Having provided information in the most accessible format possible, and after holding several meetings with the man, the clinical team found that the man could not understand information relevant to the decision. Despite being given considerable support, he was unable to describe a nursing home, or the risks and benefits associated with various alternative care arrangements, including going home. He was also unable to engage in a discussion regarding potential compromises, such as step-down rehabilitative care.

Following a number of discussions, the clinical team was concerned that the man might be avoiding engaging in the conversation in the hope that this might expedite his return home. However, when it was put to him that he could return home if he listed various risks and benefits and demonstrated an understanding of relevant information, the man still could not retain relevant information or use that information as part of the decision-making process. While he was able to communicate his decisions verbally, it was determined, on further review, that his decision-making capacity was notably impaired in relation to other decision areas too, such as finances. The support and assistance offered were insufficient to change this.

Analysis

Clinical responses in these situations vary considerably and are best facilitated through effective team working and team discussion. In this case, the health-care providers need to balance this man's rights to autonomy, health care, and appropriate shelter on the one hand, with the real, proven risk of bodily harm were he to return home for a third time. Such decisions are further impacted by the personal moral code of the individual health-care providers, the ethical guidelines set out by their profession, and constraints associated with contemporaneous legislation. Previously, assessments of capacity were commonly conducted only by medical practitioners. Affording such decisions to any one group can result in bias and the sole use of medical practitioners presents particular difficulties in the context of the so-called 'medical model', i.e. the idea that doctors view psychopathology as purely biological in nature. The Committee on the Rights of Persons with Disabilities has explicitly stated that mental capacity is not 'as commonly presented, an objective, scientific and naturally occurring phenomenon. Mental capacity is contingent on social and political contexts, as are the disciplines, professions and practices which play a dominant role in assessing mental capacity' (Committee of the Rights of Persons with Disability, 2014). Increased recognition of disability and adherence to the CRPD has resulted in demand for a broader range of practitioners being involved in such assessments.

Depending on team structure and culture, another clinical team might have taken a more conservative approach and advised strongly against discharge after the first or second admissions, considering the risks involved. This clinical team in this case, however, prioritized the man's preference to live in his own house and arranged repeated trials at home with bolstered community services. Only after two adverse outcomes did they decide to proceed to formal assessment of decision-making capacity owing to the man's apparent inability to understand information relevant to the decision about going home, including the previous adverse outcomes and the existence of alternatives.

Intervention

In this case, the conventional approach prior to Ireland's Assisted Decision-Making (Capacity) Act 2015 would have been to apply to make this man a Ward of Court. With Ireland's new capacity legislation, a decision-making assistant or co-decision-maker might have made a difference in relation to specific issues, such as accepting health-care assistants visiting the home or other elements of the homecare package. It is likely, however, that the home would have remained an unsafe environment with significant risk of further falls, even if specific elements of the care package were accepted. This risk was judged by the clinical team to exceed the limits of reasonable 'therapeutic risk-taking', especially given the man's lack of capacity to weigh up adverse outcomes. Overall, appointment of a decision-making representative appeared appropriate in this case, at least in relation to deciding about place of residence and supports to be provided. By comparison, in England and Wales, this man's diagnosis of dementia would explicitly have formed part of his capacity assessment and the Deprivation of Liberty Safeguards process might have commenced.

Case Study 2

This case study concerns a 63-year-old woman with chronic schizophrenia living in supported accommodation with two other residents and two support workers. Prior to this placement, she had been living in homeless accommodation. On this occasion, support workers raised concerns regarding the sudden appearance of a distant relative on a weekly basis. They believed that these visits were related to the woman's father's will in which he left her the family home. Support workers expressed concern regarding the risk of exploitation by this distant relative who had no contact with the woman for several decades but suddenly appeared after the woman's father died.

One of the support workers, a social worker, and a doctor on this woman's community mental health team met and discussed the matter with the woman. It was apparent to them that she needed assistance in understanding her legal position and entitlements. Firstly a significant factor in her decision-making was the fear that she would have to leave supported accommodation (where she was happy) and be forced to return to the family home. Once this fear was alleviated, the woman was better able to engage in a factual discussion regarding the will. However it remained the case that this woman would need assistance both in navigating the legal system and in making an informed decision. With clear communication and repeated conversations, she was able to understand and retain key facts, including the likely value of the house, the identity and role of the executor of her father's will, and the need for her to meet with her own solicitor without this distant relative being present. Staff at the residence facilitated this.

Analysis

In this case, the clinical team needed to weigh the risk of unnecessarily interfering with this woman's right to privacy and autonomy against the risk of possible exploitation by a newly arrived distant relative. The role of the support worker was particularly important because the first step was to inform the individual of the relevant information and her entitlements. Health professionals are in an especially responsible position in such a case, compared to relatives, on the basis that *nemo judex in causa sua* ('no person can judge a case in which they have an interest').

In this case, the support worker was an independent party who would not personally benefit from the outcome, even in an indirect manner (given that the residential care was publicly funded) and was willing to take the time to explain the situation. This facilitated an individually tailored approach that was supportive and appropriate to the person's needs. The fact that this support worker was already familiar with the woman was important, because it avoided some of the biases that might have influenced someone who did not know her already: the woman was routinely dishevelled in appearance, perseverative in speech (repeating the same concepts and phrases over and over), and had very poor baseline knowledge (grossly underestimating the value of the family home when initially asked). In addition, her fears around being removed from residential accommodation might not have been uncovered without the presence of a trusted individual such as the support worker, who provided appropriate reassurance.

There was some debate amongst the team regarding acceptable levels of interference. Those who were well acquainted with this woman felt a greater moral obligation to protect her and were less concerned with privacy. Ethically, it was agreed by all that there was a need to avoid causing harm and to achieve as just an outcome as was practicable.

Intervention

This case highlights the importance of various levels of decision-making support, rather than moving immediately to substitute decision-making. The use of functional capacity assessments facilitates a more nuanced response and promotes psychoeducation. This woman had the ability to manage her affairs but required assistance. In this scenario, the clinical team opted for the least restrictive form of assisted decision-making with the woman agreeing to a decision-making assistant who would have no legal power over her decision but would actively support her in realizing her will and preferences. In England and Wales, by way of comparison, this woman's diagnosis of schizophrenia would have formed part of the capacity assessment and she might have been referred to the 'independent mental capacity advocate service' for assistance.

Theory

Applying Moral Theories

Several moral theories apply to the concept and regulation of assisted decision-making. While beneficence, equity, and autonomy are central to rights-based legislation, there is also a role for utilitarianism, i.e. maximizing that which is good, especially when that includes protecting fundamental rights (e.g. autonomy). Consequentialism also plays an important role given the potential for negative outcomes arising from assisted decision-making. A novel process may be well intentioned and even virtuous in nature, but unintended negative outcomes can undermine its objectives or even have paradoxical effects. This could occur if a system of supported decision-making is so complex as to be unintelligible, so difficult to navigate that those who need it most cannot access it, or so expensive that some people simply cannot afford it.

In addition, Singer argues that if we know that people in war-torn countries are going to die and we do nothing, we are as responsible for their death as if we put a bullet through their heads (Singer, 1972). In light of this rather vast responsibility, one of the difficulties with assisted decision-making lies in deciding whether to tend towards errors of omission or commission, i.e. whether to ignore the fact that many people with cognitive challenges cannot make independent decisions with full capacity, or to intervene and likely prioritize safety over autonomy as well as the right to make bad decisions through potential over-involvement.

Most individuals prefer to err on the side of omission rather than intervene excessively, but health-care professionals often feel added responsibility, believing they will be held responsible for adverse outcomes. This, allied with the state's duty to intervene in certain circumstances, can tend towards errors of commission in health services, rather than errors of omission. Furthermore, health professionals are often viewed by the public as having a higher level of responsibility to intervene than the average citizen. This is not entirely unreasonable given that health professionals care for others at times of vulnerability, and it is further compounded by media reporting of an inert health system. Therefore, a cultural shift would be required to move away from this default position to act.

Kant states that we live in a world of moral responsibility and punishment (Kant, 1998). In this sense, it can be altruistic to act in another's stead and to try to navigate the line between over-involvement and under-involvement, even if this causes moral stress and self-doubt, along with the risks of not getting the balance right. On the other hand, declaring that someone lacks capacity can be confused with a desire for professional power. This would be consistent with a history of excessive medical paternalism in Ireland and elsewhere, and with Foucault's concept of the dispositive, i.e. that various administrative mechanisms and knowledge structures contrive to maintain power within the state and its institutions (Peltonen, 2004).

In this light, it is imperative that new approaches to assisted decision-making are not simply linguistic acrobatics (replacing 'substitute' with 'supported') and that legal reforms translate into meaningful change and effective altruism (in the moral sense). In Ireland, there has been undeniable change, most notably the closure of large psychiatric hospitals ('asylums'), the move towards multidisciplinary working, and a person-centred, rights-based approach to clinical care. In line with CRPD recommendations, the Irish National Clinical Programme for Disability has moved away from uni-disciplinary clinical-led advisory groups to multidisciplinary representation and an emphasis on input from those with lived experience (MacLachlan & Walsh, 2020).

Much contemporary assisted decision-making legislation, including Ireland's 2015 Act, emphasizes the importance of maximizing autonomy. Mitnick's principal-agency theory has been used to analyse the difficulties associated with state delegation, namely that inherent pitfalls arise when one person or 'agent', represents another person or group, the 'principal' (Mitnick, 2015). Mitnick states that perfect agency is rarely obtained because principals find that the marginal benefits of assuring perfect agency do not exceed the marginal costs of doing so. In other words, agency is often about the management of imperfection. For example, in Case Study 2 above, the woman in question is the 'principal' and the clinical team her 'agent'. Under previous capacity legislation, the state would have aimed to achieve perfect agency for this woman by delegating all decision-making to the judiciary through wardship. This carried marginal costs of her right to privacy and autonomy. While the provision of a decision-making assistant does less to manage the risk of exploitation and therefore does not achieve perfect agency, this measure avoids the marginal costs of breaching her right to privacy and autonomy, and better adheres to CRPD guiding principles regarding the 'freedom to make one's own choices' and 'respect for difference'.

Kant illustrates a picture of duty struggling with desire at crucial moments of choice (Kant, 1998). This conflict must not be confused with lack of capacity. Again in Case Study 2, for example, one of the woman's conflicts was the duty to honour her father's will versus her desire not to lose safe, supported accommodation. This demonstrates that exploring an individual's rationale and giving them opportunity to explain apparently 'unwise' decisions is essential for the protection of autonomy. The role of support workers and the clinical team in this case also relates to Latour's 'actor network theory', rooted in the idea that scientific knowledge is an effect of established relations between actors that form a network, rather than any entirely objective process (Callon & Latour, 1981). This theory challenges the recurrent use of 'non-human' terms for large agencies such as 'society', 'the economy', or 'the state', which are simply large networks of other actors rather than distant omnipotent entities.

This also applies to professions, where the use of group terms dehumanizes individual actors thus allowing for the manipulation of these networks to create a false sense of objectivity. This objectivity may be used to validate the actions of certain groups but equally these actions can be construed as indifferent or even malevolent in nature as a result. Assisted decision-making has traditionally been associated with certain professions, namely the legal profession and psychiatry. The new approach to assisted decision-making aims to include a range of professionals, thus broadening the network, and aims to focus on supporting actions regarding the decision at hand rather than the authority of a given entity or profession.

Latour's theory is known for highlighting the inherent contradiction between the modern, liberal ideal of the autonomous, emancipated individual and the equally modern, sociological ideal of the conditioned social agent (Muniesa, 2015). The idea of not having control over one's fate is unnerving for most people, but not as universal a fear as might be expected. Most people regularly delegate decision-making to other actors and therefore networks. Furthermore, while most people wish to respect the autonomy of others, they also have biases in relation to what makes a good or righteous decision, and face challenges regarding the extent to which others exercise their autonomy, particularly in health care (Treffert, 1973; Hilliard, 2011). (See Thought Experiments 2 and 4 for further reflection on these themes.)

Utilitarianism

Even if modern assisted decision-making can amount to a beneficent, virtuous act that promotes autonomy, does it meet utilitarianism ideals? Utilitarianism aims at maximizing what is good for all, i.e., the main goal of modern states is to maximize the wealth and welfare of the nation. Some might argue that elaborate models of assisted decision-making require the investment of considerable resources for the benefit of a small number of people. Arguably, the same could be said of many of the medical interventions and legal procedures that we currently support as a society, but which only apply to small numbers.

In Ireland, for example, there are 17,797 inpatient mental health admissions per annum, of whom 5,161 (29%) likely lack decision-making capacity regarding treatment, based on a systematic review by Okai et al. (2007). This compares with 503,000 general hospital (non-mental health) admissions per annum of which 141,000 (28%) likely lack capacity regarding treatment (Murphy et al., 2018). Of the further 25,000 nursing home residents recorded in Ireland in 2022, over 15,000 (60%) likely lack capacity regarding potential treatment options (Fitten et al., 1990). Of note, these studies were based on cross-sectional data using a variety of capacity assessment tools and the same individuals may have regained or lost capacity at various time points during their admission. This is an important consideration in the context of the new approach to assisted decision-making in which capacity refers to a specific decision at a specific point in time.

In a population of five million people (Ireland), these numbers are significant. And while patients with mental health conditions detained on an involuntary basis are afforded certain legal protections, much greater numbers in general hospitals and nursing homes might not enjoy equivalent or adequate safeguards.

As is always the case in health care, issues of equity arise, especially when there is a trade-off between efficiency and considerations of fairness regarding overall resource allocation within the state, so that other essential services are not adversely affected (Okun, 2015). In order to achieve fair access to assisted decision-making, further measures are required to meet the standards set out by the UNHCR. Policymakers need to factor socioeconomic and health-related inequalities into their decision-making to maximize the chance of success in service delivery and optimize outcomes. In Ireland, for example, the relevant court process includes a series of fees and requires a high degree of literacy. These requirements are arguably necessary to a certain extent, but they also have potential to disadvantage those with lower levels of education and lack of access to legal assistance. This in turn has the potential to reduce efficiency, diminish impact, and amplify disadvantage. In Ireland, this has been partially mitigated through stakeholder consultation (Davies et al., 2019), the Decision Support Service, and free legal aid.

These considerations also raise the issue of consequentialism, i.e. that the right action is determined by its consequences. While this is an important consideration in policymaking, it is not possible to predict all unintended consequences. In this way, consequentialism acts as a moral argument for incrementalism, where policies are built upon pre-existing policies and negative consequences can be mitigated against in that way. The intended positive consequences of assisted decision-making include greater protections for people without full capacity and promotion of their will and preference. A positive unintended consequence might be demarginalization of certain brain disorders through functional capacity assessments (i.e. a diagnosis of

Alzheimer's disease can no longer be seen as an automatic, pejorative indicator of incapacity in Ireland).

Negative consequences associated with assisted decision-making might include cost, potential for further inequity and inequality, and the risk of inadvertently sanctioning coercive practices if regulation is insufficient. For instance, under Ireland's Assisted Decision-Making (Capacity) Act 2015, a decision-making representative is still afforded full control over decision-making in a defined area of the individual's life, with a commitment that they must accord with the person's will and preference. While this is limited to specific pre-defined areas of decision-making, as compared to the previous system of wardship, full agency over another will always leave room for abuse and coercion. Of note, in their General Comment No. 1, the Committee on the Rights of Persons with Disabilities expresses the opinion that substitute decision-making of any kind contravenes the standards set out by the CRPD (Committee on the Rights of Persons with Disabilities, 2014).

Overall, the issues involved in decisions about supported decision-making involve engagement with these moral issues both at a general level (in developing law and policy) and at the level of the individual person (in assessing decision-making capacity and its consequences). This highlights the importance of reflexive practice, considering not only how we think and feel about given situations, but actively identifying strategies to help question our own attitudes. We can mitigate against the risks and against getting decisions 'wrong' by consulting widely, reflecting deeply, and reviewing a chosen course of action as the situation evolves.

Thought Experiments

1. An 18-year-old woman with anorexia nervosa is at a critically low weight and at significant risk of death if she does not receive food. The only way this can be accomplished is by placing a nasogastric tube (extending from her nose to her stomach) to restore her weight, but she refuses this. What moral issues are relevant here? If the woman's clinical situation deteriorates rapidly, should that materially change your decision?

2. A 35-year-old autistic man presents to the emergency department following an accidental paracetamol overdose of unknown quantity. He begins to scream and wave his arms when an attempt is made to take the blood tests which are immediately necessary to ascertain the concentration of paracetamol in his blood and therefore the potentially life-saving treatment that he might urgently need. There is no time to initiate the formal supports of capacity legislation, and the man's family urge you to physically restrain him to provide care. The family are hugely distressed. His elderly mother collapses to the floor in what appears to be a fainting episode. From a utilitarian perspective, how much weight do you accord to the family's distress, compared to that of the man himself?

3. A 90-year-old man with advanced dementia has been living in a nursing home for the past five years. He has nowhere else to go and his family are not able to take him into their homes. He repeatedly goes to the door of the nursing home and asks to leave. The man is not distressed when staff advise him to return to his room, and he does so without complaint. This, however, happens several times every day and often during the night. Does the man's repeated desire to leave and his lack of distress when not facilitated indicate a lack of decision-making capacity on his part? How does this management accord with his will and preference? How does the idea of consequentialism apply to this case, if at all?

4. A 35-year-old woman is diagnosed with breast cancer. As part of standard treatment, she is offered surgery followed by radiotherapy. She declines this treatment, saying that she wants to try alternative herbal treatments which do not have any systematic evidence to support them. Six months later, at medical review, her breast cancer has advanced but is still treatable. Her partner expresses concern that the woman is 'being allowed to kill herself' and says that staff at the clinic 'will have blood on their hands' if she is not 'made to accept treatment'. The woman says she would 'rather die' than have surgery, radiotherapy, or chemotherapy, even though she has two children under the age of six years. What should clinical staff do? Whose interests should they consider?

Further Reading and Listening

Gergel, T. Bound to the mast (podcast). *BBC Radio 4*, 10 June 2022. https://www.bbc.co.uk/pro grammes/m0017cmj

Murphy, V.E., Gulati, G., Whelan, D., Dunne, C.P., & Kelly, B.D. (2023). The changing face of capacity legislation in Ireland: algorithms for clinicians. *Irish Journal of Psychological Medicine, 40*(2), 109–113. https://doi.org/10.1017/ipm.2020.7

Treffert, D. A. (1973). Dying with their rights on. *American Journal of Psychiatry, 130*(9), 1041. https://doi.org/10.1176/ajp.130.9.1041

References

'AM v Health Service Executive' (2019) The Supreme Court, case 124. *Courts Service of Ireland.* https://www.courts.ie/acc/alfresco/c86d29ee-ee4e-4c18-aede-b38916adcc9d/2019_I ESC_3_1.pdf/pdf#view=fitH

'Boughton v Knight'. (1873). High Court of Chancery, LR 3 P&D 64.

Callon, M., & Latour, B. Unscrewing the big Leviathan: how actors macro-structure reality and how sociologists help them to do so. In K. Knorr Cetina, & A. V. Cicourel (Eds.), *Advances in Social Theory and Methodology: Towards an Integration of Micro- and Macro-Sociologies* (pp. 277–303). Leviathan, 1981.

Committee on the Rights of Persons with Disabilities. (2014). *General Comment No. 1 (Article 12).* New York: United Nations.

Curtis, C., Fatoki, O., McGuire, E., & Cullen, A. (2022). Moving from 'best interests' to 'will and preference': a study of doctors' level of knowledge relating to the Assisted Decision-Making (Capacity) Act 2015. *Irish Medical Journal; 115*(4), Article 585.

Davies, C., Fattori, F., O'Donnell, D., Donnelly, S., Ní Shé, É., O'Sea, M., Prihodova, L., Gleeson, C., Flynn, Á., Rock, B., Grogan, J., O'Brien, M., O'Hanlon, S., Cooney, M.T., Tighe, M., & Kroll, T. (2019). What are the mechanisms that support healthcare professionals to adopt assisted decision-making practice? A rapid realist review. *BMC Health Services Research, 19*(1), Article 960.

Department of Children, Equality, Disability, Integration and Youth. (2021). *Initial Report of Ireland under the Convention on the Rights of Persons with Disabilities.* Dublin.

Fitten, L. J., Lusky, R., & Hamann, C. (1990). Assessing treatment decision-making capacity in elderly nursing home residents. *Journal of the American Geriatrics Society, 38*(10), 1097–1104. https://doi.org/10.1111/j.1532-5415.1990.tb01372.x

Hilliard, M. T. (2011). Utilitarianism impacting care of those with disabilities and those at life's end. *Linacre Quarterly; 78*(1), 59–71. https://doi.org/10.1179/002436311803888474.

Kant, I. (1998). *Critique of Pure Reason.* Cambridge University Press.

Law Commission. (1995). *Mental Incapacity (Report no 231).* HMSO.

MacLachlan, M., & Walsh, M. (2020). *National Clinical Programme for People with Disability Governance Structure and Function.* https://www.hse.ie/eng/about/who/cspd/ncps/disabil ity/programme-governance/clinical-programme-for-disability-governance-structure-and-function.pdf

Mitnick, B. M. (2015). Agency theory. In R. James & K. Goodpaster (Eds.), *Wiley Encyclopedia of Management (Volume 2: Business Ethics)* (pp. 1–6). John Wiley & Sons, Ltd. https://doi.org/10.1002/9781118785317.weom020097

Muniesa, F. (2015). Actor-network theory. In J. D. Wright (Ed.), *International Encyclopedia of the Social and Behavioral Sciences* (2nd ed., pp. 80–84). Elsevier.

Murphy, R., Fleming, S., Curley, A., Duffy, R. M., & Kelly, B. D. (2018). Who can decide? Prevalence of mental incapacity for treatment decisions in medical and surgical hospital in-patients in Ireland. *QJM, 111*(12), 881–885. https://doi.org/10.1093/qjmed/hcy219

Okai, D., Owen, G., McGuire, H., Singh, S., Churchill, R., & Hotopf, M. (2007). Mental capacity in psychiatric patients: systematic review. *British Journal of Psychiatry, 191*(4), 291–297. https://doi.org/10.1192/bjp.bp.106.035162

Okun, A. M. (2015). *Equality and efficiency: the big tradeoff* (revised ed.). Brookings Institution Press.

Peltonen, M. (2004). From discourse to 'dispositif': Michel Foucault's two histories. *Historical Reflections/Réflexions Historiques, 30*(2), 205–219.

Singer, P. (1972). Famine, affluence, and morality. *Philosophy & Public Affairs, 1*(3), 229–243.

Treffert, D. A. (1973). Dying with their rights on. *American Journal of Psychiatry, 130*(9), 1041. https://doi.org/10.1176/ajp.130.9.1041

United Nations. (2006). *Convention on the Rights of Persons with Disabilities.* United Nations.

8

Public and Patient Involvement in Services

Time to Stop Being Patient?

Thilo Kroll

Background

'Nothing about us without us' has been the call for the active involvement of people in critical decisions about their health and lives for some time now. The disability scholar Charlton is frequently cited (Charlton, 1998) and credited for providing momentum for active people participation and involvement in decision-making across a spectrum from patient-centredness to full engagement. It is shifting from 'doing for' to a 'doing with' approach. Various terms and practices have been used over centuries of human development to denote citizen participation's value, practice, and benefit. These alternative or adjacent terms include 'patient-centred care', 'shared decision-making', 'co-production', 'citizen engagement', and 'participatory action research' (see MacFarlane, 2020; Tambuyzer et al., 2014). The collective notion of advocacy and activism is reflected in the term 'community involvement'. Public and patient involvement (PPI) is firmly rooted in fundamental democratic principles of decision-making that can be traced back to Greek philosophers and the time of the polis (Mossé, 2013). So, PPI is not a new phenomenon.

At the height of civil liberty struggles and rights-based movements, sociologist Sherri Arnstein proposed describing the level of citizen participation in decision-making as a ladder (Arnstein, 1969). The highest level is complete citizen control and power, while the lowest rung of the ladder positions the public as non-participatory objects of manipulation.

Gaber (2019) later discussed the historical context and contribution of Arnstein's work for public planning to demonstrate community agency and relationship formation for change.

Nearly four decades after Arnstein's pioneering work, the right to participate in decision-making has been firmly established in human rights law, notably in the United Nations Convention on the Rights of Persons with Disabilities (UN CRPD), ratified by 191 countries (United Nations, 2006). Article 12 of the CRPD guarantees equal legal rights, while Article 29 ensures the political rights of persons with disabilities, promoting their full and effective participation in political and public life. This includes active involvement in decision-making and access to voting procedures that are accessible, understandable, and easy to use.

Organizations with far-reaching influence, such as the Institute on Medicine (IOM) (America, 2001), the US Centers for Disease Control and Prevention (CDC) (CDC, 2011), and the World Health Organization (WHO) (Organization, 1978), have advocated for patients and the public to have a voice in decision-making.

There is mounting evidence that involving clients and the public in the design and delivery of physical and mental healthcare can improve care quality and satisfaction, and improved decision-making benefits can be achieved (Bombard et al., 2018; Funk et al., 2009; Gibbons et al., 2014; Tambuyzer & Van Audenhove, 2015; Vahdat et al., 2014). There are several additional benefits. First, it enables researchers, practitioners, and product designers to understand better complex living circumstances, patient values and preferences, and social support networks; second, it may reveal critical barriers to and disparities in accessing services or using products (e.g. medication, assistive technologies); third, it may point to disruptions or non-existence of coordinated care pathways; fourth, it provides insights into barriers and enablers of shared- and assisted decision-making; and fifth, it points to essential data variables that may modulate patient outcomes.

Finally, timely and effective PPI can also help build trust between patients, the public, and healthcare providers (Lewis et al., 2023; Ward, 2017). Trust is a critical variable which depends on how relationships and environments are formed to enable patients and members of the public to feel safe and comfortable talking about their experiences and views (Wilkins, 2018).Genuine and effective PPI requires carefully considering how collaborative working environments and processes are formed (Holmes et al., 2019). There is some concern that the use of 'patient' in PPI unduly medicalizes individuals' lives. A preference has been expressed to use 'person' or citizen instead of 'patient' in the context of PPI (Ocloo et al., 2021). It recognizes individuals as whole beings rather than solely through the lens of their health conditions. Using 'person' can help promote a more respectful and inclusive approach and underlines the intention to work in partnership. Throughout this manuscript there may be inconsistencies resulting from the language used in the literature.

Drivers of PPI

Over the past two decades, there have been several drivers of PPI (Gilfoyle et al., 2022; Tritter, 2009). One principal factor has been the desire to achieve greater utility, accountability, and transparency in clinical practice, health policy, and health-related research (Nielsen et al., 2021; Sarker & Hassan, 2010; Sleigh & Vayena, 2021; Weerakkody et al., 2017). There has been an unprecedented growth of consumer and patient advocacy organizations who also demanded better information, greater patient safety, and improvements in care coordination. Academics and advocates have also voiced criticism of the medicalization of human diversity (Correia, 2017; Richie, 2019; van Dijk et al., 2016).

The past 20 years have seen dramatic changes in information and communication technologies, which has also accelerated PPI in public and healthcare decision-making and fuelled demand for broad stakeholder engagement (Baumann et al., 2022; Bussey & Sillence, 2019; Kelly et al., 2020; Milakovich, 2010; Mossberger & Tolbert, 2008). Smartphones, mobile computing, and social media make it possible to access and share a volume of information at unparalleled speeds for previous generations. It is increasingly difficult for internet users, both on the client as well as on the professional side to discern credible, quality sources of information, and knowledge from instant, sentiment-driven content. A greater volume of information is not indicative of its usefulness and whether it ultimately contributes to knowledge and behaviour changes. As technological development accelerates, distinguishing human-generated and validated data from products compiled by artificial intelligence and bots, which may introduce biases and fake content, becomes even more challenging. On the positive side, modern knowledge, communication and data technologies have made information, in principle, more accessible and can mobilize support to challenge hitherto unquestioned orthodoxies and power relationships. Data are the currency of the 21st century. Those who collect, store, link, and analyse data are in a position of power. National governments and transnational organizations struggle to devise rules and regulations for global influence. In principle, artificial intelligence and machine learning are positioned to link different data sources, which may create new vulnerabilities and exacerbate disadvantages for those already marginalized (Leslie et al., 2021; Murdoch, 2021).

Values in PPI

Genuine PPI requires agreement on values between healthcare professionals and academics on the one hand and patients, family members, and public partners on the other. However, to begin with, healthcare professionals and patients may differ in their level of trust, perceived autonomy, and preparedness for collaboration. Healthcare professionals may be sceptical about accepting 'lay understandings' and feel more inclined to trust their professional judgment and expertise. Conversely, patients may be motivated more by intuition and experience (Fredriksson & Tritter, 2017). Patients may also prioritize decision autonomy and collaboration in the treatment process, while healthcare professionals may be primarily concerned with the service's clinical outcomes and cost-effectiveness.

The literature suggests that respect, open communication, and collaboration towards shared goals are essential (Wolf et al., 2017). Mutual respect is fundamental for the relationship (Ferguson et al., 2013).Open and transparent communication means sharing ideas, feedback, information, and criticism. Collaboration involves the ability to 'walk in each other's shoes', i.e. understand different perspectives, work towards solutions, and take critical decisions during the problem-solving process together.

Our research identified four critical values in engaging marginalized populations: respect, openness, reciprocity, and flexibility (Ní Shé et al., 2020).

Respect in community involvement means valuing the expertise and contributions of community members and making efforts to engage with them in their environments, rather than expecting them to come to healthcare or academic settings. This involves fostering openness through honest, transparent communication, allowing for the development of trust. It is essential to embrace various world views and avoid forceful confrontations to maintain openness and dialogue, which are key to exploring alternative approaches.

Reciprocity in engagement asks whether the terms and foundations of decision-making are clear and whether all parties find the rationale for decisions acceptable.

Flexibility is crucial, involving the readiness to consider alternative methods and adopt a growth mindset. This flexibility should extend to reviewing standard protocols, and adjusting the timing and location of decisions and activities. Information and procedures should be accessible in various appropriate formats to facilitate shared decision-making.

Critique of PPI and Consequences of Exclusion

While there are unquestionable benefits to PPI in health service development, health research, and health policy, several critical points also need to be highlighted. PPI thus far has been a story of relative privilege (de Graaff et al., 2021). Healthcare organizations, universities, and non-governmental charity organizations have yet to achieve equitable, diverse, and inclusive representation on their boards and decision-making bodies. Typically, advisory boards include retired academics or health professionals, predominantly of white, middle-class backgrounds. For example, many patient involvement initiatives are focused on those with higher education and income levels, meaning those in lower socioeconomic brackets are often left out of the conversation. In addition, individuals with physical or mental disabilities may not be adequately represented, as they may find it challenging to engage in the patient-provider dialogue or professionals turn to proxy informants, such as family members. It has been established that people with intellectual disabilities or limited literacy have often been excluded from the development of health evaluation instruments (Kroll et al., 2014). We have two forms of exclusion with the risk of potential bias for clinical decisions (Jahagirdar et al., 2013): explicit exclusion (intentionally not included in the sample) and implicit exclusion (no effort made to include). When we add to this picture the lack of involvement of patients from diverse backgrounds in decisions about their care, which often affects physical outcomes and social and societal participation, whatever decision is taken could be better.

Healthcare professionals often struggle to identify individuals with the appropriate skills for meaningful input in PPI, facing uncertainty about what 'meaningful' entails. This ambiguity can lead to differing perspectives on the significance of contributions between professionals and patients. Additionally, healthcare professionals may lack the training, time, or resources necessary for effectively involving patients, particularly using adapted communication methods for those with linguistic, cognitive, sensory, educational, or psychological barriers. This often results in the exclusion of individuals who cannot access standard forms of communication or are socially marginalized, such as people who are homeless, from preventive healthcare services.

Moreover, PPI can highlight cultural clashes between the structured, guideline-driven environment of clinical and academic settings and the fluid, experience-centred approach favoured by the public and patients. Professionals pressed for time may seek efficient, standardized procedures, whereas effective PPI requires transparent, trusting, and mutually beneficial relationships that are time-intensive and may deviate from conventional practices. Currently, the control and management of PPI funding by healthcare organizations and universities perpetuate power imbalances, suggesting a need for a shift in control to better involve and empower patients and the public.

The use of PPI is associated with several ethical dilemmas, which have been summarized in Box 8.1. There is emerging guidance on how these dilemmas can be made visible if not always resolved. Personal values may substantially differ within families or between individuals and professionals. Ultimately, it is important that individuals' autonomy is respected. Communication can help to explain the different positions and efforts can be undertaken to arrive at shared decisions. Coercion and persuasion are antithetical to PPI. A continuous awareness and reflection of issues of power in the decision-making process is important. If agreement cannot be reached than the willingness as well as the processes up to the point need to be examined, involving all stakeholders.

Public and Patient Involvement in Strengthening Health System Design and Evaluation

Health systems development can benefit from public engagement. Lazarus and France stated the importance of adding patient engagement to the WHO Health Systems framework in a blog post in 2014 (Lazarus & France, 2014). The close involvement of public and patient stakeholders is critical to understanding the impact health system design and policy decisions will have (Denmark & Olson, 2014; Koehlmoos et al., 2017; Sacks et al., 2018). It is also important to boost public acceptance and shared ownership of the system and that it is aligned with values and expectations. This is particularly relevant for stakeholders and communities that experience vulnerabilities. Public engagement can help identify the system's potential beneficial and

Box 8.1 Ethical Dilemmas in PPI

Balancing expertise and experience	There's an inherent tension in valuing professional expertise and the lived experience of patients and the public. Accepting that both are important and weighing up their relative contributions can be challenging but is essential for true collaborative decision-making
Tokenism	A significant ethical concern is the risk of tokenism, in that PPI is used superficially, not granting real influence and decision-making power to PPI contributors. This can hamper the integrity of PPI and the trust of participants.
Managing expectations	There is often a dilemma in managing expectations between what healthcare professionals and researchers expect from PPI and what participants think they should contribute. Aligning these expectations without disenfranchising or disappointing stakeholders requires careful handling and clear communication.
Confidentiality and privacy	Ensuring the confidentiality and privacy is critical. There is a risk that sensitive information is disclosed unintentionally, inclusion of PPI contributors as 'co-authors' requires careful consideration and discussion
Power Imbalances	Patients may feel less empowered to voice their true opinions or may believe that their contributions will not be taken seriously. Training is sometimes used about equally healthcare professionals and academics need to undertake to be skilled in using adequate communication
Equity, accessibility and affordability	Ensuring that PPI is accessible to all, including those from underrepresented or vulnerable groups, is an ethical necessity that can be difficult to achieve in practice. This includes providing appropriate support and removing barriers to participation.
PPI contributors impact on decisions	PPI contributors expect their input to significantly influence decisions, whereas professionals and academics may selectively determine what inputs to consider. Decisions must be collaboratively discussed and made transparent, which can be time-consuming and potentially frustrating. It's crucial that PPI contributors see their contributions genuinely reflected in the decision-making process.

negative impacts on the community. It may also expose sources of potential conflicts and unintended negative consequences of the system's design. It may also provide a clearer idea of the resource implications of the health system design. Ultimately, the early involvement of stakeholders and communities will contribute to a more effective and efficient implementation.

The South Central Foundation's Nuka System of Care Transformation in Alaska is a good example. A dysfunctional healthcare system was replaced through community involvement by a needs-focused system, aligned with spiritual and community values and collaboratively owned by all community members. Patients have become 'customer-owners', and they share decisions about the point of delivery of care and are actively engaged in the healthcare delivery process (Eby, 2018; Gottlieb, 2013) (Graves, 2013).

Workforce Education and Development

PPI can substantially improve system performance through inclusion in the education and training of the health workforce (Dijk et al., 2020; Gordon et al., 2020; International Federation of Medical Students' Associations, 2021; Rowland et al., 2019). Patients and family members have unique insights about their needs, preferences, living circumstances, and values to share. It is important to understand and reflect the different perspectives of all stakeholders. Parents and children, aunts and uncles, or even spouses may hold strong views, which at times may be at odds with one another. Separate conversations may be needed so that individuals are comfortable to speak freely. PPI can help current and future health professionals develop behaviours and practices that respect patients' lives. PPI can also improve communication between healthcare professionals and patients, allowing for more effective communication and collaboration. This can lead to improved patient outcomes and overall health system performance.

Technology Design and Implementation

The involvement of public and patient representatives can also provide valuable information about health technology use attitudes and habits, unmet technology needs, and preferences. In the rollout of new technologies, PPI can help professionals understand barriers to the adoption and usability of technologies (Facey et al., 2018; Hunter et al., 2018; Norburn & Thomas, 2021). For example, people with disabilities can help identify early design flaws that would have profound implications for future use by this group. They can provide information on how technologies should be introduced to patients, family members, or personal assistants, and they can suggest critical improvements after testing devices. Ultimately, they can enable designers and professionals to use technologies that will improve care quality and outcomes.

Information Systems Content and Deployment

Many health systems need help with secure, effective and integrated information systems (Ash et al., 2004; Hepworth et al., 1992; Hesse, 2008; James, 2013). Some challenges include data protection legislation, public scepticism, and slow implementation and evaluation. Any information stored or shared in healthcare must involve the public for ethical and practical reasons. The information systems must ensure that they are acceptable and usable for patients and professionals. Patients have the right to understand how these systems work and what health information is stored and processed by whom.

Moreover, they should be able to access, contribute, and provide feedback on the data systems. They can identify information gaps, errors, and difficulties in using the system. The public will only overcome scepticism if they can trust the system to be secure, user-friendly, and tailored to meet the needs of those using it. This also means that patients will have the right to exercise their right to add and remove information they consider of particular personal sensitivity and relevance.

Health Policy and Finance Prioritization

PPI is critical in shaping health policy and financial decision-making (Baumann et al., 2022; Jakab & Krishnan, 2001; Mitton et al., 2009; Souliotis, 2016). Especially in publicly or tax-funded systems, the public should play a key role in allocating resources and prioritizing services in health policy and strategies. It is essential that PPI is inclusive of marginalized and seldom-heard population groups to ensure that prioritization is based on equity principles. PPI can help monitor financial resources deployed to benefit all stakeholders, not only selected groups.

Governance and Leadership

The South Central Foundation's Nuka System of Care example has pointed to the importance of how the health system is organized. A flat hierarchy and inclusive governance and leadership through PPI can help ensure that decisions reflect community needs (Bellows et al., 2015; O'Shea et al., 2019; Pomey et al., 2016; Sharma et al., 2018). Open, continuous, and inclusive communication can help decision-makers understand communities' health and life challenges. It could help them in their outreach, engagement, and strategic planning work, and ensure timely, measured and tailored decisions. The ongoing dialogue can also help build trust and partnerships over time. Engaging the public and patients can alert health system leaders to perspectives and experiences they may not have considered otherwise. This will help them to arrive at more nuanced decisions that have a greater chance of achieving their desired outcomes. The continuous involvement of stakeholders and communities holds the promise of ultimately enhancing the quality, safety, accessibility, and equity of health systems.

PPI and Intervention Development and Evaluation

PPI has received the most attention in health-related research regarding steward-ship, financing, resources, research production, and use. There are different views about what is required to implement PPI for maximum research benefit and impact (Miller et al., 2018). The need to engage stakeholders in applied health and interven-tion research has also been reflected as the core element in the latest revision of the UK Medical Research Council (MRC) Framework for Developing and Evaluating Complex Interventions (Skivington et al., 2021). Previously, this step had been rele-gated to the implementation stage of research findings from clinical research, such as laboratory or trial research. This has been largely ineffective and costly as trials failed due to a limited understanding of the real-world circumstances in which hu-mans operate.

Systems Thinking and Design Thinking and PPI

Systems Thinking

Systems thinking and design thinking are practical and appropriate approaches that underpin, at least implicitly, many PPI initiatives (Abookire et al., 2020; Boswell, 2018; Brocklehurst et al., 2021; Holmes et al., 2019). Services need to work with the complex-ities and cultural and social dimensions that affect human lives and confront diverse challenges and 'wicked problems' that often lack clear, linear solutions (Cunningham et al., 2019; Keijser et al., 2020). Different values, views, interests, and understandings among various stakeholders, 'gravity problems' (which cannot be easily shifted) often stand in the way of meaningful problem resolutions. Systems thinking examines the interconnected elements that generate outcomes for individuals and communities. A look at the relationship between the different elements can provide avenues for inter-vention. The visualization of complex systems can provide professionals, patients, and the public with a non-verbal overview of how different life aspects affect one another. It can assist in planning interventions, and support shared decision-making processes.

Design Thinking and Collaborative Design (Co-Design)

Design thinking enjoys growing popularity in generating practice-relevant solutions in health education and service development (Aakhus & Harrison, 2015; Ku & Lupton,

2022; Valentine et al., 2017). It is not seen in opposition to evidence-based forms of intervention and service design but rather as a way of complementing these. However, design thinking typically starts with a practice rather than an academic problem. It also differs in terms of who defines this problem; according to IxDF (2016):

> Design thinking is a non-linear, iterative process that teams use to understand users, challenge assumptions, redefine problems and create innovative solutions to prototype and test. It is most useful to tackle ill-defined or unknown problems and involves five phases: Empathize, Define, Ideate, Prototype and Test

In healthcare, this means that professionals and patients would be centrally involved in the problem-solving process, not simply as data providers but as active solution developers. Design thinking can incorporate empirical literature and theoretical knowledge from the outset. Still, typically, it seeks to understand and define a problem through the experiences and perspectives of stakeholders, i.e. professionals and patients involved in the process. While there are multiple frameworks and techniques for implementing design thinking, they typically share the iterative nature of the process, which starts with gaining an in-depth understanding of the complexities of the problem (empathy) and then moves to define the specific focus for the design challenge (Auernhammer & Roth, 2021). After there is agreement on the focus, the design team brainstorms possible solutions (initially without imposing feasibility constraints), then proceeds to examine these from the perspective of stakeholders (personas) and works to build an initial prototype, which can be examined and tested in practice.

Contrary to clinical trials, there is no expectation of effectiveness but of learning from what has worked and what has not. Design thinking is associated with the 'permission to fail'. In fact, 'failure' is seen as a learning opportunity and consequently positive. The iterative nature of the design thinking approach allows us to refine the problem-solving at every stage of the cycle. An application of design thinking in healthcare is co-design. It involves the active involvement of people who use health services (patients, carers, and family members) in the planning, designing, and implementing healthcare initiatives. The Experience-Based Co-Design Field (Donetto et al., 2015) approach is a standardized format in this area but is one of many. Incorporating patient perspectives into the design process can ensure that services remain needs-focused on those receiving them. The collaborative approach fosters a sense of ownership, builds trust, and develops relationships between healthcare providers, policymakers, and the public.

Design- and systems thinking are two related approaches to solving complex problems. While systems thinking can help reveal the complex interactions of different elements in a system, e.g. how housing can affect health, well-being, employment, and social relationships, design thinking and co-design are structured but flexible ways of valuing stakeholder experiences in building collaborative solutions that are cognisant of the complexities of their lives. The combination of systems- and design thinking can generate solutions that are comprehensive and practical. The iterative nature of design thinking means solutions can be revised and tailored over time. In the next section, case examples will illustrate how design-thinking and co-design can be used as PPI tools.

Practical Applications of Systems and Design Thinking as Modalities of Public and Patient Involvement in Health and Social Care

Example 1: Co-Designing Health Services for People with Disabilities

While disability advocates have long fought—as discussed—to reframe disability from a medical to a social issue, it is also clear that people with disabilities are at greater risk for poor physical and mental health outcomes than those without disabilities. First, they may have a 'thinner margin' of health (DeJong et al., 2002) and are more vulnerable under conditions that can trigger infections; second, they face economic and structural barriers in accessing healthcare and related support in a timely and appropriate fashion. The pervasive medicalization of disability is also a chronic stressor, which may negatively impact on the mental health of people with disabilities. As a consequence, they may also have a higher rate of chronic conditions, such as diabetes, heart disease, and obesity. In terms of mental health, they may experience more social isolation and loneliness than others, may have to cope with the consequences of stigmatization and discrimination, and may be confronted with repeated frustrations due to barriers to an inappropriate provision of healthcare services and support.

The close involvement of people with disabilities and their family members can help design services that are fit for purpose. In the United States, access to primary preventative services for people with disabilities has been highlighted as an underdeveloped area for quite some time in health strategy documents such as Healthy People (2000, 2010, 2020, and 2030). Multiple studies (Kroll et al., 2006; Lofters et al., 2016; Rimmer, 1999) have documented inadequate access to health risk behaviour counselling, immunizations, and preventative health checks, such as mammograms and prostate exams. Apart from a gap in provider knowledge and skills deficits at the primary care level on how to support people with disabilities, the focus on health issues directly linked to the disability creates 'blind spots' among practitioners for other healthcare issues. Over the past two decades, innovative peer-mentoring programmes and service user manuals in the United States have been co-designed by people with disabilities to help them proactively request primary preventative services and inform practitioners (Adler et al., 2022; Haines et al., 2019; Layton et al., 2023).

The transition between care settings, especially between child and adult healthcare, is a complex challenge for many young people with disabilities. A recent work programme in Ireland included a co-design element to identify key attributes of transition services and supports for young people with cerebral palsy (CP). Five co-design workshops were conducted with a group of young people with CP who advised the research team on other study aspects and a group of parents. The Stanford D Model (Fortune et al., 2022) was used to identify and describe the transition needs of young people and their families. Iteratively, the young people and parents suggested and developed solutions to enhance the transition experience. They considered eight resources as instrumental: (1) a designated transition coordinator, (2) digital stories of transition experience, (3) written informational support, (4) a transition website, (5) transition checklists and worksheets, (6) a transition app, (7) a transition programme or course, and (8) an educational programme for health professionals (for details see (Fortune et al., 2022)).

In the UK, researchers recently used a co-design approach to capture and synthesize stroke survivor narratives and turn them into digital stories (Hall et al., 2022). The team intended to derive collective lessons that could be used to educate healthcare professionals supporting the rehabilitation process. The work programme commenced with a traditional qualitative research element with 30 stroke survivors. The information was then fed into five co-design workshops. A subset of six participants was involved in the co-design component, which comprised online workshops, a bulletin board, and an advisory committee. The team developed a framework that guided the design process and was aligned with the UK Design Council's Double Diamond method. The work was further underpinned by digital storytelling strategies and the behaviour change wheel (BCW) (Michie et al., 2011) for developing behavioural change interventions.

The co-created digital stories contain six collective lessons to enhance empathy and encourage behaviour change in healthcare professionals (HCPs) working with stroke survivors. The collective lessons were: (1) Stroke has a variety of symptoms that must all be considered; (2) Stroke can affect anyone of any age; (3) Assumptions should not be made about a survivor's lifestyle or habits; (4) It is essential to acknowledge the person behind the stroke and ensure that they are communicated with and listened to; (5) Stroke survivors can often feel unprepared for the reality of life after stroke; (6) Adapting to life after stroke is a long-term process requiring long-term support.

These examples demonstrate that co-design can be a powerful approach to integrate experiential research and service development involving people with disabilities throughout the process. The lessons learned are practical and testable.

Example 2. Co-design of Health and Support Interventions with People who Are Homeless

Homelessness is a complex challenge for many societies. There are multiple causes for and different forms of homelessness (Edgar & Meert, 2006). Media and public discourse often present a skewed picture of the homeless population, characterized by addiction and a history of criminality. Political failure to provide adequate and affordable housing is another feature often discussed but rarely resolved. The reality of homelessness is much more diverse.

In many cases of homelessness, not having a home is compounded by joblessness and physical and mental health problems, making it often difficult to establish cause and effect. People who are homeless are at greater risk for severe health problems and often lack even primary access to medical care. They are more likely to contract infectious diseases (Raoult et al., 2001), such as tuberculosis, Hepatitis B and C, or HIV/AIDS. Mental health issues such as depression, anxiety, and post-traumatic stress are common (Ayano et al., 2020). Homeless people are also at greater risk for chronic medical conditions, such as hypertension, diabetes, and asthma, as well as musculoskeletal pain (Nikoo et al., 2015).

Homeless service providers have, for some time, understood the benefits of PPI in designing their services. Organizations such as the National Health Care for the Homeless Council (NHCHC) in the United States, in their pursuit of helping homeless people get quality healthcare, have worked to ensure that homeless people have access to quality healthcare. They involved homeless clients in advocacy, resource development, and influencing legislation to improve healthcare access. In addition, homeless people are increasingly included in the decision-making process and evaluation of services. One such example is the so-called 'Speak Outs' that allows clients of service organizations in Ireland to voice their ideas, concerns, and feedback.

The involvement of homeless clients in a co-design process can be illustrated using two initiatives from Ireland (Kroll & Frazer, 2020).

The first example focuses on the fact that for individuals in Ireland who become homeless, it can be challenging to navigate the support landscape and to engage in personal development. To address this issue, a personal and organizational development training course was co-designed by four homeless clients, one member of staff of a homeless provider organization, and two academics. Six workshops, each three-hours-long, followed a design thinking structure, starting with empathy exercises and then moving to define specific life challenges related to homelessness. Solution-focused brainstorming or ideation exercises followed. The team proceeded then to build a testable 'prototype' based on the input provided by all partners. The prototype that emerged from the design sessions was a 'peer-support or buddy programme' that will be tested in one of the residential facilities of the homeless organization. The academic team members gained deep insights into the lived experience of homelessness; the client team members recognized their abilities and skills, which provided them with renewed confidence. The homeless organization got more profound insights into the client's needs and was also able to deploy a client-centred prototype.

The second example was described by Connolly et al. (2023): Young people experiencing homelessness (YPEH) face many economic, social, and psychological challenges that can impact their mental well-being. Four YPEH (aged 18–24) participated in a combined PhotoVoice and Co-Design Programme to develop a mental health service programme. Five workshops followed the five-stage Stanford D approach (empathy, define, ideate, prototype, test). The first two workshops used PhotoVoice to understand better the mental health impact and unmet needs of the YPEH. A young adult counsellor was present throughout all stages of the co-design project to provide support. The photos and group discussions in Workshops 1 and 2 highlighted the importance of nature as a source of relaxation and calm. The YPEH also pointed to the need to be seen as active and influential in their lives and not only as support recipients. Finally, the photos and interpretation by YPEH suggested a strong desire for belonging and social connection. The subsequent co-design workshops identified vital values and principles for mental health support that would be fit for purpose. Ideally, the YPEH wanted a low-threshold, informal, growth-inspiring, trauma-informed, and youth-centred MHSP programme. Trust and mutual commitment by both clients and counsellors were seen as essential. The programme prototype has since been implemented and embedded in the organization's more comprehensive mental health support. Initial feedback suggests this programme may be transformative for clients and the organization.

Practice Considerations for Public and Patient Involvement

As a small European country, Ireland has initiated to strengthen PPI in health and social care and health-related research. The government has also implemented other forms of engaging the public in shaping policies and actions of public interest (e.g. abortion rights and same-sex marriage). The public health service, the Health Service Executive (HSE), is now dedicated to strengthening PPI in services. The Health Research Board (HRB) and the Irish Research Council (IRC) have strategically invested 5 million euros in supporting the development of academic research and education systems that maximize PPI. Since 2021, seven universities and over 60 national and international partner organizations have collaborated to develop PPI education programmes and quality assurance measures and create awareness in human resource, finance, and research ethics departments for PPI as part of the National PPI Ignite Network[1]. This unique 'ecosystem' has produced several resources that inform and train academic, professional and public stakeholders in planning and conducting PPI activities. All materials are freely available on the Network's website. Ireland has been selected as an example as it is the only country where a system and nationwide approach to PPI has been taken to strengthen the public and patient voice. The work is preceded by impressive activities in other countries, including the United States (PICORI), the UK (NIHR), Canada, and Australia.

Conclusions

PPI in health service development and health-related research has gained momentum over the past decades. It responds to public pressure to dismantle

---

[1] https://ppinetwork.ie

knowledge elitism and shift from top-down forms of decision control and execution to shared decision-making. Shifting this to a more balanced form of governance, decision, and managerial control will be challenging and require innovative solutions from health organizations. The change in organization will also require changing how budgets will be allocated. Remuneration of PPI is a complex and largely undecided issue.

There is a risk of 'professionalization' or 'academization' of PPI. Public and patient collaborators are encouraged to undertake professional training to 'fit' into the world of practice and research. Conversely, academics and professionals may receive training on how to do PPI. While training and education are generally beneficial, there is a risk that only certain voices and people will be involved in partnership working, i.e. those who completed the education programme. It may cement the current problem that vocal and confident public and patient advocates serve on multiple advisory boards while the voices and lives of those less vocal, less educated, and less confident may not be heard. PPI lacks diversity of representation from underserved and seldom-heard population groups. If this issue is not tackled, there is a risk of insidious professionalization of PPI. We must ensure that relationships are refreshed, partners change, and new voices and perspectives are included.

To ensure that PPI is responsive to the changing contexts, it is important to develop learning ecosystems with broad societal support. This ecosystem should be built on shared values and principles, which help to foster collaboration and understanding between all stakeholders. The learning ecosystem should also enable stakeholders to adapt their approach to different contexts and develop bespoke working methods. This would allow for a move away from attempts to simplistic standardization. It would also encourage them to use a range of methods in their approaches, such as interdisciplinary methods, which could help to bring about more meaningful and realistic change. Finally, the learning ecosystem should enable stakeholders to measure the impact and usability of their PPI initiatives. This would demonstrate the value of PPI beyond the initial ethos and could help ensure that the impact is felt and the benefits are seen in the short and long term. It would also ensure that short-term investment cuts do not jeopardize PPI and that its commitment continues even in difficult times.

Thought Exercises

1. How do values between health professionals and patients potentially align or misalign? What could be done to achieve value transparency and agreement?
2. What are some of the practical considerations of involving people with (a) intellectual, (b) sensory, (c) behavioural or (d) physical disabilities, and (e) people with mental health conditions in health service design?
3. What are some important considerations in achieving equity in public and patient involvement?

4. What course of action would be useful if there is no agreement between PPI representatives and professionals?
5. Which ethical challenges arise when involving people considered 'vulnerable' as public and patient partners in health service design?
6. How can we avoid a 'professionalization' of PPI and refresh experiences and voices of PPI contributors?

Further Reading

Grotz, J., Ledgard, M., & Poland, F. (2020). *Patient and public involvement in health and social care research. an introduction to theory and practice*. Palgrave Macmillan.

Jameson, C., Haq, Z., Musse, S., et al. (2023). Inclusive approaches to involvement of community groups in health research: the co-produced CHICO guidance. *Research Involvement and Engagement 9*, Article 76. https://doi.org/10.1186/s40900-023-00492-9

Laidlaw, L., & Hollick, R. J. (2022). Values and value in patient and public involvement: moving beyond methods. *Future Healthcare Journal*, *9*(3), 238–242. https://doi,org/10.7861/fhj.2022-0108

Soklaridis, S., Harris, H., Shier, R., Rovet, J., Black, G., Bellissimo, G., Gruszecki, S., Lin, E., & Di Giandomenico, A. (2024). A balancing act: navigating the nuances of co-production in mental health research. *Research Involvement and Engagement*, *10*(1), 30. https://doi.org/10.1186/s40900-024-00561-7

References

Aakhus, M., & Harrison, T. R. (2015). Design thinking about communication in health system innovations. *Organizations, Communication, and Health*, *15*, Article E117.

Abookire, S., Plover, C., Frasso, R., & Ku, B. (2020). Health design thinking: an innovative approach in public health to defining problems and finding solutions. *Frontiers in Public Health*, *8*, Article 459.

Adler, R. F., Morales, P., Sotelo, J., & Magasi, S. (2022). Developing an mHealth app for empowering cancer survivors with disabilities: co-design study. *JMIR Formative Research*, Article e37706.

Arnstein, S. R. (1969). A ladder of citizen participation. *Journal of the American Institute of Planners*, *35*, 216–224.

Ash, J. S., Berg, M., & Coiera, E. (2004). Some unintended consequences of information technology in health care: the nature of patient care information system-related errors. *Journal of the American Medical Informatics Association*, *11*(2), 104–112.

Auernhammer, J., & Roth, B. (2021). The origin and evolution of Stanford University's design thinking: From product design to design thinking in innovation management. *Journal of Product Innovation Management*, *38*(6), 623–644.

Ayano, G., Solomon, M., Tsegay, L., Yohannes, K., & Abraha, M. (2020). A systematic review and meta-analysis of the prevalence of post-traumatic stress disorder among homeless people. *Psychiatric Quarterly*, *91*, 949–963.

Baumann, L. A., Reinhold, A. K., & Bruett, A. L. (2022). Public and patient involvement in health policy decision-making on the health system level–A scoping review. *Health Policy*, *126*, 1023–1038.

Bellows, M., Kovacs Burns, K., Jackson, K., & Surgeoner, B. (2015). Meaningful and effective patient engagement: what matters most to stakeholders. *Patient Experience Journal, 2*, 18–28.

Graves, B. (2013). Lower costs and better outcomes: a system of care built on relationships. *British Medical Journal, 347*, f5301.

Bombard, Y., Baker, G. R., Orlando, E., Fancott, C., & Bhatia, P. (2018). Engaging patients to improve quality of care: a systematic review. *Implement Science, 13*(1), 98.

Boswell, J. (2018). The elusive search for the public voice in health policy: the case for 'systems thinking'. *Journal of Health Services Research & Policy, 23*, 4–5.

Brocklehurst, P. R., Baker, S. R., & Langley, J. (2021). Context and the evidence-based paradigm: The potential for participatory research and systems thinking in oral health. *Community Dentistry and Oral Epidemiology, 49*(1), 1–9.

Bussey, L. G., & Sillence, E. (2019). The role of internet resources in health decision-making: a qualitative study. *Digital Health, 5*, 2055207619888073.

Clinical and Translational Science Awards Consortium, Community Engagement Key Function Committee, Task Force on the Principles of Community Engagement. (2011). *Principles of community engagement* (2nd ed.). Centers for Disease Control and Prevention/ Agency for Toxic Substances and Disease Registry. https://stacks.cdc.gov/view/cdc/11699

Charlton, J. I. (1998). *Nothing about us without us: disability oppression and empowerment.* University of California Press.

Connolly, M., Casey, S., Conroy, É., Dempsey, D., Frazer, K., Kroll, T., McDonnell Murray, R., & Walshe, P. (2023). *Co-designing a mental health support programme with young adults experiencing homelessness* [Report]. Dublin Simon Community. https://www.dubsimon.ie/ reports/researchpolicy

Correia, T. (2017). Revisiting medicalization: a critique of the assumptions of what counts as medical knowledge. *Frontiers in Sociology, 2*.

Cunningham, F. C., Ranmuthugala, G., & Westbrook, J. (2019). Tackling the wicked problem of health networks: the design of an evaluation framework. *BMJ Open, 9*(5), Article 024231.

de Graaff, B., Kleinhout-Vliek, T., & Van de Bovenkamp, H. (2021). In the works: patient and public involvement and engagement in healthcare decision-making. *Health Expectations, 24*(6), 1903–1904.

DeJong, G., Palsbo, S. E., & Beatty, P. W. (2002). The organization and financing of health services for persons with disabilities. *Milbank Quarterly, 80*(2), 261–301.

Denmark, D., & Olson, D. (2014). A communications canvas to improve and individualize patient engagement in healthcare systems redesign. *Proceedings of RSD3, Third Symposium of Relating Systems Thinking to Design,* 15–17 October 2014, Oslo, Norway. http://openresea rch.ocadu.ca/id/eprint/2073/

Donetto, S., Pierri, P., Tsianakis, V., & Robert, G. (2015). Experience-based co-design and healthcare improvement: Realizing participatory design in the public sector. *The Design Journal, 18*(2), 227–248. https://doi.org/10.2752/175630615X14212498964312

Dijk, S. W., Duijzer, E. J., & Wienold, M. (2020). Role of active patient involvement in undergraduate medical education: a systematic review. *British Medical Journal Open, 10*, Article e037217.

Eby, D. K. (2018). Customer-ownership in equity-oriented health care. *Milbank Q, 96*, 672–674.

Edgar, B., & Meert, H. (2006). *The state of homelessness in Europe: A FEANTSA study* [Report]. FEANTSA. https://www.feantsaresearch.org/download/5-20064496180 11929240409.pdf

Facey, K. M., Bedlington, N., Berglas, S., Bertelsen, N., Single, Ann N. V., & Thomas, V. (2018). Putting patients at the centre of healthcare: progress and challenges for health technology assessments. *The Patient, 11*(6), 581–589.

Ferguson, L. M., Ward, H., Card, S., Sheppard, S., & McMurtry, J. (2013). Putting the 'patient' back into patient-centred care: An education perspective. *Nurse Education in Practice*, *13*(4), 283–287.

Fortune, J., Burke, J., Dillon, C., Dillon, S., O'Toole, S., Enright, A., Flynn, A., Manikandan, M., Kroll, T., Lavelle, G., & Ryan, J. M. (2022). Co-designing resources to support the transition from child to adult health services for young people with cerebral palsy: A design thinking approach. *Frontiers in Rehabilitation Science*, *3*, Article 976580.

Fredriksson, M., & Tritter, J. Q. (2017). Disentangling patient and public involvement in healthcare decisions: why the difference matters. *Sociology of Health & Illness*, *39*(1), 95–111.

Funk, M., Lund, C., Freeman, M., & Drew, N. (2009). Improving the quality of mental health care. *International Journal for Quality in Health Care*, *21*, 415–420.

Gaber, J. (2019). Building 'a ladder of citizen participation'. *Journal of the American Planning Association*, *85*, 188–201.

Gibbons, C. J., Bee, P. E., Walker, L., Price, O., & Lovell, K. (2014). Service user- and carer-reported measures of involvement in mental health care planning: methodological quality and acceptability to users. *Frontiers in Psychiatry*, *5*, 178.

Gilfoyle, M., MacFarlane, A., Hannigan, A., Niranjan, V., Hughes, Z., & Salsberg, J. (2022). The public and patient involvement imperative in Ireland: Building on policy drivers. *Frontiers in Public Health*, *10*, 1038409.

Gordon, M., Gupta, S., Thornton, D., Reid, M., Mallen, E., & Melling, A. (2020). Patient/service user involvement in medical education: A best evidence medical education (BEME) systematic review: BEME Guide No. 58. *Medical Teacher*, *42*, 4–16.

Gottlieb, K. (2013). The Nuka System of Care: improving health through ownership and relationships. *International Journal of Circumpolar Health*, *72*, 21118.

Haines, K. J., Holdsworth, C., Cranwell, K., Skinner, E. H., Holton, S., MacLeod-Smith, B., Bates, S., Iwashyna, T. J., French, C., & Booth, S. (2019). Development of a peer support model using experience-based co-design to improve critical care recovery. *Critical Care Explorations*, *1*(3), Article e0006.

Hall, J., Kroll, T., van Wijck, F., & Bassil-Morozow, H. (2022). Co-creating digital stories with UK-based stroke survivors with the aim of synthesizing collective lessons from individual experiences of interacting with healthcare professionals. *Frontiers in Rehabilitation Sciences*, *3*, Article 877442.

Hepworth, J. B., Vidgen, G. A., Griffin, E., & Woodward, A. M. (1992). The enhancement of information systems through user involvement in system design. *International Journal of Information Management*, *12*(2), 120–129.

Hesse, B. W. (2008). Enhancing consumer involvement in health care. In J. C. Parker & E. Thorson (Eds.), *Health communication in the new media landscape* (pp. 119–141).

Holmes, L., Cresswell, K., Williams, S., Parsons, S., Keane, A., Wilson, C., Islam, S., Joseph, O., Miah, J., Robinson, E., & Starling, B. (2019). Innovating public engagement and patient involvement through strategic collaboration and practice. *Research Involvement and Engagement*, *5*, 30.

Hunter, A., Facey, K., Thomas, V., Haerry, D., Warner, K., Klingmann, I., May, M., & See, W. (2018). EUPATI guidance for patient involvement in medicines research and development: health technology assessment. *Frontiers in Medicine*, *5*, 231.

IxDF. (2016). *What is design thinking (DT)?* https://www.interaction-design.org/literature/topics/design-thinking

International Federation of Medical Students' Associations. (2021). *IFMSA policy document: Patient involvement in medical education.* https://ifmsa.org/wp-content/uploads/2021/07/Patient-involvement-in-medical-education.pdf

Jahagirdar, D., Kroll, T., Ritchie, K., & Wyke, S. (2013). Patient-reported outcome measures for chronic obstructive pulmonary disease. *The Patient, 6*, 11–21.

Jakab, M., & Krishnan, C. (2001). *Community involvement in health care financing: A survey of the literature on the impact, strengths, and weaknesses.* World Bank Discussion Paper No. 28884. World Bank. https://openknowledge.worldbank.org/handle/10986/13706

James, J. (2013). Patient engagement. *Health Affairs Health Policy Brief, 14.*

Keijser, W., Huq, J.-L., & Reay, T. (2020). Enacting medical leadership to address wicked problems. *BMJ Leader, 4*, 12–17.

Kelly, J. T., Campbell, K. L., Gong, E., & Scuffham, P. (2020). The internet of things: impact and implications for health care delivery. *Journal of Medical Internet Research, 22*(11), Article e20135.

Koehlmoos, T., Kimsey, L., Bishai, D., & Lane, D. (2017). The imperative for a health systems approach to global health engagement. *Joint Force Quarterly, 84*, 107.

Kroll, T., & Frazer, K. (2020), Designing for growth and development – a co-designed course for homeless people. *European Journal of Public Health, 30*, Article ckaa165.1271.

Kroll, T., Jones, G. C., Kehn, M., & Neri, M. T. (2006). Barriers and strategies affecting the utilisation of primary preventive services for people with physical disabilities: a qualitative inquiry. *Health & Social Care in the Community, 14*(4), 284–293.

Kroll, T., Wyke, S., Jahagirdar, D., & Ritchie, K. (2014). If patient-reported outcome measures are considered key health-care quality indicators, who is excluded from participation. *Health Expectations, 17*(5), 605–607.

Ku, B., & Lupton, E. (2022). *Health design thinking: creating products and services for better health.* MIT Press.

Layton, N., Harper, K., Martinez, K., Berrick, N., & Naseri, C. (2023). Co-creating an assistive technology peer-support community: Learnings from AT Chat. *Disability and Rehabilitation: Assistive Technology, 18*, 603–609.

Lazarus, J. V., & France, T. (2014). *A new era for the WHO health system building blocks?* https://healthsystemsglobal.org/news/a-new-era-for-the-who-health-system-building-blocks/

Leslie, D., Mazumder, A., Peppin, A., Wolters, M. K., & Hagerty, A. (2021). Does 'AI' stand for augmenting inequality in the era of covid-19 healthcare. *British Medical Journal, 372*, n304.

Lewis, R., Boydell, N., Blake, C., Clarke, Z., Kernaghan, K., & McMellon, C. (2023). Involving young people in sexual health research and service improvement: Conceptual analysis of patient and public involvement (PPI) in three projects. *BMJ Sexual & Reproductive Health, 49*(2), 76.

Lofters, A., Guilcher, S., Maulkhan, N., Milligan, J., & Lee, J. (2016), Patients living with disabilities: the need for high-quality primary care. *Canadian Family Physician, 62*, Article e457–e464.

MacFarlane, A. E. (2020). Optimising individual and community involvement in health decision-making in general practice consultations and primary care settings: a way forward. *European Journal of General Practice, 26*(1), 196–201.

Michie, S., van Stralen, M., & West, R. (2011). The behaviour change wheel: a new method for characterising and designing behaviour change interventions. *Implementation Science, 6*, Article 42.

Milakovich, M. (2010). The internet and increased citizen participation in government. *eJournal of eDemocracy & Open Government, 2*(1), 1–9.

Miller, F. A., Patton, S. J., Dobrow, M., & Berta, W. (2018). Public involvement in health research systems: a governance framework. *Health Research Policy and Systems, 16*(1), Article 79.

Mitton, C., Smith, N., Peacock, S., Evoy, B., & Abelson, J. (2009). Public participation in health care priority setting: a scoping review. *Health Policy, 91*(3), 219–228.

Mossberger, K., & Tolbert, C. (2008). *Digital citizenship: the internet, society and participation.* MIT Press.

Mossé, C. (2013). The demos's participation in decision-making: Principles and realities. In J. P. Árnason, K. A. Raaflaub & P. Wagner (Eds.), *The Greek polis and the invention of democracy: A politico-cultural transformation and its interpretations* (pp. 260–273). Wiley-Blackwell.

Murdoch, B. (2021). Privacy and artificial intelligence: challenges for protecting health information in a new era. *BMC Medical Ethics, 22*, 122.

National Academy of Medicine. (2001). *Crossing the quality chasm: A new health system for the 21st century.* National Academies Press.

Ní Shé, É., Cassidy, J., Davies, C., De Brún, A., Donnelly, S., Dorris, E., Dunne, N., Egan, K., Foley, M., Galvin, M., Harkin, M., Killilea, M., Kroll, T., Lacey, V., Lambert, V., McLoughlin, S., Mitchell, D., Murphy, E., Mwendwa, P., ... O'Philbin, L. (2020). Minding the gap: identifying values to enable public and patient involvement at the pre-commencement stage of research projects. *Research Involvement and Engagement, 6*, Article 46.

Nielsen, J., Eckstein, L., Nicol, D., & Stewart, C. (2021). Integrating public participation, transparency and accountability into governance of marketing authorisation for genome editing products. *Frontiers in Political Science, 3*, Article 747838.

Nikoo, N., Motamed, M., Nikoo, M. A., Neilson, E., Saddicha, S., & Krausz, M. (2015). Chronic physical health conditions among homeless. *Journal of Health Disparities Research & Practice, 8*, Article 17.

Norburn, L., & Thomas, L. (2021). Expertise, experience, and excellence. Twenty years of patient involvement in health technology assessment at NICE: an evolving story. *International Journal of Technology Assessment in Health Care, 37*, Article e15.

O'Shea, A., Boaz, A. L., & Chambers, M. (2019). A hierarchy of power: the place of patient and public involvement in healthcare service development. *Frontiers in Sociology, 4*, Article 38.

Ocloo, J., Garfield, S., Dean Franklin, B. D., & Dawson, S. (2021). Exploring the theory, barriers and enablers for patient and public involvement across health, social care and patient safety: a systematic review of reviews. *Health Research Policy and Systems, 19*, Article 8.

Pomey, M.-P., Morin, E., Neault, C., Biron, V., Houle, L., Lavigueur, L., Bouvette, G., St-Pierre, N., & Beaumont, M. (2016). Patient advisors: how to implement a process for involvement at all levels of governance in a healthcare organization. *Patient Experience Journal, 3*(2), 99–112.

Raoult, D., Foucault, C., & Brouqui, P. (2001). Infections in the homeless. *The Lancet Infectious Diseases, 1*(2), 77–84.

Richie, C. S. (2019). Not sick: liberal, trans, and crip feminist critiques of medicalization. *Journal of Bioethical Inquiry, 16*(3), 375–387.

Rimmer, J. H. (1999). Health promotion for people with disabilities: the emerging paradigm shift from disability prevention to prevention of secondary conditions. *Physical Therapy, 79*(5), 495–502.

Rowland, P., Anderson, M., Kumagai, A. K., McMillan, S., Sandhu, V. K., & Langlois, S. (2019). Patient involvement in health professionals' education: a meta-narrative review. *Advances in Health Sciences Education, 24*(3), 595–617.

Sacks, E., Morrow, M., Story, W. T., Shelley, K. D., Shanklin, D., Rahimtoola, M., Rosales, A., Ibe, O., & Sarriot, E. (2018). Beyond the building blocks: integrating community roles into health systems frameworks to achieve health for all. *BMJ Global Health, 3*(Suppl 3), Article e001384.

Sarker, A., & Hassan, M. (2010). Civic engagement and public accountability: an analysis with particular reference to developing countries. *Public Administration, 15*(2), 381–417.

Sharma, A. E., Huang, B., Knox, M., Willard-Grace, R., & Potter, M. B. (2018). Patient engagement in community health center leadership: how does it happen. *Journal of Community Health, 43*(6), 1069–1074.

Skivington, K., Matthews, L., Simpson, S. A., Craig, P., Baird, J., Blazeby, J. M., Boyd, K. A., Craig, N., French, D. P., McIntosh, E., Petticrew, M., Rycroft-Malone, J., White, M., & Moore, L. (2021). A new framework for developing and evaluating complex interventions: update of Medical Research Council guidance. *British Medical Journa (Clinical research ed.), 374*, Article n2061.

Sleigh, J., & Vayena, E. (2021). Public engagement with health data governance: the role of visuality. *Humanities and Social Sciences Communications, 8*, Article 149.

Souliotis, K. (2016). Public and patient involvement in health policy: a continuously growing field. *Health Expectations, 19*, 1171–1172.

Tambuyzer, E., Pieters, G., & Van Audenhove, C. (2014). Patient involvement in mental health care: one size does not fit all. *Health Expectations, 17*(1), 138–150.

Tambuyzer, E., & Van Audenhove, C. (2015). Is perceived patient involvement in mental health care associated with satisfaction and empowerment? *Health Expectations, 18*(4), 516–526.

Tritter, J. Q. (2009). Revolution or evolution: the challenges of conceptualizing patient and public involvement in a consumerist world. *Health Expectations, 12*, 275–287.

United Nations. (2006). *United Nations Convention on the Rights of Persons with Disabilities.* https://social.desa.un.org/issues/disability/crpd/convention-on-the-rights-of-persons-with-disabilities-crpd

Vahdat, S., Hamzehgardeshi, L., Hessam, S., & Hamzehgardeshi, Z. (2014). Patient involvement in health care decision making: a review. *Iran Red Crescent Medical Journal, 16*, Article e12454.

Valentine, L., Kroll, T., Bruce, F., Lim, C., & Mountain, R. (2017). Design thinking for social innovation in health care. *The Design Journal, 20*, 755–774.

van Dijk, W., Faber, M. J., Tanke, M. A., Jeurissen, P. P., & Westert, G. P. (2016). Medicalisation and overdiagnosis: what society does to medicine. *International Journal of Health Policy and Management, 5*(11), 619–622.

Ward, P. R. (2017). Improving access to, use of, and outcomes from public health programs: the importance of building and maintaining trust with patients/clients. *Frontiers in Public Health, 5*, Article 22.

Weerakkody, V., Irani, Z., Kapoor, K., Sivarajah, U., & Dwivedi, Y. K. (2017). Open data and its usability: an empirical view from the citizen's perspective. *Information Systems Frontiers, 19*, 285–300.

Wilkins, C. H. (2018). Effective engagement requires trust and being trustworthy. *Medical Care, 56*(10 Suppl 1), S6–S8.

Wolf, A., Moore, L., Lydahl, D., Naldemirci, Ö., Elam, M., & Britten, N. (2017). The realities of partnership in person-centred care: a qualitative interview study with patients and professionals. *BMJ Open, 7*, e016491.

World Health Organization. (1978). Declaration of Alma-Ata: International Conference on Primary Health Care, Alma-Ata, USSR, 6–12 September 1978.

9
The Politics of Diagnosis and Alternatives
The Power Threat Meaning Framework

Trudy Meehan, Emma Hickey, Cian Aherne, and Sarah Robinson

Introduction

There is growing recognition that mental health is intricately linked to our social, economic, and physical environments (e.g. Johnstone & Boyle, 2018; Office of the High Commissioner for Human Rights, 2023; Pickett & Wilkinson, 2010). Experiences of adverse environments can be causal, and create emotional distress (Boyle, 2022; Read et al., 2006; Pickett & Wilkinson, 2010). Psychology and psychiatry, however, have struggled to move beyond a 'disorder' based conceptualization of emotional distress or what Gergen (1997) called the 'discourse of deficit.'

The UN Special Rapporteur, Dainius Puras (2017) has stated that '[r]eductive biomedical approaches to treatment that do not adequately address contexts and relationships can no longer be considered compliant with the right to health' (p. 17). Despite this, mental health difficulties are growing (Brinkmann, 2016; Dooley & Fitzgerald, 2012; Dooley et al., 2019), and research which indicates that social determinants play a (often causal) role in distress, the biomedical model (which focuses on diagnosis, medication, and reducing 'symptoms') predominates in many mental health services (Brinkmann, 2016; Davies, 2021; Farrell & McMahon, 2021; Hari, 2018; Dooley & Fitzgerald, 2012; Dooley et al., 2019; Office of the High Commissioner for Human Rights, 2023). The dominance of the biomedical model despite arguments about the negative impacts of psychiatric drugs (Bentall, 2009; Davies & Read, 2019; Hutton et al., 2013; Kirsch, 2009; Kirsch et al., 2008; Moncrieff, 2008; Read & Sacia, 2020; Read & Williams, 2019), and documented increases in stigma from mental health campaigns that reify ideas of mental health being 'an illness like any other' (e.g. Albee & Joffe, 2004; Malla et al., 2015, & Read et al., 2006).

In this chapter we suggest that the 'inertia to the "biomedical" installed base', a term we borrow from science and technology studies to describe 'the organizational, institutional, regulatory, sociotechnical arrangements that are already in place' (Aanestad et al., 2017, p. 29), creates ethical dilemmas and difficulties for practice and the young people we work with.

As practitioners, educators and researchers, we are concerned with the dominance of the biomedical single story and, how it impacts to young people. In this chapter, we introduce an alternative, evidence-based, and non-stigmatizing framework called the Power Threat Meaning Framework (PTMF) for understanding and working with emotional distress that is non-diagnostic and offers some suggestions to help practitioners and academics navigate the transition to a more contextual understanding and practice of care. Through a fictional case study of a young woman called Olivia, we demonstrate the ethical and moral challenges that the privileging of biomedical approaches in contemporary psychological organizational structures create and discuss implications for policy and practice. We take a pragmatist approach in exploring some of the ethical tensions Olivia's case highlights and draw on reflections made by Dylan and Caoimhe (Youth Advocates from Jigsaw) to pose some core ethical questions for us as researchers and practitioners in this space.

Reflexive Statement

As co-authors of this chapter Emma and Cian both work as clinical psychologists in Jigsaw, the National Centre for Youth Mental Health in Ireland and apply the Power Threat Meaning Framework (PTMF) in practice. Sarah is a researcher who is interested in how diagnostic culture impacts and shapes experiences, and how technology can reify diagnostic understandings and influence young people's meaning-making about emotions. Trudy worked as a senior clinical psychologist in the Child and Adolescent Mental Health Services in the Irish public health service. She is currently a lecturer and researcher in the Centre for Positive Health Sciences, Royal College of Surgeons in Ireland University of Medicine and Health Sciences. Trudy is also a user of mental health services and is neurodivergent. We had input on the case study and discussion regarding psychiatric diagnoses from two Jigsaw Youth Advocates. Caoimhe and Dylan are young people who have an interest in youth mental health and who also happen to have used mental health services in the past. They met with us to discuss the case study and support our check as to whether it was reflective of young people's experiences. In addition, they discussed their experiences of and opinions on diagnosis. We realized that the issue of diagnosis constantly shifted and morphed, depending on what subject position we were speaking from. As present and historical clients of mental health services, Trudy, and Dylan and Caoimhe, vacillated between advocating for getting rid of psychiatric diagnoses (as per DSM-5, Guha, 2014) and at other times speaking about the practical reality of needing a label to access supports. It led to interesting discussions and challenges around how to adequately represent all the 'voices' that contributed to the writing of this chapter. Finally, when referring to psychiatric diagnoses throughout this chapter, we acknowledge that this model is mainly practised and used by psychiatrists, psychologists, and general practitioners in the healthcare system. Next, we introduce the PTMF.

The Power Threat Meaning Framework

The PTMF is a co-produced project with people who have used mental health services, psychologists, and other mental health professionals, published by the British Psychological Society (BPS). The framework brings together evidence about the ways in which power influences people's lives, the impact that the misuse of power has on emotional well-being, and the ways we have learned to respond (otherwise referred to as 'threat responses'). In a biomedical approach these are often described as 'symptoms'. The framework acknowledges the influence of biological/genetic and epigenetic/evolutionary factors in mediating and enabling (rather than necessarily *causing*) these threat responses or coping mechanisms. It emphasizes relational, social, cultural, and material factors in shaping the emergence, persistence, experience, and expression of threat responses.

The PTMF also suggests that we pose four core questions when considering one's emotional well-being journey: 'What happened to you?' (or How does power operate in your life?): 'How did it affect you?' (or 'What kind of threats does this pose?'); 'What sense did you make of it?' (or 'What is the meaning of these situations and experiences to you?') and 'What did you have to do to survive?' (or 'What kinds of threat responses are you using?') (Johnstone et al. 2018, p. 9). It argues for a contextual understanding of the person, considering how they make meaning of their experiences and the functions of their threat responses.

Some of the common forms of power that the PTMF highlights include ideological power, which can be understood as the messages we get from powerful systems, such as the media and the government, which can have a positive and negative impact on us (Aherne & Hickey, 2022). For example, psychiatric diagnoses can be considered a form of ideological power if given without consent. Even when given with consent, compliance may reflect submission to ideological power. Other forms of power can be interpersonal (e.g. the power to care or not care or withdraw/withhold love; (Johnstone & Boyle, 2018) and coercive power (e.g. intimidation or violence scare or force people into compliance; (Johnstone & Boyle, 2018).

Jigsaw has moved towards working with contextual lenses of understanding, such as the PTMF, with young people as it endeavours to offer a trauma-informed approach that is non-pathologizing and enables dialogue with young people about their experiences. Figure 9.1 outlines the flow of a PTMF conversation that someone working as a practitioner at Jigsaw (2021) might use with a young person.

Olivia's Case Study

We now present a fictional case study of a young woman called Olivia that was made by drawing various true but anonymized stories together. In totality it is fictional but each of the elements are drawn from real-life examples of therapeutic interventions and aim to offer a case study that illustrates the concrete situated dilemmas that Cian and Emma navigate in clinical practice. We presented this case study to two Jigsaw Youth Advocates, Caoimhe and Dylan, and spoke with them to ask them if they feel the case is representative of a young person's experience. They reflected that it was. Dylan and Caoimhe both felt that it is common for many young people to experience multiple challenges or adversities. We also asked them to give us their reflections on the potential diagnosis which we share more of towards the end of the chapter in the section on ethical dilemmas and reflections. In this case study, we try to adopt a pragmatist ethical pathway for the person at the centre of the intervention using the PTMF as a lens in therapeutic practice.

Initial Information A young woman (Olivia), aged 17, was referred to a youth mental health service. The referral information and initial screening unveiled a pattern of suicidality and self-harm. Furthermore, Olivia had been told by the psychiatrist in a previous mental health service that she is 'emotionally unstable'. She had been prescribed medication, which she had been told would decrease the severity of her distress and had been advised to seek a psychiatric assessment/diagnosis in Adult Mental Health Services when she turns 18. The clinical psychologist that she worked with in the same service mentioned to her that she would likely receive a diagnosis of 'borderline personality disorder' given her unstable relationships, feelings of abandonment, and impulsive and risky behaviour including self-harm.

Working with Olivia through the Lens of the PTMF

Getting to know Olivia: Olivia was slow to open-up in her initial sessions. She explained that she finds it difficult to trust people and that her experiences of mental health services to date had been negative. Olivia's engagement with services had drawn on a deficit-based narrative which positioned Olivia as beyond help and complex. Olivia described experiences of being told at various stages that she is both 'not unwell enough' and 'too unwell' to receive support from services. Olivia's concerns about side effects of medication (e.g. weight gain) were also dismissed when brought to review appointments in other services. The first sessions were spent building rapport with Olivia while listening to her experiences and collaborating with her to piece the story together in a coherent meaningful way. Some initial strengths identified included Olivia's interest in dance and performance art.

Previous Service Experiences: Due to Olivia's previous experiences of help-seeking with mental health services, it was likely that she had experienced iatrogenic harm (harm from the service that was being used for support). This harm was particularly in relation to not feeling heard, not being supported with concerns about the side effects of medication, and being told that it is likely that her challenges could be best explained by a psychiatric diagnosis (rather than any attempts being made to understand the context of her experiences). This obfuscated any potential other exploration of what may have been affecting Olivia's mental health and did not allow for further discussions to emerge regarding Olivia's life experiences.

Integrating the PTMF Questions in Therapy

Olivia reported a childhood fear associated with witnessing her parents arguing a lot when she was growing up. Oliva's parents were no longer together at the time of the intervention and Olivia was living permanently with her father, his partner, and her half-sibling. Pre-adolescence, Olivia had shared some brief experiences of homelessness when in the care of her mother. Contact with mum was inconsistent and limited due to ongoing ruptures in their relationship without attempts at repair. Olivia's mother had been given a diagnosis of 'borderline personality disorder'. Olivia outlined that she is aware other family members have varied mental health diagnoses and she was very conscious of how this family history may impact her. Olivia described her current relationship with her dad as 'up and down'; she acknowledged that he has a temper which can lead to regular arguments and clashes at home. See Figure 9.1 for a suggested guide on how the PTMF questions and worksheets might be used in sessions with young people.

Olivia also talked about the pressure she has experienced in school to do well in her State Exams. Olivia described this pressure as coming entirely from within and was quite self-critical about her ability to cope with daily pressure, stress, and anxiety. Upon her previous service's conclusions (that Olivia was 'emotionally unstable'), Olivia had looked up her 'symptoms' on the internet. Given her family history, she was certain she must have a disorder. In therapy, Olivia explained that she 'always knew there was something wrong with me' and that, from some searches on Google, she felt her symptoms fit in line with 'borderline personality disorder'. Olivia spoke about sometimes cutting herself when she feels emotionally overwhelmed and that she drinks to excess most weekends. Olivia acknowledged that drinking alcohol can sometimes magnify feelings of hopelessness, sadness, and anxiety. Olivia asserted that she would like the therapy sessions to focus on helping her understand her emotions better and to be able to cope better with them daily.

After several sessions, when trust had been built and the therapist was assured that Olivia saw the therapy room as a safe space, the therapist suggested using a particular framework (the PTMF) to help put a shape on Olivia's story to gain a deeper understanding of how she was feeling. Olivia agreed that this was something she would like to do. The therapist explained that one of the main questions of the framework is "what happened to you?" and that this is asked with the understanding that lots of things that happen to us can have an impact on our mental health. When the therapist asked Olivia what things had happened to her that might have affected her mental health, Olivia initially talked about her experiences of her parents and academic pressure but then suddenly became tearful and upset. The therapist slowed the session down at this point with some space for silence and asked Olivia what she was thinking of. Olivia then disclosed that she had been sexually assaulted at a house party when she was fourteen. She acknowledged that this may be an important aspect of her story but that she finds it hard to speak about this experience due to intense feelings of shame. Olivia also reported that she shared what happened at the time with her

Using the worksheets

Please use any vocabulary that you and the young person find helpful. The questions overlap, and therefore so will the responses - they are not expected to fit neatly under specific questions. The following are some suggested instructions for how one might approach using the PTMF questions in sessions:

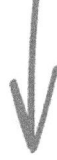

What has happened to you?
This may be easier for some young people to identify than others and some forms of power are easier to identify than others. The information sheets on ideological power are intended to be used at this point as a way of exploring some of the more subtle, or hidden forms of power that may have contributed towards feelings of distress. Sometimes young people find these more subtle messages difficult to identify, and as a result can internalise feelings of distress.

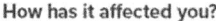

How has it affected you?
Once different experiences and associated power structures have been explored, the impact on physical, social and emotional-well being is looked at with the young person. Talk through step one again, and its connection with the impact on wellbeing to help with clarity. Sometimes young people have found it helpful for this question to specifically focus on emotions.

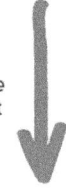

What sense did you make of it?
Sometimes young people may have answered some of this question in their response to the first two questions. In simply asking the question, however, they tend to give it a rethink and add further detail. Sometimes asking, 'What did you learn about yourself/other people/the world as a result of this experience?', can help. Again, it is worth talking through the responses to the first two questions to add cohesion to the response to this question.

What did you have to do to survive?
It can be helpful to use the second handout (entitled 'Threat responses') when talking through this question. Ultimately looking at the function of young people's threat responses is important. Again, it is helpful to review the first three questions, and then ask, 'Now, thinking through all of that, how did you survive what happened?'

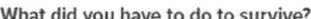 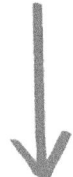

What are your strengths?
This can feel like a respite from the depths of the other questions. It gives the young person a chance to reflect on all that they've done to get through the challenges, and the protective factors they may have. It can be helpful to rephrase this question in different ways if the young person is not particularly comfortable talking about 'strengths'.

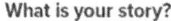 

What is your story?
Young people can sometimes feel like their previous answers have sufficiently covered their story (particularly in session). This question gives them an opportunity to take away what they've reflected upon, and use a blank page to review it all in their own words.

Figure 9.1 Using Jigsaw's Worksheets about the PTMF in practice, taken from (Aherne & Hickey, 2022).

mother, a close friend, and her boyfriend. She recalled that they all explained to her, in different ways, that she must be exaggerating or making up what happened and that they blamed her for ending up in a situation where this could happen. She reported that she was encouraged to move on from this experience and not to dwell on it. Olivia became silent in the session following this disclosure and it appeared as though she had been brought back to this time of being blamed and silenced. The therapist let

Olivia know that they were here when she was ready to talk again and gave her the option of returning to this topic, pausing the session to take a break, or ending the session a bit early, depending on what Olivia felt she needed. The therapist also positively reinforced Olivia's disclosure and acknowledged the courage this took based on previous help-seeking experiences.

PTMF Reflections

It is evident that coercive power and interpersonal power have been operating negatively in Olivia's life in several ways—her autonomy and choice have been violated through her experiences of sexual assault, and denial and silencing of this experience by her family, friend, and boyfriend. A trauma-informed approach to working with Olivia would mean providing her with a different relational template than she had met with so far (Treisman, 2016). It would mean providing a space that is safe, collaborative, and empowering. As Olivia had been silenced and dismissed by her attacker, her mother, her friend, her boyfriend, and prior mental health services, it will take time for Olivia to feel empowered. Giving Olivia choice and control over elements of her care, therefore, is vital. Examples of this include choice regarding the gender of the clinician, the agenda for sessions, the trajectory and pace of sessions, the time of appointments, and choice of clinic room. We mention giving Olivia choice about the listed factors because in the service discussed, these are the factors that a client can have some choice about. Ideally, she should have choice about ethnicity (Coleman, Wampold, & Casali, 1995), socioeconomic background (Balmforth, 2009; Trott & Reeves, 2018), sexual orientation (Liddle, 1996), personality, empathy, and other factors that may be relevant to her. While Olivia's choices are limited by the reality of scarce resources, it is still worth offering choice where we can. Providing choice and improving therapeutic alliance is an ethical issue as it directly feeds into the quality of the therapeutic experience and potential outcomes (Flückiger et al., 2018; Horvath & Symonds,1991). In the context of choosing healthcare providers, the principles of Article 25 (Health) of the United Nations Convention of Rights of People with Disabilities (UNCRPD) (United Nations, 2006) stress the importance of autonomy, including the freedom to make one's own choices, and independence of persons. While the convention may not explicitly state the right to choose a specific healthcare provider, the overall emphasis on non-discrimination, accessibility, and respect for the individual autonomy and decision-making of persons with disabilities implies that they should be able to choose their treatment and providers as part of their rights to healthcare. Similarly, The United Nations Principles for the Protection of Persons with Mental Illness and the Improvement of Mental Health Care (United Nations, 1991) support the rights of persons to personal autonomy and treatment that is suited to their cultural background. Choice is both a right and a cornerstone of evidence-based practice in psychology, fostering informed consent, and allowing clients to align their therapy with personal values and needs (APA, 2005).

In addition, it will be important to explore with Olivia the function behind some of her threat responses (such as self-harm) and to help her develop meaning in relation to the challenges that she has faced. Another important aspect of interpersonal power at play for Olivia was the emphasis placed on her family history of mental health diagnoses and the impact of this on Olivia's identity or understanding of herself and others in her life. There was a deterministic path mapped out for Olivia by previous practitioners indicating a diagnosis was almost inevitable given her presenting behaviours and family history.

Olivia's Experiences in the Context of Ethics and Rights

As practitioners, educators and researchers, we draw on a pragmatist ethical framework inspired by Cornish and Gillespie's (2009) approach to the problem of knowledge in health psychology. Pragmatism is not concerned with realist questions such as, what knowledge is the truth? Or in our instance, whether diagnostic approaches or the PTMF represent the truth. It acknowledges the *pluralities of knowledge* in our postmodern world, where grand narratives have been called into question (Cornish & Gillespie, 2009) and critically asks, does knowledge serve our purposes rather than whether knowledge reflects the 'truth'. Pragmatism also acknowledges the diversity of interests and purposes that different knowledges serve.

We would like to highlight some of the associated challenges that have come with the conventional biomedical approach to Olivia's experiences. In keeping with our pragmatist approach, we ask whose interests are being served? Does medication solve the real-world problems that Olivia faces and bring her closer to understanding what is happening or does it numb her to the challenges she faces? Olivia wants to understand why she is drawn to self-harm and why her emotions are overwhelming. Through exploring her adversities, she is attuned to the influences of her environment and how power has operated in her life. In our case study, we suggest that traditional approaches did not serve Olivia's ultimate preferences. We consider Olivia's case study generative rather than generalizable (Cornish, 2020) in the sense that it generates new ways of approaching other cases like Olivia's.

Furthermore, Olivia's right to informed consent regarding prescription of medication and the application of a potential lifelong diagnosis of personality disorder had not been honoured. She was given no information of the medication's side effects or efficacy or about the implications of potentially receiving a diagnosis of borderline personality disorder. For mental health practitioners, the central ethical principle must be to first, do no harm. In keeping with the WHO QualityRights initiative that advocates for a rights-based approach to mental health, Olivia should have been presented with information on what psychiatric diagnoses mean, information on other lenses through which to understand her distress (i.e. a formulation-based approach), on the medication prescribed, on side effects that may occur and on potential withdrawal effects once medical intervention ends. Olivia was not presented with different pathways of choice for her therapeutic intervention during her time with her first mental health service, further disenfranchising her in the process of formal help-seeking. Any medical or psychological intervention used by a professional in Olivia's care involves a commitment to the ethical principle of transparency. This means including Olivia as an active agent in her care and committing to a 'doing with not doing to' approach to therapeutic intervention (Treisman, 2016). It is important to note that any lens or approach used coercively rather than collaboratively runs the risk of causing harm to the person in distress.

While Olivia has been abused, her belief that there was something wrong with her, was confirmed through practitioners' emphasis of an impending diagnosis, rather than supporting Olivia to make sense of her experiences and responses to abuse and threat in her life. Clarity, consistency, collaborative meaning-making, and narrative building with the PTMF were important elements of Olivia's intervention to attempt to repair harmful messages that Olivia received and internalized about her distress through a biomedical rather than a complex holistic contextualized response.

Ethical Considerations for Practitioners

We pose some 'questions' below as challenges to generate reflection and open our thinking about broader ethical issues in our work posed by the case study of Olivia. We want to focus on issues where practitioners can intervene in their current work, rather than simply give a theoretical, abstract critique, or suggest that the only relevant change is a massive cultural and societal shift. While all of us work towards and advocate for structural change in mental health systems and our society, we are conscious that many find the pace of change disheartening and can argue that it is pointless or hopeless to try to make changes. We can make changes in our day-to-day practice, and we have an ethical and moral obligation to do so (Kidd et al., 2022).

Do we have an ethical duty to understand whose interests the biomedical installed base currently serves? And to offer pragmatist alternatives that better support the interests of people in distress?

Within this case study we have hinted at the impact 'the biomedical installed base' has had on Olivia, the language of 'disorder', medication as first line of treatment, online resources which confirm her fears that there is something 'wrong' with her in biomedical terms and the practitioners who unwittingly reified these understandings and indicated an inevitability of 'disorder' at 18. However, it is also important to understand how biomedical power is ingrained in the systems in which we work, research, and teach. As MacLachlan (2023) has elsewhere pointed out, 'Of course, we have some brilliant, open, participative, and progressive psychiatrists who willingly background both themselves and "medical-model" thinking and promote psychosocial interventions. But we should not have to wish for exceptional individuals; we should design the system the way we want it to work.'

As researchers and practitioners, we are heartened by the growing numbers of individual practitioners who are taking a more wholistic approach and moving away from biomedical formulations of their patients. However, we continue to be confounded by the inertia of the biomedical installed base in the mental health service as a system, which involves the everyday embeddedness of biomedical approaches through conventions of practice, uses of diagnostic manuals, the time afforded clients, the treatments suggested, and even as Pretorius, McCashin & Doyle (2022) find information young people find in their google searches.: Mental health literacy as an approach has also arguably promoted a cultural shift in how lay people understand emotional distress, with Brinkmann (2016) now suggesting we live in a diagnostic culture.

We recognize the value of receiving a diagnosis as currently one of the only pathways to access care, for many people. However, for Olivia, none of these ways of making sense of her distress enabled her to process the trauma she had previously experienced nor to recognize the ways in which power has operated in her life. They lead to disempowerment and threat responses that enabled Olivia to numb the ongoing pain of her traumatic childhood, family adversities, and abuse. A helpful alternative might be working with the therapeutic alliance and the use of the PTMF. This relationship facilitates personal meaning-making, a sense of empowerment and agency. By making the ingrained systemic practices of internalizing and pathologizing distress, visible with service users, we can enable them to navigate the challenges it poses, and to find alternative more supportive ways to make sense of their experience and distress. We argue more on this point in our final question below, but for now we need to say that it is not enough for practitioners to make visible the functions and potential harms of the biomedical discourse and practice that exist within our health care institutions.

We must work in ways that support the people who attend our services, to become fully knowledgeable about the languages and practices that can be imposed on their experiences. To do this effectively, we must work in ways that respect and actively look for the lived experiential knowledge of the people who consult with us as, positioning them as valued knowers and co-constructors of mental health practice and systems. This is no longer a choice on the part of individual clinicians, we are mandated to empower our clients when we embrace a rights-based approach to mental health as outlined by WHO (2019) QualityRights Initiative. For clinicians in Ireland, the Mental Health Commission and the Health Service Executive have pledged to support the QualityRights Initiative. The initiative promotes changes in both individual practice and institutional culture and processes in favour of respecting the right to informed consent, the promotion of autonomy and choice, and supporting a recovery model, set in the person's own community. Training in the QualityRights Imitative is available on the WHO website (https://www.who.int/teams/mental-health-and-substance-use/policy-law-rights/qr-e-training) and is intended for those in power who make institutional-wide changes, individual practitioners, and people who use mental health services. The WHO and the UN published a guidance document titled

Mental Health, Human Rights and Legislation: Guidance and Practice (OHCHR, 2023) where the implications of a rights-based approach to mental health is explored in detail.

Do we have an ethical duty to use language and practices that bring people into community and connection and away from isolation?

In her first encounter with mental health services, Olivia's experiences were narrated to her in internalizing, medicalized, pathologizing, and individualizing language. She was told that she needed to attend adult mental health services when she turns 18 so that she can get an appropriate psychiatric diagnosis and it was indicated to her that she would likely receive a diagnosis of borderline personality disorder. Such language has the consequence of concealing the social, political, and contextual factors of her experience. It also functions to individualize Olivia as an object of medical intervention. This is a common experience for those who attend psychiatric services where this kind of language is used. Young Irish adults have expressed feelings of not being adequately 'seen' or 'understood' by the mental health professionals with whom they work, and that practitioners are 'exclusively interested in a process of diagnosis, followed by medication' (Farrell & Mahon, 2021, p. 42). The young adults reported feeling that the prevailing model of understanding their suffering was individualistic and biomedical based on problem/solution. They said that what was lacking was an acknowledgment of their suffering and unique experience of that suffering *in* context. This is an urgent issue of finding belonging and connection (United States, Office of the Surgeon General, 2023) through recognition of their experiences and the ability to join with others in shared meaning making about their experiences.

Both Caoimhe and Dylan must hold the tension between the dangers of pathologizing labels and the absence of a shared label or concept if we move away from labels entirely. Dylan explained that when you are 'already feeling isolated, being told (you) are not alone can help'. Caoimhe agreed with Dylan explaining, 'if there's no label, then you feel like there's no one like me'. She demonstrated the importance of shared concepts for community building and support saying, 'I can go online to ask my community for help and advice'. Staying with the complexity of shared labels, Caoimhe went on to say, 'if you believe your label too much, you will be consumed'. There is a role for shared concepts in allowing us to escape isolation and find ourselves in community and connection. However, psychiatric diagnostic systems do not feel like the most helpful nor appropriate concepts to do this for Caoimhe and Dylan and for us as practitioners. The technologies of psychiatric power inevitably function to internalize and individualize problems and to take people out of connection and community. This leads us to our next ethical question below.

Do we have an ethical duty to do more than just provide an alternative? Do we need to open new knowledge and practices and provide cultural critique?

One might ask which we should change first, our language, our practice, or the person's ability to resist power in their daily lives. The answer is that we need to address all three as they are intertwined. As Youth Advocate, Dylan explained, "it's the social outlook on the label that is the problem, not just the label" as knowledge mediates social action (Cornish & Gillespie, 2009). We need to critique the knowledge framework that comes with the label, not just the diagnostic label itself. This means further national and international discussion and dialogue within and between professions about how the current dominant knowledge framework on mental health cannot be separated from the vested interests at play to maintain power and privilege within teams that are predominantly hierarchical in nature.

In the case of Olivia, we need to consider the role of psychiatric diagnosis in her life. Consideration needs to be given to the impact of the power imbalance in mental health services on Olivia's, and others, subjective understanding of distress, personal identity, and on future help-seeking behaviours. The meaning of distress has been imposed upon Olivia (through a psychiatric diagnosis) rather than co-constructed together (person and clinician) as a collaborative experience to create a coherent understanding for more empowering outcomes. To become empowered, we first need to have the experience of being listened to, validated, and understood, which are at the heart of Rogerian, person-centred principles. However, Winsdale (2013) points out that even Rogers was aware that positive regard alone was not enough to support empowerment. We need to also afford the people we work with the possibility to interrogate and deconstruct the normalizing judgements and the political ramifications inherent in psychiatric diagnoses.

Adding the lens of the PTMF and other kinds of deconstructive approaches that draw on the work of Foucault and Derrida (e.g. Narrative Therapy), we see that Olivia and the people we work with need both nonjudgement *and* the opportunity to learn the skills and knowledges to recognize, evaluate, and if they choose resist the psychiatric practices and language that can be imposed upon them. By supporting Olivia and others to make sense of their experience in their terms and to join them and support these ways of talking and narrating their experiences, we can start to undo some epistemic injustices that people attending mental health services are faced with. An epistemic injustice is an injustice 'done to someone specifically in their capacity as a knower' (Fricker, 2007, p. 1). In this case it is a harm done to Olivia by inhibiting her capacity to know the history and consequences of the psychiatric knowledge that is being applied to her. It is also done to her by diminishing her status as knower or expert on her own experiences.

Our moral and ethical duties then are multiple. To support Olivia and others, we must both give them adequate knowledge to either choose or deconstruct the psychiatric labels applied to them and value their experience not just descriptions of their experiences. To do this requires that we educate ourselves about the 'epistemic biases' that are 'built into the concepts of mental disorder' that we work with (Kidd et al., 2022, p. 13). We need to be knowledgeable about potential harms to identity that could be enacted when categorical psychiatric diagnoses, language, and practices are used to define a person's distress. Distress exists on a continuum and current DSM psychiatric descriptions and diagnoses fail to accurately represent this idea. Secondly, with this awareness we need to have available to us alternative ways of talking and practicing that can avoid or at least minimize these harms. We already have ways of thinking and practicing available in the form of PTMF and earlier deconstructive approaches like Narrative Therapy that can have useful and functional alternatives. Practitioners have suggested alternative ways to formulate experiences and offer language that are more aware of the social embeddedness of mental health experiences (Aherne & Hickey, 2022; Johnstone & Boyle, 2018). We have no more reasons to not change our practices, yet despite evidence and broad acceptance of basic principles such as collaborative and respectful care and shared decision making, researchers have found that there remain attitudinal and intuitional barriers (Bee et al., 2015; Coulter, 2017; Slade, 2017).

Conclusion

It is time to provide pathways for resistance and alternative knowledges. We have become too reliant on the tools of the natural sciences, taking things apart and separating them into their component parts, fixing them for study, and labelling them to reduce them to fixed objects within a self-contained, decontextualized individual. This is the opposite to the interconnected (Gergen, 2009), contextually embedded reality in which we live and experience our health and mental health. Our health and mental health exist as contextual events within a wider social, political, and ecological landscape in which there is ever increasing levels of interconnection and interdependence for our 'one health' (WHO, 2023). The United Nations Principles for the Protection of Persons with Mental Illness and the Improvement of Mental Health Care (UN, 1991) support this embedded and interdependent concept of the patient as a person with autonomy who has a right to receive culturally appropriate care in their community. We can embrace the PTMF as a feasible and legitimate option in the wider context of trauma-informed working and authentic person-centred care. We can even go beyond it (Gergen et al., 1996) and become better at deconstructing psychiatric and psychologizing practices, educate ourselves about epistemic biases and harms (Fricker, 2007), and share these skills and knowledge to the people who come into our offices. We must also respect those we work with as authoritative and valuable knowers and work with them to develop our practices and understandings going forward. Using PTMF we can generate new knowledges and practices to make real-world changes, rethinking mental health and our practices within the field.

Questions

1. In what way does the power you hold as a mental health professional show up in your practice? How, if at all, do you reflect on and acknowledge this?

2. How do the principles outlined in this chapter of choice, collaboration, and transparency fit within your current team culture?

3. How does the power of the biomedical installed base influence your practice? How does the taken-for-granted, the norms of psychology and psychiatry unwittingly lead to harm? How can this be made visible and challenged?

Further Reading

Aherne, C., & Hickey, E. (2022). *Using the Power Threat Meaning Framework with Young People: A Suggested Guide Booklet.* https://cms.bps.org.uk/sites/default/files/2022-09/Jigsaw%20-%20using%20the%20PTMF%20with%20young%20people.pdf

Boyle, M. (2022). Power in the power threat meaning framework. *Journal of Constructivist Psychology, 35*(1), 27–40. https://doi.org/10.1080/10720537.2020.1773357

Johnstone, L., & Boyle, M. (2018). The power threat meaning framework: An alternative nondiagnostic conceptual system. *Journal of Humanistic Psychology, 65*(4) https://doi.org/10.1177/0022167818793289

Kidd, I. J., Spencer, L., & Carel, H. (2022). Epistemic injustice in psychiatric research and practice, *Philosophical Psychology, 38*(2), 503–531. doi: 10.1080/09515089.2022.2156333

Office of the High Commissioner for Human Rights (representing the WHO and the UN). (2023). *Mental health, human rights and legislation: guidance and practice.* World Health Organization and the United Nations (represented by the Office of the United Nations High Commissioner for Human Rights). https://waps.ohchr.org/sites/default/files/documents/publications/WHO-OHCHR-Mental-health-human-rights-and-legislation_web.pdf

References

Aanestad, M., Grisot, M., Hanseth, O., & Vassilakopoulou, P. (2017). Information infrastructures and the challenge of the installed base. In M. Aanestad, M. Grisot, O. Hanseth & P. Vassilakopoulou (Eds.), *Information infrastructures within European health care: Working with the installed base* (pp. 25–33). Springer.

Aherne, C., & Hickey, E. (2022). *Using the Power Threat Meaning Framework with Young People: A Suggested Guide Booklet.* https://cms.bps.org.uk/sites/default/files/2022-09/Jigsaw%20-%20using%20the%20PTMF%20with%20young%20people.pdf

Albee, G. W., & Joffe, J. M. (2004). Mental illness is NOT 'an illness like any other.' *Journal of Primary Prevention, 24,* 419–436.

American Psychological Association (APA). (2005). Policy statement on evidence-based practice in psychology. https://www.apa.org/practice/guidelines/evidence-based-statement

Balmforth, J. (2009). 'The weight of class': Clients' experiences of how perceived differences in social class between counsellor and client affect the therapeutic relationship. *British Journal of Guidance & Counselling, 37*(3), 375–386. https://doi.org/10.1080/03069880902956942

Bee, P., Price, O., Baker, J., & Lovell, K. (2015). Systematic synthesis of barriers and facilitators to service user-led care planning. *British Journal of Psychiatry, 207*(2), 104–114. doi:10.1192/bjp.bp.114.152447

Bentall, R. (2009). *Doctoring the mind: Why psychiatric treatments fail.* Penguin.

Boyle, M. (2022). Power in the power threat meaning framework. *Journal of Constructivist Psychology, 35*(1), 27–40.

Brinkmann, S. (2016). *Diagnostic cultures: A cultural approach to the pathologization of modern life*. Routledge.

Coleman, H. L. K., Wampold, B. E., & Casali, S. L. (1995). Ethnic minorities' ratings of ethnically similar and European American counsellors: A meta-analysis. *Journal of Counselling Psychology, 42*, 55–64.

Cornish, F. (2020). Towards a dialogical methodology for single case studies. *Culture & Psychology, 26*(1), 139–152.

Cornish, F., & Gillespie, A. (2009). A pragmatist approach to the problem of knowledge in health psychology. *Journal of Health Psychology, 14*(6), 800–809.

Coulter, A. (2017). Shared decision making: everyone wants it, so why isn't it happening? *World Psychiatry, 16*, 117–118. doi:10.1002/wps.20407

Davies, J., & Read, J. (2019). A systematic review into the incidence, severity and duration of antidepressant withdrawal effects: Are guidelines evidence-based? *Addictive Behaviours, 97*, 111–121.

Davies, J. (2021). *Sedated: How modern capitalism created our mental health crisis*. Atlantic Books.

Dooley, B., & Fitzgerald, A. (2012). *My world survey. National Study of Youth Mental Health in Ireland*. https://www.myworldsurvey.ie/full-report

Dooley B., O'Connor, C., Fitzgerald A., O'Reilly, A. (2019). *My world survey two: The National Study of Youth Mental Health in Ireland*. https://www.myworldsurvey.ie/content/docs/My_World_Survey_2.pdf

Farrell, E., & Mahon, Á. (2021). Understanding student mental health: difficulty, deflection, and darkness. *Ethics and Education, 16*(1), 36–50.

Flückiger, C., Del Re, A. C., Wampold, B. E., & Horvath, A. O. (2018). The alliance in adult psychotherapy: A meta-analytic synthesis. *Psychotherapy, 55*(4), 316–340. https://doi.org/10.1037/pst0000172

Fricker, M. (2007). *Epistemic injustice: Power and the ethics of knowing*. Oxford University Press.

Gergen, K. J., Hoffman, L., & Anderson, H. (1996). Is diagnosis a disaster? A constructionist trialogue. In F. W. Kaslow (Ed.), *Handbook of relational diagnosis and dysfunctional family patterns* (pp. 102–118). Wiley.

Gergen, K. J. (1997). The place of the psyche in a constructed world. *Theory & Psychology, 7*(6), 723–746.

Gergen, K. J. (2009). *Relational being: Beyond self and community*. Oxford University Press.

Guha, M. (2014). Diagnostic and statistical manual of mental disorders: DSM-5. *Reference Reviews, 28*(3), 36–37.

Hari, J. (2018). *Lost connections: Uncovering the real causes of depression-and the unexpected solutions*. Bloomsbury Publishing.

Harper, D. J. (2023). De-medicalising public mental health with the *Power Threat Meaning Framework*. *Perspectives in Public Health, 143*(3), 151–155. doi:10.1177/17579139231157531

Horvath, A. O., & Symonds, B. D. (1991). Relation between working alliance and outcome in psychotherapy: A meta-analysis. *Journal of Counselling Psychology, 38*, 139–149.

Hutton, P., Weinmann, S., Bola, J., & Read, J. (2013). Antipsychotic drugs. In J. Read & J. Dillon (Eds.), *Models of madness: Psychological, social and biological approaches to psychosis* (2nd Ed., pp. 105–124). Routledge.

Jigsaw. (2021). *Start Making Sense*. https://www.jigsaw.ie/wp-content/uploads/2023/01/Start-Making-Sense.pdf

Johnstone, L., & Boyle, M. (2018). The power threat meaning framework: An alternative nondiagnostic conceptual system. *Journal of Humanistic Psychology, 65*(4). https://doi.org/10.1177/0022167818793289

Kidd, I. J., Spencer, L., & Carel, H. (2022). Epistemic injustice in psychiatric research and practice. *Philosophical Psychology, 38*(2), 503–531. doi: 10.1080/09515089.2022.2156333

Kirsch, I. (2009). *The emperor's new drugs: Exploding the antidepressant myth.* The Bodley Head.

Kirsch, I., Deacon, B. J., Huedo-Medina, T. B., Scoboria, A., Moore, T. J., & Johnson, B. T. (2008). Initial severity and antidepressant benefits: a meta-analysis of data submitted to the Food and Drug Administration. *PLoS Medicine, 5*(2), e45. doi: 10.1371/journal.pmed.0050045

Liddle, B. J. (1996). Therapist sexual orientation, gender and counselling practices as they relate to ratings on helpfulness by gay and lesbian clients. *Journal of Counselling Psychology, 43*(4), 394–401.

MacLachlan, M. (2023, 22 May). *Mental Health Services must be prised from the grip of psychiatry,* The Irish Times. https://www.irishtimes.com/opinion/2023/05/22/mental-health-services-must-be-prised-from-grip-of-psychiatry/

Malla, A., Joober, R., & Garcia, A. (2015). 'Mental illness is like any other medical illness': a critical examination of the statement and its impact on patient care and society. *Journal of Psychiatry and Neuroscience, 40*(3), 147–150.

Manthei, R. J. (1983). Client choice of therapist or therapy. *Personnel and Guidance Journal, 61,* 334–340.

Manthei, R. J. (2006). What can clients tell us about seeking counselling and their experience of it? *International Journal for the Advancement of Counselling, 13*(5), 541–555.

Maskey, S. (2022). Report on the look-back review into child & adolescent mental health services, HSE, Dublin. https://www.hse.ie/eng/services/news/newsfeatures/south-kerry-camhs-review/report-on-the-look-back-review-into-camhs-area-a.pdf

Moncrieff, J. (2008). *The myth of the chemical cure.* Palgrave Macmillan.

Office of the High Commissioner for Human Rights (representing the WHO and the UN). (2023). *Mental health, human rights and legislation: guidance and practice.* World Health Organization and the United Nations (represented by the Office of the United Nations High Commissioner for Human Rights). https://waps.ohchr.org/sites/default/files/documents/publications/WHO-OHCHR-Mental-health-human-rights-and-legislation_web.pdf

Pickett, K., & Wilkinson, R. (2010). *The spirit level: Why equality is better for everyone.* Penguin.

Pretorius, C., McCashin, D., & Coyle, D. (2022). Supporting personal preferences and different levels of need in online help-seeking: a comparative study of help-seeking technologies for mental health. *Human–Computer Interaction, 39*(5–6), 288–309.

Puras, D. (2022). Report of the Special Rapporteur on the right of everyone to the enjoyment of the highest attainable standard of physical and mental health. *Philippine Law Journal, 95,* 274.

Read, J., Haslam, N., Sayce, L., & Davies, E. (2006). Prejudice and schizophrenia: a review of the 'mental illness is an illness like any other' approach. *Acta Psychiatrica Scandinavica, 114*(5), 303–318.

Read, J., & Sacia, A. (2020). Using open questions to understand 650 people's experiences with antipsychotic drugs. *Schizophrenia Bulletin, 46*(4), 896–904.

Read, J., & Williams, J. (2019). Positive and negative effects of antipsychotic medication: an international online survey of 832 recipients. *Current Drug Safety, 14*(3), 173–181.

Slade, M. (2017). Implementing shared decision making in routine mental health care. *World Psychiatry, 16,* 146–153. doi:10.1002/wps.20412

Treisman, K. (2016). *Working with relational and developmental trauma in children and adolescents.* Taylor & Francis.

Trott, A., & Reeves, A. (2018). Social class and the therapeutic relationship: The perspective of therapists as clients. A qualitative study using a questionnaire survey. *Counselling and Psychotherapy Research, 18*(2), 166–177. https://doi.org/10.1002/capr.12163

United Nations. (1991). The Principles for the Protection of Persons with Mental Illness and the Improvement of Mental Health Care. https://www.ohchr.org/en/instruments-mechanisms/instruments/principles-protection-persons-mental-illness-and-improvement

United Nations. (2006). United Nations Convention on the Rights of Persons with Disabilities.https://www.un.org/development/desa/disabilities/convention-on-the-rights-of-persons-with-disabilities/convention-on-the-rights-of-persons-with-disabilities-2.html

United States, Office of the Surgeon General. (2023). *Our epidemic of loneliness and isolation: The U.S. Surgeon General's advisory on the healing effects of social connection and community.* U.S. Department of Health and Human Services. https://www.hhs.gov/sites/default/files/surgeon-general-social-connection-advisory.pdf

White, M., & Epston, D. (1990). *Narrative means to therapeutic ends.* WW Norton.

Winsdale, J. (2013). From being 'non-judgemental' to deconstructing normalising judgement. *British Journal of Guidance and Counselling, 41*(5),1–12. http://dx.doi.org/10.1080/03069885.2013.771772

World Health Organization. (2019). *QualityRights materials for training, guidance and transformation.* World Health Organization. https://www.who.int/publications-detail/who-qualityrights-guidance-and-training-tools

World Health Organization. (2023). *One health fact sheet.* World Health Organization. https://www.who.int/news-room/fact-sheets/detail/one-health

10

Codes of Ethical Conduct for Psychiatrists and Their Inclusion of Human Rights

Rachel Brown, Ikenna D. Ebuenyi, and Malcolm MacLachlan

Introduction

Psychiatry as a branch of medicine focuses on conditions relating to human mental life, such as mental health conditions, neurodevelopmental conditions, and those associated with aging, such as dementia and other psychosocial disabilities (Bloch & Pargiter, 2002). Due to this specific focus psychiatrists 'deal with unique ethical dilemmas and complexities arising from psychiatric practice' (Bloch et al., 2022, p. 1201). Up until the 1970s, general medical codes of ethics were used by the profession to manage and guide ethical issues. However, due to the distinct nature of the discipline's scope of practice, specific psychiatric ethical codes of conduct were developed by professional psychiatric organizations. This reflects the special role that psychiatrists have in terms of ethics associated with the human condition, and in particular ethics that pertain to human rights (Fiorillo et al., 2016). Psychiatry as a discipline has faced heavy criticism for human rights offences (Harding, 1989) often relating to the person's/patient's right to privacy, informed consent, involuntary placement and treatment, and the use of coercive practices (Steinert & Henking, 2022). Due to these issues, there have been consistent calls for psychiatric codes of ethics to be reviewed, updated, and revised, not only to reflect the changing morality of society (Blach & Pargiter, 2002), but to be more in line with human rights legislation (Pathare, 2003). Yet, how current codes represent human rights is difficult to determine, as is how these codes can be effective guides for human rights-based practice (Bloch et al., 2022). In what follows, we explore the extent to which professional psychiatric organization's codes of ethical conduct represents key concepts of human rights based on Pope's (2018) five connections between human rights and sciences, as has been similarly applied to psychological codes of ethics, such as Huminuik's (2024) 'The Five Connections: A human rights framework for psychologists'.

The Importance of Human Rights for Psychiatry

The nature of psychiatry requires psychiatrists to work within specific settings where human rights are central to those they provide services to. Fiorillo et al. (2016) state the 'practice of psychiatry requires clear moral and ethical frameworks based on preservations of human rights'. Yet, many criticisms have been made regarding the extent to which psychiatrists promote, protect, or at least respect human rights as well as the degree of power and responsibility psychiatrists have been given in regard to the human rights of the individuals they provide services to (Pérez Pérez et al., 2024). Devitt and Kelly (2019) refer to 'close links between clinical ethics, human rights and the lived experience of mental illness and mental health care' (p. 47). They state that a change in attitudes and culture within psychiatry is needed with strong ethical codes and practice guidelines that are human-rights centred. By doing so the lived experience of those receiving services from psychiatrists may be improved and their human rights better protected and respected. In this way, human rights can be at the forefront of services provided by psychiatrists.

Power and Responsibility

Psychiatrists often deal with individuals who are experiencing difficulties and need support, care and are given treatments such as medication or psychotherapy (Fiorillo et al., 2016). For people who receive services from psychiatrists, there is potential for service users to be in a position of diminished power particularly in terms of their human rights due to circumstances which make them vulnerable to power imbalances (Harding, 1989). The psychiatrist on the other hand has power in many forms. They have direct power of involuntary placement and the power to determine treatment. Occasionally, they can use coercive measures to persuade persons/patients to take medications, undergo electroconvulsive therapy (ECT), and attend for psychological therapies (Faissner & Braun, 2023). This expert power can also be used to persuade public opinion and in the role of expert witnesses within legal cases (Channaveerachari et al., 2022). While these are generally done with a genuine commitment to the well-being of the person and the public, in many jurisdictions a psychiatrist has the power to act without informed consent. Fiorillo et al. (2016) suggest the powers psychiatrists have generate ethical challenges with the 'need to balance three different and often controversial interests: 1) the basic human rights of the persons concerned; 2) public safety; 3) the need for adequate treatment of the patients' (p.449). This demonstrates the complexity of the ethical dilemmas psychiatrists encounter while conducting their practice.

The powers that psychiatrists have also endows them with a significant responsibility to act in ways that are inline not only with the Hippocratic Oath 'treatment according to the patient's best interests (beneficence), avoiding harm (non-malfeasance)'

(Marzanski et al., 2006), but also within the guidelines of human rights documents, treaties, and conventions (Harding, 1989). However, Bloch et al. (2022) states it is not clear if these codes function effectively as guides for ethical practice that is human-rights based, as they often do not include reference to such documents, treaties, and conventions. This is problematic as psychiatrists have both power and responsibility. So how they use this to benefit those in receipt of their services in a manner that is in line with codes of ethics, legislation, and human rights is very important and can be very challenging (Radden, 2002).

Settings of Practice

Not only are the activities in which psychiatrists conduct their practice prone to challenges regarding ethics and human rights, but also the settings in which psychiatrists conduct their work are often problematic as they are key sites where human rights offences may be committed (Harding, 1989). For example, psychiatrists often work within general and mental health hospitals, in care homes for older adults and those with psychosocial disability, in schools, prisons, and within the military. In these settings, power structures operate in ways that may influence or even constrain the psychiatrist from acting ethically to protect not only the human rights of those in their care, but their own rights too (Strauss, 2017). For example, a psychiatrist who may witness human rights abuses may not be able to effectively report these without fear of dismissal or retribution and the loss of their job/income. Psychiatrists may also have a vested interest in the activities of the institution that is committing human rights offences (Fava, 2010). Finally, the challenges of these settings may have a damaging effect on the well-being and mental health of psychiatrists themselves, and their own human rights in this regard need to be protected (Jovanovic et al., 2016). As such, having rights-informed ethical codes that are applicable to the settings in which psychiatrists provide services is essential to protect the human rights of both the psychiatrist and those they provide services to.

Case Study

To illustrate how a lack of incorporation of a human rights-based framework in ethical codes can affect psychiatric practice we have provided the following case study. XY is a young psychiatrist with interest in social psychiatry. Since completing their specialist training in general adult psychiatry, they have been exploring opportunities of a niche area to build their career. This interest led them to volunteer to provide mental health services for asylum seekers. They were particularly interested in this population as they wanted to compare their observations with their work in prison mental health services, where they spent some time working alongside their supervisor. They started their volunteer service in high spirits in the hope of providing care for the asylum seekers in need of mental health services. However, soon their interaction with the asylum seekers revealed a 'new truth' for them. Increasingly, they doubted the usefulness of the anti-depressants and anxiolytics they were prescribing for many of the people whom they felt were battling stressful life events and current situations. XY also developed doubts about whether talk therapy could really be effective if it fell short of promising a pathway to residency status, a roof, a warm bed, and a home for the asylum seekers. XY also had doubts if some of the asylum seeks/patients they saw really desired the care they were providing, or were only accepting it in the hope it would further their asylum claims.

Following completion of the World Health Organization (WHO) training on QualityRights XY increasingly reflected on the scope of patients' rights and became convinced that the asylum seekers they saw were in fact deprived of many rights. XY decided to identify some other colleagues from both psychiatry and other mental health disciplines, to support an initiative which provided a structured group for asylum seekers to link their lack of human rights to their mental health conditions. XY established a 'Right Mental Health' which they led and was co-led by an asylum seeker. The group's work helped to authenticate the reasonableness of the group members' distress (mental health conditions), given the unreasonableness of their living circumstances. This group also reached out to a local politician who—after some time—attended one of the group meetings. In time the members of the group felt that they were doing something to at least try and address the causes of their distress, and this allowed them to choose more freely if they also wished to accept medication or talk therapy as potentially contributing to helping them. Ultimately XY advocated within their own national psychiatric association for guidance on human rights advocacy to be incorporated in the professions code of ethics.

Human Rights and Current Psychiatric Codes of Ethical Conduct

In the previous section, we outlined some of the situations and setting in which human rights are central to the practice of psychiatry. These 'realities are a constant reminder that the practice of psychiatry requires clear moral and ethical frameworks based on preservations of human rights' (Fiorillo et al., 2016. p.4). Current professional psychiatric codes of conduct should act as the moral and ethical framework that supports human rights, yet these are criticized by Bloch et al. (2022) as being insufficient in terms of incorporating human rights. Also, these codes are infrequently revised, and supplementary materials are often needed as guidance for effective practice and when used for disciplinary processes.

Radden (2002) suggests that the values and norms associated with mental health conditions are culturally bound, and so we can assume that the production of psychiatric codes is also bound to cultural beliefs and practices (MacLachlan, 2006). The codes we have examined in this chapter are from English-speaking countries, which suggests that they have been influenced by 'westernized' cultural concepts, at least to some extent. This could be problematic when the westernized norms of the profession are incongruent to that of the persons they seek to serve. While cultural specificity may be beneficial to codes, Sonsone et al. (2024) found that when comparing the European Psychiatric Association (EPA) and World Psychiatric Associations (WPA) codes, there were key differences, but also key fundamental similarities and that the inalienable human rights of all people should be the basis of any ethical code.

While human rights documents can be critiqued for their westernized values, these documents, conventions, and treaties provide the basis for the ethical and moral treatment of humanity, regardless of defining characteristics such as sex, race, nationality, language, or religion. Additionally, they establish that humans not be subject to such offences as torture or slavery and that all humans are entitled to basic rights, such as freedom of travel, a fair public trail, and the right to seek asylum (see Chapter 1 for a discussion of the cultural foundations of human rights). The document most associated with human rights is the United Nations' Universal Declaration of Human Rights (UDHR) (UN General Assembly, 1949). The United Nations outlines the following qualities of human rights: universality and inalienability, indivisibility, interdependence and inter-relatedness, equality and non-discrimination, participation and inclusion, and accountability and rule of law (UN General Assembly, 1949; see also Chapter 1). Huminuik (2024) argues that inclusion of human rights documents within professional codes of ethics in psychology, gives clarity and credence that those who abide by the code will foster, promote, and protect human rights. This is equally applicable to the discipline of psychiatry. Perhaps if a human rights ethos had been included as part of the professional ethics training of XY's, then they might have been better prepared to deal with and confront the human rights challenges of the asylum seekers who also had significant mental health conditions.

The Five Connections Framework

Claude (2002) developed a framework of 'connections' which aimed to encourage a link between science and human rights. Building on this, Huminuik (2024) applied these 'connections' to the work of psychologists and their ethics codes. Here we extend Claude's framework to psychiatry in a similar way with the same conviction that 'assiduous adherence to ethics codes by professionals can support the protection of human rights, but unless they are *fully integrated with human rights principles, ethics codes do not provide sufficient protections against human rights violations*' (Huminuik, 2024, p.4, emphasis added). While Huminuik applied this framework to the activities of psychologists, it is equally applicable to other human sciences and services, such as psychiatry. The 'five connections' of the human rights framework are: (1) psychiatrists possess human rights by virtue of being human as well as specific rights essential to their profession and discipline; (2) psychiatrists apply their knowledge and methods to the greater realization of human rights; (3) psychiatrists respect human rights and oppose the misuse of psychiatric science, practice, and applications and their negative impact on human rights; (4) psychiatrists ensure access to the benefits of psychiatric science and practice; and (5) psychiatrists advocate for human rights.

Aim of Analysis

The aim of this analysis was to examine the extent to which Claude's (2002) 'five con-nections' relating to human rights are represented in the ethical codes of psychiatric organizations from five English speaking countries. We aimed not only to provide an evaluation of the codes' ability to foster, promote and protect human rights, but high-light ways in which the codes can be revised to be human rights informed. We feel that by doing so it will not only allow better protection and promotions of human rights but provide a clearer and more effective guide for psychiatric practice that will benefit not only service users/patients, but also psychiatrists and potentially other service providers too.

Method

Materials and Selection Process

Five codes were identified as suitable for this study with a rationale for preventing in-terpretive challenges and the need for translation. As such we selected codes that were available in English and free to access online. The five codes came from professional psychiatric organizations from six countries as displayed in Table 10.1 (Australia and

Table 10.1 Country, professional psychiatric organisation, and abbreviate used in relation to ethical codes of conduct reviewed

County	Professional psychiatric organization	Abbreviation	Reference
United States of America (USA)	American Psychiatric Association	APA	APA (2013)
Australia New Zealand/ Aotearoa	Royal Australian and New Zealand College of Psychiatrists	RANZCP	RANZCP (2018)
Canada	Canadian Psychiatric Association	CPA	CPA (1996)
Ireland	College of Psychiatrists of Ireland	CPI	CPI (2019)
United Kingdom (UK)	Royal College of Psychiatrists	RCPSYCH	RCP (2016)

Note. South Africa was not included as the South African Society of Psychiatrists do not have their own code and utilize a general medical code (please see 'Materials and Selection Process' section above for an explanation)

New Zealand/Aotearoa have a combined code of ethics). Please note that while South Africa was eligible for inclusion based on being an English-speaking County, the South African Society of Psychiatrists do not have their own code of ethics and use a general code from the Health Professional Council of South Africa. For this reason, they were not included in this study as their code was not specific to the profession of psychiatry.

Data Analysis

The Five Connections Framework provided the basis for analysis of specific themes based on the underlying concepts which foster, promote, and protect human rights. An *additional theme (concept: 6)* focused on the extent to which the codes use rights-specific language and referenced human rights conventions, treaties, and documents, such as the UDHR. It is essential for codes of ethics to include specific reference to human-rights documents to provide clarity and specificity when referring to human-rights-based language (Huminuik, 2024). Table 10.2 presents the six concepts that were analysed in the respective codes of ethics, and a one-word summary concept for ease of exposition. Codes were read several times and text was analysed for the six conceptual themes. For each psychiatric organization's code of ethical conduct relevant sections of text were catalogued based on the core concepts as well as how the code referenced human rights. The scores were first made by RB and then reviewed for inter-rater reliability for one of the codes by IDE. The score for each rater rating were within one point on each of the six scales.

Table 10.2 Criteria used to evaluate the presence of key concepts of human rights

1.	*Self:* The ethics code indicates that psychiatrists possess rights themselves, by virtue of being human, as well as specific rights relevant to their profession and discipline. Protection of psychiatrist's human rights.
2.	*Realization:* The ethics code indicates that psychiatrists actively apply their knowledge and methods to the greater realisation of human rights. Active promotion of human rights by the discipline.
3.	*Infringements:* The ethics code indicates that psychiatrists respect human rights and actively oppose the misuse of psychiatric science. Psychiatrists will not commit and will seek to actively prevent human rights offences.
4.	*Access:* The ethics code indicates that psychiatrists promote access by all persons to the benefits of psychiatric science and practice. Equality of human rights and preventing discrimination.
5.	*Advocacy:* The ethics code indicates that psychiatrists actively advocate for human rights. Advocacy role of psychiatrists
6.	*Incorporation:* The ethics code indicates how and where human rights documents/treaties/conventions have been incorporated in the code. Promotes clarity of commitment and direct links to human rights legislation.

Scoring of Codes

Codes were scored on a scale of 0 to 6 based on the presence of the core concept/theme as displayed in Table 10.3. The rating scale was based on Equiframe (Amin et al., 2011) and EquIPP (Huss & MacLachlan, 2016) frameworks developed for systematic policy analysis for the inclusion of core concepts such as human rights and vulnerable groups. This approach to policy analysis was developed in an international project on social inclusion (EquiFrame) and subsequently elaborated in a UNESCO-funded project (EquIPP); and these are now both available from UNESCO's Inclusive Policy Lab, under their Management of Social Transformation (MOST) programme. These frameworks have been used in numerous countries across Europe, Asia and Africa (see e.g. McVeigh et al., 2024; Ebuenyi et al., 2021). While category 6 (incorporation) was scored on the same 0 to 6 point scale, separate criteria were used based on the frequency and specificity of language and reference to specific human rights documents, as opposed to inclusion of concepts/themes. The rationale for rating category six can be seen in Table 10.3. The scores for each code of ethics scores from the six concepts were added to produce a final score with a possible top score of 36. Final scores were ranked on the representation of human rights within the code as low (0–12 points), moderate (13–27 points), or high (28–36 points).

Table 10.3 Scoring criteria for presence of human rights concepts in ethics codes of conduct

---

Scoring of concepts 1–5

0 Core concept *not present.*
1 Core concept can be *inferred but no explicit mention of it.*
2 Core concept explicitly *mentioned (regardless of terminology used).*
3 Core concept explicitly mentioned and *explained/defined.*
4 Core concept explicitly mentioned/defined and indication of *action to be taken* to achieve the concept.
5 Concept clearly mentioned/defined including actions to be taken and methods of *monitoring specified.*
6 Concept clearly mentioned/defined including actions to be taken and methods of monitoring specified, and procedures for *addressing violations indicated.*

Scoring of concepts 6: Incorporation

0 Does not refer to human rights either directly or inferred.
1 Language used infers human rights
2 Uses rights-based language and terms, but not specifically uses term human rights.
3 Specifically refers to human rights.
4 Specifically refers to human rights and specified rights (*rights of patients/children*)
5 Specifically refers to human rights and supporting documents/treaties.
6 Specifically refers to human rights and supporting documents/treaties with specific detail of documents referenced.

Results

Table 10.4 shows the ratings of ethics codes of conduct for professional psychiatric organizations of the USA, Australia New Zealand/Aotearoa, Canada, and the UK, with both individual and totalled concept/theme scores and ratings. (See Table 10.1 for identification of the organizations considered.) There are considerable variations thematically across scores within codes, yet most codes total score clustered around a mean of 15. Two codes, APA and CPA scored in the low range, while the remaining codes—RANZCP, CPI, and RCPSYCH—scored moderately; with RANZCP having the top total score of 20 out of 36. Concept 1 *Self* and concept 2 *Realization* had the lowest combined score of 5 out of 36, while concept 4 *Access* had the highest total score of 20 out of 36. Within individual codes there was a wide range of scores across concepts such as the RANZCP code which scored 1 in concepts, 1 *Self* and 2 *Realization,* while scoring 5 in concept 6 *Incorporation.* While some codes did score highly in individual concepts none of the codes scored within the high range due to low scoring in other concepts/themes. It is important to note that low scores resulted from the lack of the concept being clearly described and unclear language being used making the presence of the concept ambiguous or absent. Overall results suggest that while some codes have made some efforts to foster, promote, and protect human rights, there is room for improvements.

Discussion

The findings of this study suggest that while some psychiatric organizations codes of ethical conduct contain elements of the concepts related to human rights, there is significant room for improvement if these codes are to foster, promote, and protect the human rights of both psychiatrists and those they serve. This is in line with Bloch et al. (2022) who suggests greater specificity and clarity is needed when it comes to human rights in psychiatric ethics codes. Not only in terms of inclusion of human rights documents, conventions, and treaties, but greater clarity and specificity of language used throughout the codes. Doing so may help to prevent or at least increase awareness of human rights offences and promote more rights-informed practices in future.

The case study example and the experience of XY highlight the opportunity to provide a stronger human rights ethos in psychiatric practice. It is also important that a stronger rights perspective recognizes the dilemma's psychiatrists may find themselves in with regard to upholding rights, and the ensuing moral stress and injury they may experience in their practice, as shown in Chapter 1 of this book. For example, a stronger rights-informed approach may help to balance the ethical dilemma between basic human rights, public safety, and the need for adequate treatment of patients (Fiorillo et al, 2022). While codes performed moderately in terms of concept 3, codes could be strengthened by more clearly specifying the consequences of infringements

Table 10.4 Total and subscale scores for presence of human rights concepts in ethics codes of conduct by national psychiatric organization

Psychiatric organization	Concept 1 *Self*	Concept 2 *Realisation*	Concept 3 *Infringements*	Concept 4 *Access*	Concept 5 *Advocacy*	Concept 6 *Incorporation*	Total 00/36	Rating
APA	1	1	4	4	1	1	12	Low
RANZCP	1	1	4	4	5	5	20	Moderate
CPA	1	1	2	4	1	2	11	Low
CPI	1	1	4	4	4	3	17	Moderate
RCPSYCH	1	1	4	4	2	3	15	Moderate
Concept/ theme total	5	5	18	20	13	14	M=15	

Note. Australia and New Zealand/Aotearoa use the same code.

of ethics codes. This not only would function as expert guidance, but also give a precedent that future infringements could be evaluated against. However, care should be taken when comparing one case of infringements of codes to another, as all instances will have situational cultural and temporal specificity as will the codes that they are subject to (MacLachlan, 2006).

One of the key areas that all codes were lacking in was in concept 1: Self. This is problematic because of the power and responsibility that comes with the role of the psychiatrist. For example, the CPI code states in section 10.2 'Psychiatrists should have an awareness of the health and well-being of colleagues, including trainees and students, with whom they work, and the effect this could have on the patients they come into contact with.' This suggests that the psychiatrists should monitor their colleagues for infringements to the code, which if it does refer to UDHR, then human rights as well. However, how this would be implemented is unclear as it suggests only to have an 'awareness' regarding their colleagues, demonstrating the ambiguousness of the language used in this code. Another example is from the CPA code that state in section E43, 'Recognize that you cannot serve patients, society, and the profession well if you do not care for your own physical and emotional health and well-being.' Again, this suggests the responsibility lies with the individual psychiatrist but does not cite any human rights legislation. In both of these examples the human rights of the psychiatrists themselves are weakly inferred. Improvements could be made by directly outlining that the rights of psychiatrists are protected with reference to human rights documents, conventions and treaties. This is an important balance because often psychiatrists may feel that rights-based approaches are only critical of their work, rather than also affirming their own rights as individuals and practitioners.

Most codes performed moderately in concept 4: Access. This was because codes strongly outlined guidelines in terms of discrimination based on gender, race, ethnicity, religion, etc. The RANZCP code had special inclusion of rights if indigenous populations. Other codes could also benefit from such statements specifically where there has been a history of discrimination of indigenous population such as the 'First Nations' Americans in the United States (Gone, 2004). Giving codes cultural and/or historical specificity strengthens their ability to provide not only access to marginalized groups whose circumstances may place them in greater need of services, but that services provided are culturally sensitive and appropriate (Ranjbar et al., 2020).

Recommendations

As a result of this exploration of human rights concepts within this sample of psychiatric organizations ethical codes of conduct we have several key recommendation. First and foremost, is the inclusion of, and regular reference to, human rights documents such as the UDHR. The World Health Assembly and the WHO's Comprehensive Mental health Action Plan 2013–2020 strongly suggest the inclusion of other group specific human rights documents including but not limited to: Principles for the Protection of Persons with Mental Illness and the Improvement of Mental Health Care (MI Principles) (UN General Assembly, 1991), United Nations Convention on the Rights of Persons with Disabilities (UNCRPD)(UN General Assembly, 2008), United Nations Convention on the Rights of the Child (UNCRC) (UN General Assembly, 1989), and the United Nations Declaration on the Rights of Indigenous Peoples (UNDRIP) (UN General Assembly, 2006).

Inclusion of human rights documents, conventions, and treaties such as these can provide clarity and specificity when human-rights-based language is used within the codes. It will also provide greater clarity and guidance not only for practice but in legal settings if human rights offences do occur, as argued by Steinert and Henking (2022). However, it will not in itself address conflicts between what human rights documents require and what national laws or individual morality require of psychiatrists. The extent to which international or 'parent' codes such as those of the EPA and WPA can incorporate human rights (Sansone et al., 2024) whilst remaining context and culturally sensitive, is still unclear.

National psychiatric professions should regularly revise their codes of ethics and in doing so should consider: (1) the inclusion of documents, conventions, and treaties relating to human rights such as the MI Principles, UNCRPD, and UNCRC as well as the UNDRIP; (2) greater clarity and specificity in overall language and specifically language used when referring to human rights with reference to the previous documents, conventions, and treaties; (3) inclusion of consequences for infringements of the codes; (4) regular revision of codes to reflect social changes in morality and values, but also technological developments, such as artificial intelligence; (5) inclusion of service users as guides in the generation and revisions of codes. Of course other improvements are possible and will be contextually adapted. These recommendations when implemented would enable codes to operate not only as codes of conduct, but also as documents that protect and promote human rights of both those providing and receiving psychiatric services, and as practical guidance for psychiatrists.

Limitations

As the sample of psychiatric organization's codes of ethical conduct analysed were limited to English speaking countries, the extent to which we can generalize findings is questionable. As these codes were from countries that could be considered westernized codes are also likely associated with western cultural values and again undermine the generalizability to non-western cultures. Additionally, the inalienable human rights described in the UDHR have been criticized for being of the same westernized values and primarily relevant to WEIRD populations (western, educated, industrialized, rich, and democratic) (Henrich et al., 2010). However, we feel that the value of comparative ratings is less in terms of ranking countries or cultures norms but more so exploring how other ethics codes seek to address human rights.

Conclusion

To conclude, human rights must inform the ethical codes of psychiatry, and to a much greater extent than is the case presently. This is necessary due to the unique ethical issues that psychiatrists encounter in their practice and the nature of their work. Making human rights central to psychiatric ethical codes of conduct will also make it central to the ethos of the profession and motivate and guide psychiatrists to promote human rights principles within their profession and the community, and hopefully navigate conflicting demands, such as national laws which do not comply with human rights. According to Morrissey (2020), completion of the WHO QualityRights training programme can foster substantial improvement in attitudes towards human rights amongst service providers. Codes need to specifically and clearly outline what is expected in terms of the ethical conduct of psychiatrists to protect the human rights of themselves and others, but professional psychiatric organizations need to have clear repercussions for those who break the ethical codes and commit human rights offences, or break national laws. Doing so will ensure that those in receipt of services form psychiatrists will have their human rights protected and establish greater equality of power between the psychiatrist and those that they serve.

Questions and Thought Exercises

1. What elements of psychiatric practice align best with a human-rights-informed approach to mental health?
2. How can codes of ethics delineate the best way for psychiatrists to address possible conflicts between individual's morality, professional obligations, national laws and international human rights?
3. How is it possible to promote a person's human rights and at the same time admit them involuntarily to institutionalized care?
4. How should psychiatrists engage with human rights advocacy organizations in planning service developments.

Further Reading

Devitt, P., & Kelly, B. D. (2019). A human rights foundation for ethical mental health practice. *Irish Journal of Psychological Medicine, 36*(1), 47–54. https://doi.org/10.1017/ipm.2016.44

Huminuik, K. (2024). The five connections: A human rights framework for psychologists. *International Journal of Psychology, 59*(2), 218–224. https://doi.org/10.1002/ijop.12908

Gill, N., & Sartorius, N. (Eds.) (2024). *Mental health and human rights: challenges of the United Nations Convention on the Rights of Persons with Disabilities to mental health care.* Springer. https://link.springer.com/book/10.1007/978-3-031-52179-9

Herrman, H., Galderisi, S., Allan, J., Rodrigues, M. (2024). Human Rights and Mental Health Care: A Perspective from the World Psychiatric Association. In N. Gill & N. Sartorius (Eds.) *Mental Health and Human Rights. Sustainable Development Goals Series* (pp. 169–171). Springer, Cham. https://doi.org/10.1007/978-3-031-52179-9_12

References

American Psychiatric Association (APA). (2013). The principles of medical ethics; with annotations especially applicable to psychiatry. https://www.psychiatry.org/getmedia/3fe5eae9-3df9-4561-a070-84a009c6c4a6/2013-APA-Principles-of-Medical-Ethics.pdf

Amin, M., MacLachlan, M., Mannan, H., El Tayeb, S., El Khatim, A., Swartz, L., Munthali, A., Van Rooy, G., McVeigh, J., Eide, A. H., & Schneider, M. (2011). EquiFrame: A framework for analysis of the inclusion of human rights and vulnerable groups in health policies. *Health and Human Rights Journal, 13*, 82. http://hdl.handle.net/11070/2605

Bloch, S., & Pargiter, R. (2002). A history of psychiatric ethics. *Psychiatric Clinics, 25*(3), A509–A524. https://doi.org/10.1016/S0193-953X(02)00003-5

Bloch, S., Kenn, F., & Lim, I. (2022). Codes of ethics for psychiatrists: past, present and prospect. *Psychological Medicine, 52*(7), 1201–1207. https://doi.org/10.1017/S0033291722000125

Canadian Psychiatric Association (CPA). (1996). The 1996 CMA Code of Ethics annotated for psychiatrists. https://cpa.ca/docs/File/Ethics/CPA_Code_2017_4thEd.pdf

Channaveerachari, N. K., Manjunatha, N., Mukesh, J., Damodharan, D., & Dass, G. P. (2022). The psychiatrist as an expert witness. *Indian Journal of Psychiatry, 64*(Suppl 1), S42–S46. doi: 10.4103/indianjpsychiatry.indianjpsychiatry_721_21

Claude, R. P. (2002). *Science in the service of human rights.* University of Pennsylvania Press.

College of Psychiatrists of Ireland (CPI). (2019). Professional Ethics for Psychiatrists. https://irishpsychiatry.ie/wp-content/uploads/2019/05/CPsychI-HRE-Professional-Ethics-for-Psychiatrists-FINAL.pdf

Devitt, P., & Kelly, B. D. (2019). A human rights foundation for ethical mental health practice. *Irish Journal of Psychological Medicine, 36*(1), 47–54. https://doi.org/10.1017/ipm.2016.44

Ebuenyi, I. D., Smith, E. M., Munthali, A., Msowoya, S. W., Kafumba, J., Jamali, M. Z., & MacLachlan, M. (2021). Exploring equity and inclusion in Malawi's national disability mainstreaming strategy and implementation plan. *International Journal for Equity in Health, 20*, 1–7. https://doi.org/10.1186/s12939-020-01378-y

Faissner, M., & Braun, E. (2023). The ethics of coercion in mental healthcare: the role of structural racism. *Journal of Medical Ethics, 50*(7), 476–481.https://doi.org/10.1136/jme-2023-108984

Fava, G. A. (2010). Conflicts of Interest. In H. Helmchen & N. Sartorius (Eds.), *Ethics in Psychiatry. International Library of Ethics, Law, and the New Medicine* (Vol. 45). Springer, Dordrecht. https://doi.org/10.1007/978-90-481-8721-8_4

Fiorillo, A., Volpe, U., & Bhugra, D. (2016). Role and responsibilities of psychiatrists. In A. Fiorillo, U. Volpe & D. Bhugra (Eds.), *Psychiatry in practice: education, experience, and expertise* (pp. 1–10). Oxford University Press. http://ndl.ethernet.edu.et/bitstream/123456789/3063/1/339.pdf#page=26

Fiorillo, A., Ventriglio, A., Sampogna, G., & Falkai, P. (2022). Innovations in psychiatry: challenges and future directions. *International Review of Psychiatry, 34*(7–8), 659–662. https://doi.org/10.1080/09540261.2022.2153011

Gone, J. P. (2004). Mental health services for Native Americans in the 21st century United States. *Professional Psychology: Research and Practice, 35*(1), 10. https://psycnet.apa.org/doi/10.1037/0735-7028.35.1.10

Harding, T. W. (1989). The application of the European Convention of Human Rights to the field of psychiatry. *International journal of law and psychiatry, 12*(4), 245–262. https://doi.org/10.1016/0160-2527(89)90017-4

Henrich, J., Heine, S. J., & Norenzayan, A. (2010). The weirdest people in the world? *Behavioral and Brain Sciences, 33*(2-3), 61–83. https://doi.org/10.1017/S0140525X0999152X

Huminuik, K. (2024). The five connections: A human rights framework for psychologists. *International Journal of Psychology, 59*(2), 218–224. https://doi.org/10.1002/ijop.12908

Huss, T., & MacLachlan, M. (2016). *The EquIPP Manual*. Global Health Press.

Jovanovic, N., Fiorillo, A., & Rössler, W. (2016). Managing self: time, priorities, and well-being. In A. Fiorillo, U. Volpe & D. Bhugra (Eds.), *Psychiatry in practice: education, experience, and expertise* (pp. 33–44). Oxford University Press.

Fiorillo, A., Volpe, U., & Bhugra, D. (2016). Role and responsibilities of psychiatrists. In A. Fiorillo, U. Volpe & D. Bhugra (Eds.) *Psychiatry in practice: education, experience, and expertise* (pp. 1–10). Oxford University Press. http://ndl.ethernet.edu.et/bitstream/123456789/3063/1/339.pdf#page=26

MacLachlan, M. (2006). *Culture and health: a critical perspective towards global health*. Wiley.

Marzanski, M., Coupe, T., & Musunuri, P. (2006). Attitudes of mental health practitioners to the Hippocratic Oath: tradition and modernity in psychiatry. *Psychiatric Bulletin, 30*(9), 327–329. https://doi.org/10.1192/pb.30.9.327

McVeigh, J., Mannan, H., Ebuenyi, I. D., & MacLachlan, M. (2024). Inclusive and equitable policies: EquiFrame and EquIPP as frameworks for the analysis of the inclusiveness of policy content and processes. In L. Ned, M. R. Velarde, S. Singh, L. Swartz & K. Soldatić (Eds.), *The Routledge International Handbook of Disability and Global Health* (pp. 60–74). Routledge.

Morrissey, F. (2020). An evaluation of attitudinal change towards CRPD rights following delivery of the WHO QualityRights training programme. *Ethics, Medicine and Public Health, 13*, Article 100410. https://doi.org/10.1016/j.jemep.2019.100410

Pathare, S. (2003). *Mental Health Legislation & Human Rights* (Vol. 5). World Health Organization. https://www.ohchr.org/sites/default/files/documents/publications/WHO-OHCHR-Mental-health-human-rights-and-legislation_web.pdf

Pérez Pérez, B., Pujol i Llombart, M., & Mora, E. (2024). Human rights and psychiatric power in dispute. Towards a radicalization of democracy? *Revista Direito e Práxis, 15*, e65459. https://doi.org/10.1590/2179-8966/2022/65459i

Pope, K. S. (2018). A human rights and ethics crisis facing the world's largest organization of psychologists. *European Psychologist, 24*(2), 180–194. https://doi.org/10.1027/1016-9040/a000341

Radden, J. (2002). Psychiatric ethics. *Bioethics, 16*(5), 397–411. https://doi.org/10.1111/1467-8519.00298

Ranjbar, N., Erb, M., Mohammad, O., & Moreno, F. A. (2020). Trauma-informed care and cultural humility in the mental health care of people from minoritized communities. *Focus, 18*(1), 8–15. https://doi.org/10.1176/appi.focus.20190027

Royal Australian and New Zealand College of Psychiatrists (RANZCP). (2018). Code of Ethics. https://www.ranzcp.org/getmedia/2e090981-cdd2-4dee-a317-f8718bc7dc47/Code-of-Ethics-Aug-2025.pdf

Royal College of Psychiatrists (RCP). (2016). Good Psychiatric Practice: Code of Ethics. https://www.rcpsych.ac.uk/docs/default-source/improving-care/better-mh-policy/college-reports/college-report-cr186.pdf

Sansone, N., Tyano, S., Melillo, A., Schouler-Ocak, M., & Galderisi, S. (2024). Comparing the World Psychiatric Association and European Psychiatric Association codes of ethics: discrepancies and shared grounds. *European Psychiatry, 67*(1), e38, 1–6 https://doi.org/10.1192/j.eurpsy.2024.1748.

Steinert, T., & Henking, T. (2022). Law and psychiatry—current and future perspectives. *Frontiers in Public Health, 10,* 968168. https://doi.org/10.3389/fpubh.2022.968168

Strauss, A. L. (2017). *Psychiatric ideologies and institutions.* Routledge.

United Nations General Assembly. (1949). *Universal declaration of human rights* (Vol. 3381). Department of State, United States of America. https://www.un.org/sites/un2.un.org/files/2021/03/udhr.pdf

United Nations. (1989). Convention on the Rights of the Child. https://www.ohchr.org/sites/default/files/crc.pdf

Assembly, U. G. (1991). Principles for the protection of persons with mental illness and the improvement of mental health care. *Adopted on, 17.*

United Nations. (2006). United Nations Declaration on the Rights of Indigenous Peoples. https://www.un.org/development/desa/indigenouspeoples/wp-content/uploads/sites/19/2018/11/UNDRIP_E_web.pdf

United Nations. (2008). United Nations Convention on the Rights of Persons with Disabilities.https://nda.ie/disability-policy/uncrpd

11

Task Shifting/Sharing as a Panacea to the Dearth of Human Resources for Mental Health

Baher Ibrahim and Ikenna D. Ebuenyi

Introduction

'How many global mental health students does it take to deliver a community mental health intervention? None, because they task shift all the work.' The intention behind this light hearted joke, which was common during our MSc in Global Mental Health at King's College London and the London School of Hygiene and Tropical Medicine, is facetious, but the sentiment is a real one. It is hard not to get the impression that task shifting, or task sharing, is often touted as a panacea to the dearth of human resources not only in global mental health but in global health generally. 'Task shifting' or 'task sharing' entails the shifting of tasks usually performed by individuals with specialized training to non-specialized health workers, including primary health care workers and community workers. The aim of this is to make better use of available resources and allow 'all providers to work at the top of their scope of practice' (Purgato et al., 2020, p. 2). It is an approach that has arisen in response to the lack of human resources necessary for health service provision. In the particular case of mental health, 'the responsibility for providing mental health screening, referrals, management, and follow-up is shared between trained non-specialized health workers and specialists'. This paradigm 'allows the efficient use of non-specialists, who exist in greater numbers than specialists and are often already embedded in the health system' (Rebello et al., 2014, p. 310). This paradigm, or rather the exercise of attempting to define it, raises new questions: What exactly does it mean to practice at the top of one's scope? Does it refer to what other workers cannot or will not do? Does it refer more to conceptual knowledge or the application of skills? 'Top' also strongly implies a hierarchical model of knowledge that privileges narrow specialism at the expense of holistic coverage. Definitional issues aside, task shifting has received good press in diverse global contexts: it has been demonstrated to be effective in detecting and diagnosing depression in Makueni County, Kenya (Musyimi et al., 2017; Musyimi, 2017) and cost-saving in treating depressive and anxiety disorders in primary care in Goa, India (Buttorff et al., 2012).

The idea of task shifting in global health can formally be traced back to the 1970s, though it has a longer history in colonial medicine. Immediately before the Alma Ata declaration of 1978, the World Health Organization (WHO) published a report entitled 'Mental Health Collaborative Study for Strategies on Extending Mental Health Care', which proposed integrating mental health care into the duties of community health workers. Task shifting began to take on a central role with the increased funding made available for combating human immunodeficiency virus/acquired immunodeficiency syndrome (HIV/AIDS), malaria, and tuberculosis (Vitoria et al., 2009). These approaches in turn contributed to WHO's mental health Gap Action Program (mhGAP), which emphasizes task shifting in global mental health (Kohrt & Mendenhall, 2016). The field of global mental health formally started in 2007 with the publication of the *Lancet* series, and mhGAP took shape in 2008. By 2020, a systematic review by Galvin and Byansi could claim that 'task shifting has proven to be a valuable tool to increase access for mental health services in low- or middle-income countries (LMICs), and particularly in sub-Saharan Africa' and that 'non-specialist workers that can be trained to provide mental healthcare represent a largely untapped pool of treatment supporters' that promotes sustainability and cost-effectiveness because they are less mobile than higher cadre health workers and so more likely to remain in their communities. They concluded that lay mental health workers 'currently represent the future of mental health services for many in the developing world' (Galvin & Byansi, 2020, p. 357). A 2017 systematic review by Seidman and Atun similarly found that 'task shifting can help achieve cost savings and improve efficiency', but most of this evidence was in the context of tuberculosis and HIV/AIDS (Seidman & Atun, 2017, p. 9). Despite the recency of these interventions and studies, these ideas have a much longer history, as we demonstrate below using the example of the introduction of mental health into medical humanitarianism in Cambodian refugee camps over 30 years ago.

Though the terms 'task shifting' and 'task sharing' are often used interchangeably, Efendi et al. (2022) emphasize that it must be a matter of sharing and collaboration with adequate supervision and appropriate legal frameworks. If not done carefully, task shifting or task sharing becomes in effect 'task dumping', the issue alluded to in the joke above. If it does become task dumping, it runs numerous risks: non-specialized health workers may experience 'a disruption of their selves as they feel incompetent to address issues from an expert's vantage point', leading to 'blaming and stigmatizing service-users and their family members as a result of feelings of incompetence' (Kohrt & Griffith, 2015, p. 585).

There is also the risk of non-experts missing what a biomedical approach categorizes as important signs and symptoms. This is problematic insofar as non-specialized workers are trained in a medical model that privileges expert knowledge. Charging task shifting with training inadequate cadres of workers that may 'miss' what physicians calls symptoms and signs also obscures the central issue here: how much does one need to know in order to perform a particular job effectively? Does knowing more automatically translate into doing better? A review by Deimling Johns, Power, and

MacLachlan (2018) on task shifting in community mental health interventions in low- and middle-income settings found that 'length of training does not seem to demonstrate an association to evidence of effectiveness', and that the humanistic theory forming the 'base for many psychological interventions being used by highly trained professionals' may constitute a 'very appropriate base for nonprofessional interventionists' (p. 222).

There are also ripple effects in the wider community when community workers are trained to view psychosocial problems through a biomedical lens: the 'induction of community volunteers in the language of formal mental health impedes their freedom to work outside biomedical discourse, thereby taking away locally available and valued solutions to human distress' (Kottai & Ranganathan, 2020, p. 539). Finally, community health workers and volunteers who have usually not been involved in the planning of interventions are 'prone to unfair employment practices and exploitation at the hands of the program managers' (Philip & Chaturvedi, 2018, p. 105). Padmanathan and De Silva's systematic review concluded that 'for task-sharing to be successful and sustainable a number of factors need to be considered: distress experienced by the task-sharing workforce; their self-perceived level of competence; the acceptance of the workforce by other health care professionals; and the incentives provided to ensure retention of the workforce' (Padmanathan & De Silva, 2013, p. 82).

The promotion of task shifting in LMICs also has colonial overtones that should not be ignored. European colonial regimes sought to deliver medical care in the African nations they colonized by creating 'sub professional medical schools and qualifications'. Variously known as 'African doctors', 'native medical auxiliaries', and 'assistant medical officers', they were used to deliver health care on the cheap and were seen as a solution to the lack of European doctors, something newly independent African states sought to reverse (Clark & Toshner, 2023).

Finally, we must question the degree to which neoliberal logic pervades global health initiatives such as task shifting, which is attractive to policymakers precisely because it promises cost-effectiveness, efficiency, and rapid scalability to the maximum number of 'consumers'—privileging fiscal over moral concerns (Keshavjee, 2014). The common rationale and justification for its use is that it offers an alternative to healthcare where nothing exists; yet this sophistry leaves out the cost and unintended consequences of care provision based on limited or inappropriate knowledge. The relevant ethical questions here are: what is the minimum training required in order to provide effective interventions for as many people as possible, and at what point does mandating longer training begin to be about indulging professions rather than about ensuring safety and quality of services?

The philosophical schools that are relevant to ethical dilemmas in global health are utilitarianism, deontology, and consequentialism. Utilitarianism argues for the maximum possible good, deontology argues for an ethical code of rules, and consequentialism evaluates an action based on its effect (Katz, Lahey, & Campbell, 2014). An example of how these can be applied to particular contexts will be illustrated using the introduction of mental health into medical humanitarianism and post-conflict society in Cambodia in the 1980s and 1990s. By examining a historical case study from which we have sufficient critical distance, we can better think about some of the ethical challenges facing us in global mental health today.

Historical Case Study: Community Mental Health in Cambodian Refugee Camps

The fall of the Khmer Rouge in 1979 was followed by an exodus of Cambodians towards the Thai border. From 1979 to 1993, hundreds of thousands of Cambodians lived in unsafe, militarized refugee camps on the border. The Cambodian border crisis was a seminal moment in the history of medical humanitarianism, and the first time since the post-war era in Europe that practices and technologies of mental health were introduced in a setting of crisis (Taithe, 2016). The mental health experience amassed by practitioners there, particularly around the concept of 'trauma', set the stage for the expansion of trauma-focused humanitarian mental health interventions in the 1990s, particularly in the former Yugoslavia (Pupavac, 2002).

At the forefront of the mental health challenge posed by Indochinese displacement was a group of professionals in Boston who founded the Indochinese Psychiatry Clinic in 1981, which became the Harvard Program in Refugee Trauma (HPRT) in 1988. Despite the presence of a significant Indochinese patient population presenting to public health services, very few of them ever presented to mental health services. At a time when 'trauma' was in the ascendancy as a cultural phenomenon in Western consciousness (Fassin & Rechtman, 2009), Indochinese refugees—alongside Holocaust survivors, Vietnam veterans, and victims of rape—were an ideal patient population. In addition to providing clinical care, the HPRT clinicians attempted to engage the local Cambodian community through the conduction of oral history interviews, which led to a deeper engagement with the cultural meaning behind the loss and trauma experienced by their patients. HPRT was at the forefront of the development of a new science of refugee trauma (Mollica, 2009).

In 1988, the knowledge and experience forged with resettled Cambodians in the US served as the launchpad for a humanitarian mission to the Thai-Cambodian border camps. Led by Dr Richard Mollica, co-founder of HPRT, a team sponsored by the World Federation for Mental Health (WFMH) arrived in Site 2, the largest camp on the border, to conduct a mental health survey. The resulting report by Richard Mollica and Russell Jalbert, 'Community of Confinement: The mental health crisis in Site 2' (Mollica & Jalbert, 1989), was simultaneously a technical and political document, recommending specific mental health interventions alongside calling for a political solution that would enable the encamped Cambodians to return home. No artificial dichotomy between mental health and political solutions was made. A 16% prevalence of post-traumatic stress disorder (PTSD) and 20% prevalence of depression were estimated, and camp mental health services were judged to be lacking and deficient. Indigenous Cambodian healing traditions were found to be 'fragmented and disintegrated', 'relegated to a limited cultural role and an almost non-consequential mental health role', justifying the conclusion that the Khmer people 'must look to Western non-Buddhist providers for protection and material comfort'. Though influential in the history of humanitarian mental health and refugee trauma, Mollica informed me in an interview in 2017 that it was never published in a mainstream scientific journal at the time due to its focus on human rights, which was then quite a novelty in mental health and psychiatry.

Following this fact-finding mission, the team from HPRT followed up with another visit to Site 2 in 1989, producing a report entitled 'Turning Point in Khmer Mental Health: Immediate Steps to Resolve the Mental Health Crisis in the Khmer Border Camps', which was submitted to the UN Border Relief Operation (UNBRO), the UN body created to administer the camps (Mollica et al., 1989). In addition to advocating for a political resolution to the conflict and proposing measures to address social determinants of mental health, it recommended a six-month training programme for Khmer lay mental health workers, to be integrated into existing structures. It was anticipated that this would provide a cadre of Khmer mental health workers that would assist in Cambodia's recovery and post-conflict reconstruction upon repatriation—this continued into the 1990s through the Harvard Training Program in Cambodia. The report also advocated collaboration with local refugee-led mental health initiatives set up in the camps, such as Nuon Phaly's Khmer People's Depression Relief Unit (KPDR) and Meas Nee's Mental Health and Traditional Healing Center (MHTH). This collaborative model was described by Svang Tor (1996) as the 'KCBM model'— 'Krou Khmer, Counseling, Buddhism, Medication', where 'Krou Khmer' refers to Buddhist monks and literally means 'teachers of the Khmer'.

This model of training and task shifting was not without its detractors, not only for task shifting per se, but because of the assumptions of Western biomedicine its detractors charged it with harbouring and imposing. One such critic was Sister Joan Healy, an Australian nun and social worker who worked closely with Meas Nee in the MHTH (Healy, 2016). Healy was present during the visits of the HPRT team in 1989, and had sharp words for the Turning Point report. The first problem she noted was the very definition: what was happening in the border camps was not a mental health problem, she declared, but one of sociopolitical problems and human rights violations. To portray the Cambodian people as mentally ill, Healy argued, was to perpetuate another injustice and further violate their human rights. Healy's criticisms anticipated Derek Summerfield's (1999) well known criticisms of trauma and PTSD around the medicalization and individualization, and thereby neutralization, of social and political problems, which are recast as health issues amenable to technical solutions. The second problem Healy identified was that the recommendations of the Turning Point report were largely based on experience amassed with Cambodian refugees in resettlement who had a wholly different set of problems than their compatriots trapped in the border camps. She quoted a resident in Site 2 who said to a Cambodian American mental health worker who was a member of the visiting team: 'Your people suffer in paradise. Our people suffer in hell' (Healy, 1990).

Joan Healy's criticisms provide food for thought for reflecting on the impact of the introduction of Western psychiatric methods to the Cambodian border camps and subsequently Cambodia, and the philosophical underpinnings of such interventions. 'We may not be able to solve the human rights problem overnight, but that is no reason to let conditions at Site 2 fester' Mollica told the *Los Angeles Times* in 1990 (Getlin, 1990). 'If you're bleeding badly, even a Band-Aid is better than nothing.' This assumption—that producing some good is better than not producing any good at all—is a utilitarian one. It is an assumption that pervades much of global mental health discourse in its focus on cost-effective, rapidly scalable interventions (Marseille & Kahn, 2019). It becomes problematic for two reasons: when the Band-Aid, introduced as a stopgap measure, becomes the goal; and when unintended harm is caused by the Band-Aid solution.

Healy's criticisms can also be critiqued, however. The charge of applying biomedical paradigms and technical solutions to political problems carries weight because of the implication that technocratic solutions are being used to neutralize and delegitimize human suffering, and the concomitant righteous anger directed at injustice. It carries with it, perhaps unintentionally and sometimes intentionally, a charge of complicity with power structures. However, pragmatism dictates that any health intervention will be designed and delivered within the prevailing power structures. We would never get anything done otherwise, it could be argued. The HPRT actors neither ignored nor refuted the political dimension of their work: lobbying for mental health care to help the sufferers went with advocating for a political solution that would end their encampment. This criticism also carries the assumption that there is a value difference between political suffering and medicalized distress, potentially revealing more about the assumptions and values of the persons making the charge than the object of its critique.

Another philosophical underpinning underlying the HPRT intervention and humanitarian interventions in general is deontological—the duty to intervene to alleviate suffering. Where this sense of duty comes from must be made explicit. For example, James Lavelle, co-founder of HPRT, spoke of the 'collective guilt for messing up Southeast Asia in the first place' that provided part of the motivation for engaging with Indochinese refugee mental health (Haines, 1988). It is important to acknowledge these motivations because they are actualized in the asymmetrical power relations between humanitarians and beneficiaries. Western humanitarians brought their own experience of guilt and reckoning with the Holocaust to the Thai-Cambodian border, where they 'encountered genocide victims afresh with the intellectual tools and historical baggage arising from the European experience of the Holocaust' (Taithe, 2016. p. 338).

Finally, consequentialism is illustrated by Joan Healy's critique. She did not doubt that the recommendations outlined in the Turning Point report were motivated by altruism and compassion, but argued that there would be unintended consequences that argued against intervention in the manner suggested.

Contemporary Case Study: Mental Health and Psychosocial Support in Syrian Humanitarian Settings and Refugee Camps

The conflict in Syria that began with the 'Arab Spring' in 2011 ended in 2024 with the fall of the Assad regime. As this chapter goes to press, it remains to be seen how it will fare under the new regime. Prior to the start of the conflict, Syria was classified as a middle-income country with a robust public sector national health system, a growing private sector, and little reliance on civil society and charity organizations (Akik et al., 2020). Since the start of the conflict, over 13.4 million people in Syria have been displaced, about half of that total internally. Syrians account for 1 in 5 refugees globally, with 6.5 million refugees registered in 131 countries. At the end of 2024, sixty-nine per cent of Syrian refugees were registered in neighbouring Lebanon, Jordan, and Turkey; further afield, Germany is host to a sizable population (UN High Commissioner for Refugees, 2024). Reviews on research into the mental health of forcibly displaced populations reveal a substantial burden of mental health problems, though there remains a lack of high-quality data (Cratsley, Brooks, & Mackey, 2021). Meta-analyses have demonstrated high rates of PTSD and depression (Blackmore et. al, 2020). Like the Cambodian border crisis in the 1980s, the Syrian crisis is a 'humanitarian setting characterized by protracted conflicts, lack of governance and dependence on international aid for health service delivery' (Habboush, Ekzayez, & Gilmore, 2023, p. 1). Unlike in the 1980s, however, there is recognition of the pressing need for mental health services in humanitarian settings, as well as a number of guidelines and policy frameworks.

The Inter-Agency Standing Committee (IASC) guidelines on Mental Health and Psychosocial Support (MHPSS), developed in 2007, provide a guiding framework. The MHPSS pyramid (Figure 11.1) suggests that the majority of support—the base of the pyramid—should be devoted to basic safety and security (Level 1) and the strengthening of community supports (Level 2). The next level is focused non-specialized supports such as psychological first aid (Level 3)—this is where task shifting fits in. Specialized mental health services—the tip of the pyramid (Level 4)—are required by a much smaller number of people (Inter-Agency Standing Committee, 2007). Initiatives that focus on individualized interventions for those who meet the criteria for a psychiatric diagnosis will consequently miss most of the population in need of support. WHO's mhGAP-Humanitarian Intervention Guide (mhGAP-IG) (World Health Organization & UNHCR, 2015) offers guidelines on the delivery of MHPSS services by non-specialized health workers in humanitarian settings. In such contexts, task shifting has emerged as a creative response and adaptation to the exodus of healthcare workers from Syria, alongside other strategies such as outreach activities to increase access to health services, remote management, and operating in 'underground' facilities to mitigate the risk of attack (Akik et al., 2020). Bou-Orm et al. (2023) have investigated the provision of MHPSS in Northwest Syria and found

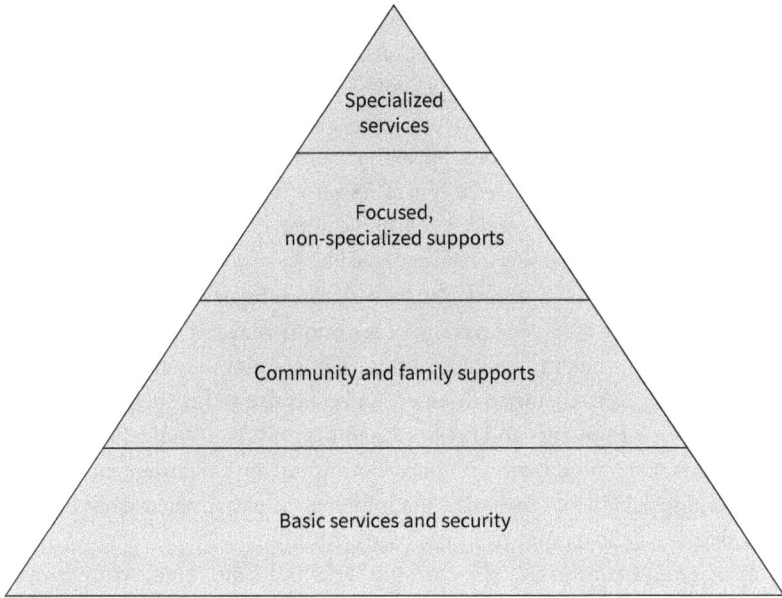

Figure 11.1 Inter-Agency Standing Committee Pyramid for MHPSS.

that task shifting was a promising approach to improve service delivery, but identified gaps in the sustainability and scalability of services.

It would be disingenuous to suggest that task shifting should *not* be used in a situation such as present day Syria and its neighbouring countries when it may constitute the only method of providing services that would otherwise be unattainable. However, when do we move beyond the 'doing something is better than doing nothing' stage? Task shifting interventions should be planned and delivered with a view towards 'what next?' rather than perpetuating the status quo with repeated interrupted cycles of short-term funding. Woodward et al. (2023) examined the delivery of a task sharing psychological intervention called Problem Management Plus (PM+) to Syrian refugees in Jordan as part of the Syrian REfuGees MeNTal HealTH Care Systems (STRENGTHS) project. The aim of STRENGTHS was to examine and enhance the effectiveness and scalability of the mental health systems of eight countries hosting Syrian refugees in Europe and the Middle East through the introduction of novel psychological interventions. Developed by WHO for use with adults experiencing depression, anxiety, grief, and PTSD, PM+ consists of five sessions of psychoeducation, behavioural activation, and problem-solving techniques. Woodward et al. (2023) found that despite the potential of task shifted interventions like PM+ to 'effectively increase access to psychological support for communities with high mental health needs, such as refugees', there were major barriers to scaling up and integration into existing systems, limiting the potential for sustainability.

Further pitfalls in delivering MHPSS to refugees, such as lack of cultural acceptability and a tendency to individualize interventions, have been highlighted by Kerbage et al. (2020), who investigated MHPSS service provision at Levels 3 and 4 of the IASC pyramid to Syrian refugees in Lebanon. Their study provides important food for thought on how *not* to deliver MHPSS interventions. Speaking to Lebanese providers, programme co-ordinators, and policy-makers, Kerbage et al. found a perception that Syrian culture was an obstacle to mental health service provision ('illiteracy', 'traditional', 'lack of education') and that MHPSS interventions were considered a means to *educate* Syrian refugees about mental health. Contrast this with Syrian refugees' perceptions of MHPSS provision: emotional distress was a result of environmental and psychosocial stressors, not a mental health problem amenable to clinical intervention; symptoms of emotional distress were a normal rather than diseased, and collective rather than individual, reaction to a build-up of stressors and pressure; and the only 'true and definite' solution to the problems facing refugees was a political, not clinical, one: resettlement. The chances of success and scalability of a mental health intervention where perceptions of providers and beneficiaries are so diametrically opposed are minimal.

Comparing and contrasting the cases of Syria and Cambodia, many similarities are apparent that offer lessons for MHPSS service provision in humanitarian settings or settings with a dearth of human resources for mental health services. There is, first of all, the definition of the problem: defining a problem as *either* a political *or* health issue creates an inaccurate and unhelpful binary. We would do better to retain both explanatory paradigms and the different kinds of understanding they offer, while acknowledging that their relative utility vis-à-vis one another differs across time and situations. Second, there is the issue of scope: is this a problem best addressed by individualized mental health interventions delivered to those with the most distressing experiences, or could resources be used more efficiently and equitably by providing and strengthening basic social services and community supports? Again, such a binary is limiting, and it would be better to retain both perspectives and judge situations on a case-by-case basis, recognizing that there will be trade-offs in every situation. Third, there is the issue of cultural sensitivity, contextual relevance, and acceptability— not only to the recipients of non-specialist delivered interventions, but to the non-specialists themselves. Finally, there is the issue of sustainability: what happens when humanitarian organizations withdraw or when research funding cycles end? One way to conceptualize how we might approach these questions is to imagine an analogous situation of task shifting, albeit more formalized, in the Global North: the expansion of allied health professionals such as physician associates (PAs) and nurse practitioners (NPs) to respond to increasing demand for health care services.

Thought Experiments and Conclusion

The use of non-specialized workers in the Global South has been touted as a measure to address the perennial unmet need of physical and mental health services. Research on examples of these measures and the use of non-specialized workers across Africa and Latin America has suggested that these cadres of non-specialized community health care workers are as effective as traditional highly trained mental health care providers (Rocha et al., 2021). A study in Kenya reported a 79% positive predictive value in diagnosing and detecting major depressive disorders (Musyimi, 2017; Musyimi et al., 2017). An economic evaluation of task shifting interventions for common mental health problems in India concluded that it was not only cost-effective, but also cost-saving (Buttorff et al., 2012). This narrative may be appealing to governments of LMICs because it offers an opportunity to utilize stop gap measures as a substitute for years of infrastructural neglect. 'Perhaps it is time to reconsider the investments traditionally reserved for the training of psychologists, psychiatrists and other mental health practitioners!', policymakers might say. This invites the question of whether they are being used as temporary measures or as ends in themselves. As one Lancet (2019) editorial put it, 'they need to consider at what point do they stop providing temporary solutions and define their end goal'. This neoliberal logic is not exclusive to LMICs—it also underlies the drive to shift duties traditionally in the domain of physicians to PAs and NPs in high-income countries.

What is often left unsaid in the discourse on task sharing in LMICs is the limited training, lack of formal structure and supervision, and precarious employment of non-specialized workers. In Nigeria, several of these cadres of workers were used for TB/HIV programmes, and traditional birth attendants for maternal health programmes, because they were cheaper and more expedient (Oyebode et al., 2021; Ajisegiri et al, 2023). According to Iwu and Holzemer (2017), task shifting is associated with excessive workload, job dissatisfaction, and may worsen existing HIV-related workforce challenges. These cadres and forms of care pervade most public facilities used by the 'common people' in most low-resource settings. In sharp contrast, the PAs and NPs being increasingly used in Europe and North America have formal training, a defined scope of practice, and more clearly defined roles in the public health service. Although the quality of service has come under scrutiny, and has prompted concern regarding the blurring of boundaries between PAs/NPs and physicians—as a recent case raised in the British Parliament (House of Commons, deb. 6 July 2023) illustrates—there exists a better supporting systems infrastructure for these cadres in high-income countries. These differences invite us to explore what we would do in the following situations:

1. If we had a child with a severe mental health problem, would we trust their care to a non-specialized worker or would we prefer a psychologist/psychiatrist?
2. If one, or one's family member, is pregnant, would we prefer that she receive care from a traditional birth attendant or an obstetrician?
3. If we are stranded in an area in a resource-poor country where non-specialized workers with limited training have largely replaced surgeons, would we agree to have them perform an appendectomy, or would we rather book a flight to the capital, or to a country in the Global North, to have the surgery?

4. What are the available strategies to promote task sharing/shifting as a time-limited stopgap measure to ensure that policy-makers in low resource settings do not abandon the efforts towards funding and resources to train specialist mental health providers?

5. Is it better to provide an effective and excellent mental health service to 30% of a population or an effective but only minimally adequate service to 100% of the population?

6. If research indicates that a either a psychologist, a psychiatrist, a social worker or a community health worker would all be equally effective in providing a service for your mental health condition, what factors would influence our choice of who to seek a service from?

Further Reading

Ager, A. (2021). Creative tensions in the framing of MHPSS. *Forced Migration Review*, (66), 5–8.

Ibrahim, B. (2024). Medicalizing the refugee experience: Fractured continuities and claims of novelty in the psychiatric study of forced migration. *Yearbook of Transnational History, 7*, 147–170.

Musyimi, C. W., Mutiso, V. N., Nyamai, D. N., Ebuenyi, I. D., & Ndetei, D. M. (2019). Integration of traditional birth attendants into mental healthcare: a multistakeholder qualitative study exploration. *BioMed Research International, 2019*(1), Article 8195267.

Pupavac, V. (2006). Refugees in the 'sick role': Stereotyping refugees and eroding refugee rights (Research Paper No. 128). http://www.unhcr.org/en-us/research/working/44e198712/refugees-sick-rolestereotyping-refugees-eroding-refugee-rights-vanessa.html

References

Ajisegiri, W. S., Abimbola, S., Tesema, A. G., Odusanya, O. O., Peiris, D., & Joshi, R. (2023). 'We just have to help': Community health workers' informal task-shifting and task-sharing practices for hypertension and diabetes care in Nigeria. *Frontiers in Public Health*, 11, Article 1038062.

Akik, C., Semaan, A., Shaker-Berbari, L., Jamaluddine, Z., Saad, G. E., Lopes, K., Constantin, J., Ekzayez, A., Singh, N.S., Blanchet, K., DeJong, J., & Ghattas, H. (2020). Responding to health needs of women, children and adolescents within Syria during conflict: intervention coverage, challenges and adaptations. *Conflict and Health*, 14, Article 37.

Blackmore, R., Boyle, J. A., Fazel, M., Ranasinha, S., Gray, K. M., Fitzgerald, G., Misso, M., & GibsonHelm, M. (2020). The prevalence of mental illness in refugees and asylum seekers: A systematic review and meta-analysis. *PLoS medicine, 17*(9), Article 1003337.

Bou-Orm, I. R., Moussallem, M., Karam, J., deLara, M., Varma, V., Diaconu, K., Apaydin, M. C. B., Van den Bergh, R., Ager, A., & Witter, S. (2023). Provision of mental health and psychosocial support services to health workers and community members in conflict-affected Northwest Syria: a mixed-methods study. *Conflict and Health, 17*, Article 46.

Buttorff, C., Hock, R. S., Weiss, H. A., Naik, S., Araya, R., Kirkwood, B. R., Chisholm, D., & Patel, V. (2012). Economic evaluation of a task-shifting intervention for common mental disorders in India. *Bulletin of the World Health Organization, 90*(11), 813–821.

Clark, H., & Toshner, M. (2023). *Physician associates: a solution for healthcare staff shortages or a colonial throwback?* https://theconversation.com/physician-associates-a-solution-for-hea lthcare-staff-shortages-or-a-colonial-throwback-214424

Cratsley, K., Brooks, M. A., & Mackey, T .K. (2021). Refugee mental health, global health policy, and the Syrian crisis. *Frontiers in Public Health, 9*, Article 676000.

Deimling Johns, L., Power, J., & MacLachlan, M. (2018). Community-based mental health intervention skills: task shifting in low- and middle-income settings. *International Perspectives in Psychology: Research, Practice, Consultation, 7*, 205–230, Article 4.

Efendi, F., Aurizki, G. E., Yusuf, A., & McKenna, L. (2022). 'Not shifting, but sharing': stakeholders' perspectives on mental health task-shifting in Indonesia. *BMC Nursing, 21*(1), Article 165.

Fassin, D., & Rechtman, R. (2009). *The empire of trauma: an inquiry into the condition of victimhood.* Princeton University Press.

Galvin, M., & Byansi, W. (2020). A systematic review of task shifting for mental health in sub-Saharan Africa. *International Journal of Mental Health, 49*(4) 336–360.

Getlin, J. (1990). Treating the tormented: in an Asian refugee camp, pilot mental health program seeks to ease the despair" *Los Angeles Times,* 4 January. https://www.latimes.com/archi ves/la-xpm-1990-01-04-vw-486-story.html

Habboush, A., Ekzayez, A., & Gilmore, B. (2023). A framework for community health worker optimisation in conflict settings: prerequisites and possibilities from Northwest Syria. *BMJ Global Health, 8*(7), Article 011837.

Haines, H. (1988). Interview: Richard Mollica and James Lavelle. *Mental Health News August/ September 1988, Mental Health Foundation of New Zealand,* 13–15.

Healy, J. (1990). A dialogue on Khmer Mental Health from Site 2/Thai-Cambodian Border (January 18th, 1990). *Refugee Studies Centre, Forced Migration Online, RSC/EK61 HEA.* http://repository.forcedmigration.org/show_metadata.jsp?pid=fmo:563

Healy, J. (2016). *Writing for Raksmey: A story of Cambodia.* Monash University Publishing.

Iwu, E. N., & Holzemer, W. L. (2017). HIV task sharing between nurses and physicians in Nigeria: examining the correlates of nurse self-efficacy and job satisfaction. *The Journal of the Association of Nurses in AIDS Care, 28*(3), 395–407.

House of Commons, Physician Associates Deb (6 July 2023). 735, col. 1025. http://www.publi cations.parliament.uk/pa/hcdeb1990

Inter-Agency Standing Committee. (2007). Guidelines on mental health and psychosocial support (MHPSS) in emergency settings. https://www.mhpss.net/toolkit/mhpss-and-eie/resou rce/iasc-guidelines-on-mental-health-and-psychosocial-support-in-emergency-settings

Katz, C. L., Lahey, T. P., & Campbell, H. T. (2014). An ethical framework for global psychiatry. *Annals of Global Health, 80*(2), 146–151.

Kerbage, H., Marranconi, F., Chamoun, Y., Brunet, A., Richa, S., & Zaman, S. (2020). Mental health services for Syrian refugees in Lebanon: perceptions and experiences of professionals and refugees. *Qualitative Health Research, 30*(6), 849–864.

Keshavjee, S. (2014). *Blind spot: How neoliberalism infiltrated global health.* University of California Press.

Kohrt, B. A., & Griffith, J. L. (2015). Solving global mental health praxis. In L. J. Kirmayer, R. Lemelson & C. A. Cummings (Eds.), *Re-visioning psychiatry: Cultural phenomenology, critical neuroscience, and global mental health* (pp.544–574). Cambridge University Press.

Kohrt, B., & Mendenhall, E. (2016). *Global mental health: Anthropological perspectives.* Routledge.

Kottai, S. R., & Ranganathan, S. (2020). Task-shifting in community mental health in Kerala: tensions and ruptures. *Medical Anthropology, 39*(6), 538–552.

Marseille, E., & Kahn, J. G. (2019). Utilitarianism and the ethical foundations of cost-effectiveness analysis in resource allocation for global health. *Philosophy, Ethics, and Humanities in Medicine, 14*, Article 5.

Mollica, R. F. (2009). *Healing invisible wounds: Paths to hope and recovery in a violent world.* Vanderbilt University Press.

Mollica, R. F., Lavelle, J., Tor, S., & Elias C., (1989). Turning point in Khmer Mental Health: Immediate steps to resolve the mental health crisis in the Khmer border camps. *World Federation for Mental Health, Committee on Refugees and Migrants.*

Mollica, R. F., & Jalbert, R. R. (1989). Community of confinement: The mental health crisis in Site Two (displaced persons camps on the Thai-Kampuchean border), *World Federation for Mental Health, Committee on Refugees and Migrants.*

Musyimi, C. W. (2017). *Mental health care in rural Kenya: Improving quality of life and mental health through evidence-based mental health interventions in the informal sector.* [PhD thesis]. Vrije Universiteit Amsterdam.

Musyimi, C. W., Mutiso, V. N., Musau, A. M., Matoke, L. K., & Ndetei, D. M. (2017). Prevalence and determinants of depression among patients under the care of traditional health practitioners in a Kenyan setting: Policy implications, *Transcultural Psychiatry, 54*(3), 285–303.

Oyebode, T. A., Hassan, Z., Afolaranmi, T., Auwal, M., Shehu, M., Kelechi, N., Oche, A., Sagay, S., Gwamna, J., Okonkwo, P., & Kanki, P. (2021). Improving PMTCT coverage and access in communities with unmet needs in Jos, Nigeria by adopting task shifting and task sharing strategies. *European Journal of Preventive Medicine, 9*(3) 83–93.

Padmanathan, P., & De Silva, M. J. (2013). The acceptability and feasibility of task-sharing for mental healthcare in low and middle income countries: A systematic review. *Social Science & Medicine, 97,* 82–86.

Philip, S., & Chaturvedi, S. K. (2018). Musings on Task Shifting in Mental Health. *Journal of Psychosocial Rehabilitation and mental health, 5*(2) 103–107.

Pupavac, V. (2002). Pathologizing populations and colonizing minds: International psychosocial programs in Kosovo. *Alternatives, 27*(4), 489–511.

Purgato, M., Uphoff, E., Singh, R., Thapa Pachya, A., Abdulmalik, J., & van Ginneken, N. (2020). Promotion, prevention and treatment interventions for mental health in low- and middle-income countries through a task-shifting approach. *Epidemiology and Psychiatric Sciences, 29,* e150–e150.

Rebello, T. J., Marques, A., Gureje, O., & Pike, K. M. (2014). Innovative strategies for closing the mental health treatment gap globally. *Current Opinion in Psychiatry, 27*(4), 308–314.

Rocha, T. I. U., Aschar, S. C. de A. L. Hidalgo-Padilla, L., Daley, K., Claro, H. G., Martins Castro, H. C., Dos Santos, D. V. C., Miranda, J. J., Araya, R., & Menezes, P. R. (2021). Recruitment, training and supervision of nurses and nurse assistants for a task-shifting depression intervention in two RCTs in Brazil and Peru. *Human Resources for Health, 19,* Article 16.

Seidman, G., & Atun, R. (2017). Does task shifting yield cost savings and improve efficiency for health systems? A systematic review of evidence from low-income and middle-income countries, *Human Resources for Health, 15*(1), Article 29.

Summerfield, D. (1999). A critique of seven assumptions behind psychological trauma programmes in war-affected areas. *Social Science & Medicine, 48*(10), 1449–1462.

Taithe, B. (2016). The cradle of the new humanitarian system? International work and European VOLUNTEERS at the Cambodian BORDER CAMPS, 1979–1993. *Contemporary European History, 25*(2), 335–358.

The Lancet. (2019). Task sharing: stopgap or end goal?, *The Lancet Psychiatry, 6*(2), 81.

Tor, S. (1996). A model called KCBM. In J. Lavelle, S. Tor, R. F. Mollica, K. Allden, & L. Potts (Eds.), *Harvard guide to Khmer mental health by Harvard Program in Refugee Trauma* (pp. 7–14). Harvard University.

UNHCR. (2022). Global Trends: Forced Displacement in 2024. https://www.unhcr.org/global-trends-report-2024

Vitoria, M., Granich, R., Gilks, C. F., Gunneberg, C., Hosseini, M., Were, W., Raviglione, M., & De Cock, K. M. (2009). The global fight against HIV/AIDS, tuberculosis, and malaria: Current status and future perspectives. *American Journal of Clinical Pathology*, *131*(6), 844–848.

WHO & UNHCR. (2015). mhGAP Humanitarian Intervention Guide (mhGAP-HIG) Clinical management of mental, neurological and substance use conditions in humanitarian emergencies. https://www.who.int/publications/i/item/9789241548922

Woodward, A., Sondorp, E., Barry, A. S., Dieleman, M. A., Fuhr, D. C., Broerse, J. E. W., Akhtar, A., Awwad, M., Bawaneh, A., Bryant, R., Sijbrandij, M., Cuijpers, P., & Roberts, B. (2023). Scaling up task-sharing psychological interventions for refugees in Jordan: a qualitative study on the potential barriers and facilitators. *Health Policy and Planning*, *38*(3), 310–320.

12

Moving Upstream

Developing Theories of Change to Address Human Rights and Wrongs

Holly Wescott, Malcolm MacLachlan, and Hasheem Mannan

Introduction

The World Report on Disability (World Health Organization & World Bank, 2011) estimates that more than one billion people—about 15% of the world's population—live with some form of disability; and that in comparison to non-disabled people, they have higher rates of poverty, less economic, political, and cultural participation, lower educational achievements, poorer health outcomes, increased dependency, and less legal protection. In 2006, the United Nations General Assembly adopted the Convention on the Rights of Persons with Disabilities (CRPD, the Convention) (UN General Assembly, 2006). It acknowledges the historic and contemporary pervasive discrimination, exclusion, and marginalization of people with disabilities. It also specifies the duty of States Parties to take all appropriate measures to promote, protect and ensure the full and equal enjoyment of all human rights and fundamental freedoms, by all persons with disabilities. The CRPD is the most widely and rapidly adopted human rights instrument in history; and 185 of the 193 UN Member States have ratified the Convention with 100 of these also ratifying the Optional Protocol. The CRPD complements the commitment to the principle of non-discrimination enshrined in the Universal Declaration of Human Rights, and addresses it in the specific context of disability, moving decisively to a rights-based model of disability.

Psychosocial sciences have made significant contributions to understanding and addressing challenges associated with a wide range of disabilities (Goodley & Lawthom, 2006); however, this has often been from more of an individual/medical-model perspective, rather than from a social or human rights-model perspective. We have argued that barriers to implementation of the CRPD are embedded within longstanding social structures and attitudes that do not give way easily. Often such discriminatory practices—even when not necessarily intentional—are nonetheless 'protected' because of the advantages that accrue to others 'the advantage of keeping things as they are, of maintaining the status quo' (MacLachlan & Mannan, 2016, p. 102). Such attitudes and practices may seem 'natural,' or 'just the way things are', effectively 'othering' those with disability and making them separate to those without disability. Individuals' attitudes and social structures co-construct each other. Social structures are patterned social relationships mediated through social institutions, such as schools or health services, policies or laws, norms or conventions (Westcott, 2024).

A United Nations Programmatic Response

The UN Partnership to Promote the Rights of Persons with Disabilities (UNPRPD) is a unique collaborative effort that brings together UN organizations, governments, civil society—including organizations of persons with disabilities—and other partners to promote the rights of persons with disabilities through implementation of the CRPD (UNDP, 2020). The UNPRPD is funded through a Multi-Partner Trust Fund with contributions from a range of donor countries. The fund and the partnership were established explicitly to address structural barriers to realizing disability rights; and from 2014 to 2019 worked across 38 countries (see Figure 12.1) and with two regional networks (the Pacific Disability Forum and the African Disability Forum) (UNDP, 2016).

It is important to remember international instruments of law do not in themselves ensure the implementation of disability rights or the success of stated goals. Indeed, the expansion of human rights tools has been criticized: de Waal (2003, p. 254) states, 'This proliferation of laws is a problem. Many are impractical. Some cannot realistically be implemented. Others have been signed by governments that do not have the

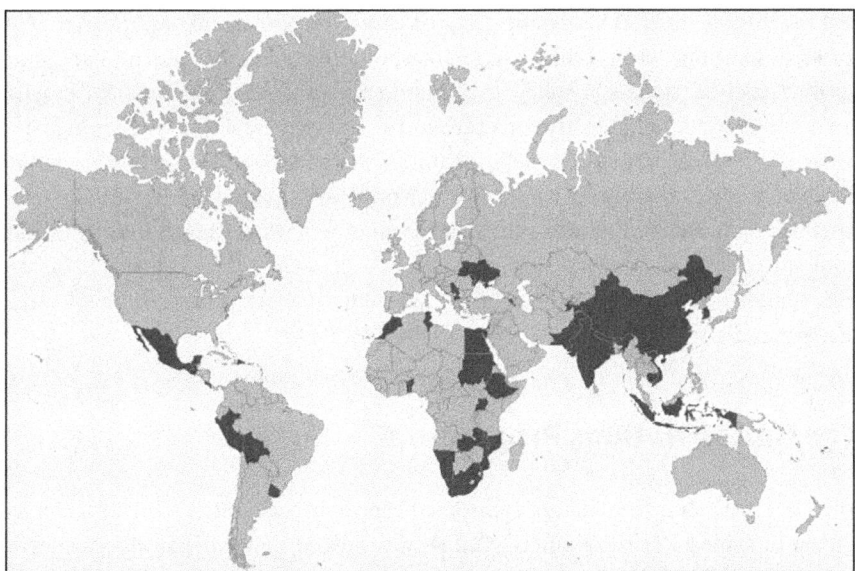

Figure 12.1 The 38 Countries (highlighted in green) in which the UNPRPD had projects through the first three funding rounds of the programme.

capacity or the will to implement them. This is actually a sign of disrespect for the rule of law.' The specific experience of marginalization and oppression facing persons with disabilities make the CRPD both an important paradigm shift and equally difficult to action within existing structures that privilege the maintenance of systems based on older models of disability.

There are two main paradigms that function as both a definition of disability, as well as a model for understanding the implications of disability. The first considers disability as a deficit or problem strictly within and concerning the individual (Marks, 1997; Levitt, 2017; Winance, 2016). This paradigm has been called *the medical model*, as the attempts to address disability have largely been 'cure' oriented (Marks, 1997; Levitt, 2017; Winance, 2016). The medicalization of disability is only part of the lens. Terminology such as 'wheelchair-bound' or 'hearing impaired' inextricably link the person to notions of limitation and are often used to label or define people and groups. Exclusion of people with disabilities may be addressed by making the body 'normal' (homogeneous, or able bodied), conforming the individual to narrow and relatively fixed social norms.

An alternative approach to disability is *the social model* which regards the problem as being external to the individual and relational to the environment (Marks, 1997; Levitt, 2017; Winance, 2016). Aspects of the environment (also known as *structures*) were built for some people/bodies to participate, but not all (Power, Lord, & deFranco, 2013). The classic example is a wheelchair user crossing a street without a dropped kerb. This model of disability aims to suggest the dropped kerb is prohibiting the individual from crossing the street, rather than the capacity of the person with mobility difficulties. Had that dropped kerb been installed, the individual would have full access to cross the street. A kerb ramp design is easy to recognize and requires a straightforward solution, while other barriers—especially structural barriers—are more abstract, such as barriers in policy or education practices. So 'environmental' barriers are not necessarily tangible structures around us, but also the abstract structures comprised of networks, attitudes, beliefs, institutional practices, and larger social systems. The *human rights model* of disability—which build in the social model—understands disability as individuals entitled to rights as all others, where interventions include both environmental and structural changes, as well as rights to access health-related interventions with dignity and having the inherent value of the person upheld, rather than a paradigm of solely adjusting the disabled individual.

The United Nations Programme

The UNPRPD identified factors considered central in facilitating structural change, shown in Table 12.1. The KnowUNPRPD was the knowledge management component of the UNPRPD and it incorporated a range of activities: provision of intensive introductory training and subsequent review, one-week long workshops; personal coaching; a Help Desk providing analysis and feedback for draft applications to the

Table 12.1 Factors central in facilitating structural change according to the UNPRPD programme

Enabling factor	Thematic priority
Enabling legislation and policy frameworks	Promote the ratification of the CRPD whenever relevant, and the development (or reform) of legislation and policies (disability-specific and not) as well as strategies and action plans
Empowering cultural norms	Reverse stigma, prejudices and negative stereotypes while promoting supportive and empowering attitudes
Access to services (mainstream and targeted)	Enhance access to mainstream as well as targeted services by improving their design and delivery modalities, and by promoting measures that will increase availability and affordability
Access to justice	Increase access to justice for persons with disabilities and the capacity of the justice sector to appropriately respond to the specific circumstances of persons with disabilities
Application of accessibility standards	Promote the application of accessibility standards to products, environments and processes, including non disability-specific interventions undertaken by development partners
Adequate access to rehabilitation, habilitation including assistive technology	Improve access to rehabilitation and habilitation—including assistive technology—by strengthening the availability and affordability of services and improving the design of assistive technologies
Adequate data and evidence	Improve disability-specific data and support research on different aspects of disability as well as the codification of evidence

fund; and conducting programmatic research and sometimes providing additional technical and research support (MacLachlan & Mannan, 2016). The essence of the knowledge management programme was to help participants understand how best to think about disability in a rights-based way (re UNCRPD) and how best to change social structures (laws, institutions, professions) that did not reflect such an understanding of disability.

Social order and their underlying forces often organize into hierarchies in which some groups are dominant and others subordinate. Social dominance theory explores how inequality and dominance are maintained through legitimizing myths, or cultural ideas strong and widespread enough to either legitimize one group or delegitimize another, resulting in meaningful resource divisions (Sidanius et al, 1994). Race, gender, and disability have been subject to delegitimization based on cultural myths so pervasive as to become the status quo. Myths that uphold the existing dominant understanding of 'othered' groups are considered hierarchy-enhancing, according to social dominance theory (Pratto & Steward, 2012). Alternatively, hierarchy-attenuating myths offer another explanation for such beliefs. For example, the social and rights-based model of disability advocates for a paradigm shift in the dominant myths about disability.

Theory of Change

Theory of Change (ToC) is a theory-based approach to planning, implementing, or evaluating change at any level (individual, organizational, or community). It articulates explicitly how an initiative is intended to achieve outcomes through actions, while considering its context (Ling & Todd, 2015). Thus, it is the end result of a series of critical thinking exercises that aim to provide detailed understanding of the immediate and mid-term changes required for a particular community to achieve a long-term goal (Harris, 2005). ToC is a fundamentally participatory process, involving active engagement by key stakeholders (Taplin & Clark, 2012). Participants articulate their long-term goals, identify the actions that they believe are required for the achievement of these goals, and identify which actions each participant will take responsibility for producing (Harris, 2005). Connell & Kubisch (1998) have noted that high quality ToCs have three defining characteristics: plausibility (evidence and common sense suggest that activities will lead to desired outcomes); feasibility (economic, technical, political, institutional, and human resources will be available to carry out the initiative); and testability (it is specific and complete enough for an evaluator to track its progress in credible and useful ways). These three qualities help to ensure that a ToC can realistically affect change in a particular setting.

ToC is distinct from sociological or psychological theories, which describe why change occurs, although these may be used to inform the ToC (De Silva et al. 2014). De Silva et al. (2014) have illustrated how ToC can aid the development of interventions by providing a framework for enhanced stakeholder engagement and by explicitly designing an intervention that is embedded in the local context.

There is a very limited literature on programmatic disability initiatives, particularly around the development of stakeholder partnerships as enshrined in the CRPD. In one study Asada et al. (2019) found early engagement activities such as alliance strengthening, capacity building, and overall readiness for change to be critical factors, prompting revisions to their initial ToC framework, especially given short programmatic timelines. Findings highlighted the programmatic need to address readiness for change as an evolving state throughout the project lifecycle and create a distinction between organizational capacity and individual leadership or technical expertise.

Application of Theory of Change

A ToC provides a framework for realistic and flexible planning by applying critical thinking to the design, implementation, and evaluation of programmes intended to instigate change in a specific context (Vogel, 2012). Fundamentally, ToCs focus on *how* an intervention will work, rather than whether an intervention will work (Rogers, 2014). ToC is useful both as a planning tool and for carrying out monitoring and evaluation (Taplin & Clark, 2012). A ToC can be used to develop a project plan, and this can in turn be used as a reference point for evaluation of the project (Rogers, 2014). During the development stage, outcomes are explicitly defined, and each outcome is assigned one or more specific indicators of success, which can then be assessed as implementation proceeds (Taplin & Clark, 2012).

Case Study 1—A Global Theory of Change

One of the components of the KnowUNPRPD workshops was to help each participant draft a ToC for the UNPRPD implementation in their own country. Having completed 6 weeks of training workshops with participants from three separate rounds of the programme, we have evolved a global ToC for the KnowUNPRPD. These participants were mostly drawn from United Nations agencies, although the first round also involved a government representative, and each round involved some representation from civil society. On average there were more female than male participants and they ranged from being newly appointed with limited or no knowledge of disability, to senior people with considerable experience and expertise in the disability sector.

At one of our final workshops, we dedicated a session to co-developing a Global Theory of Change which incorporated the essential common features of different country ToCs (omitting specific contextual differences and variations). This also prompted participants to think reflexively about what they are doing, their position, and what their role is in the change process. In doing so, participants were given sticky notes to identify key variables in the UNPRPD process of project implementation, and collaboratively discuss and locate each variable at the appropriate stage of activities. Once all 10 UNPRPD project representatives reached consensus, we further presented this Global ToC to participants in the third round of the UNPRPD for further comment and validation of its relevance to their own country ToC development.

Starting at the far left of the ToC, the CRPD is the United Nations Convention on which the UNPRPD is predicated; the Partnership provides human and financial resources, which are justified on evidence (data) informed arguments for the need for structural change in countries which ally to the programme. Moving to the right of the ToC, each country is required to adopt a tripartite partnership between several UN agencies (minimum of three), a number of government departments (more for cross-sectoral projects), and a number of civil-society agencies (which ideally includes an organization of persons with disabilities and may also include other community or international non-governmental organizations). These country-level partnership projects generally involve some aspect of capacity enhancement (awareness, knowledge, skills about disability), some aspect of advocating for structural change, and a strong element of participatory consultation with rights-holders (people with disabilities) as well as duty bearers (usually governments). Again, evidence (data) on disability, including prevalence, types, discrimination in employment, access to health or education, and so on is used to support these initiatives.

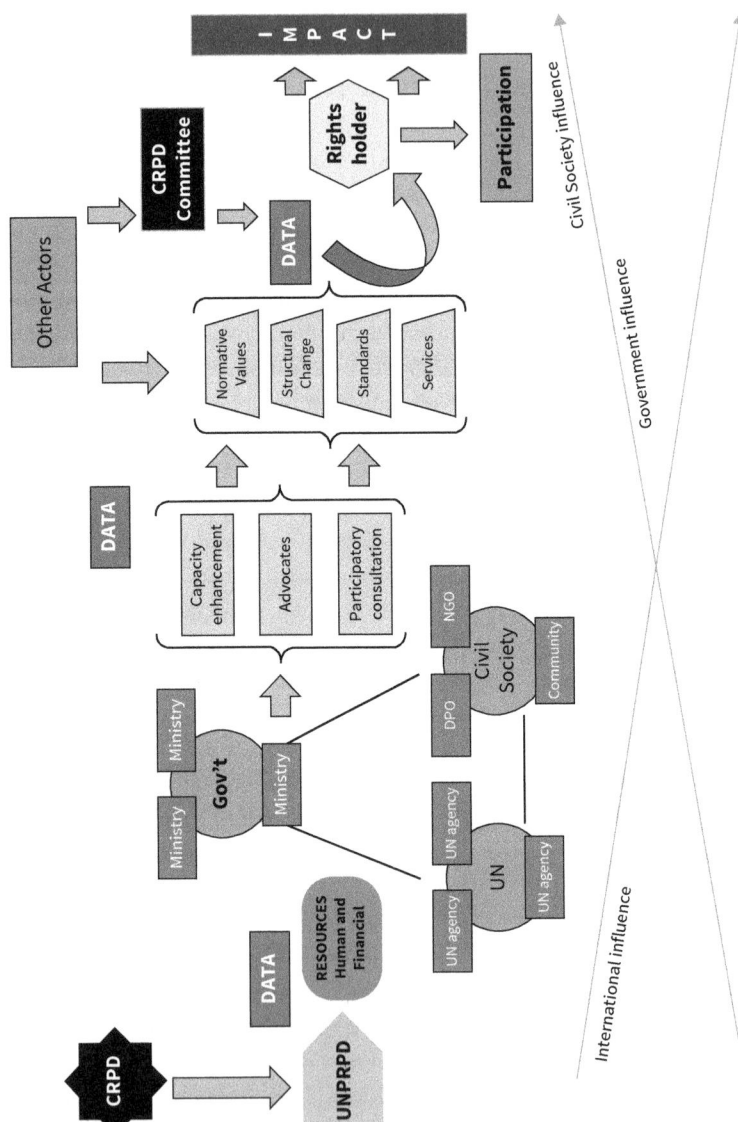

Figure 12.2 The KnowUNPRPD Global Theory of Change.

Normative values and social structures are identified as sites of action and need for change, which may involve changing acceptable standards and how services are accessed or delivered. This is likely to involve other actors in these spheres—including businesses, professional organizations, unions, and religious groups. These actions should produce further data—ideally compared to a previous baseline—allowing for the testing of assumptions through evaluating indicators of change (e.g. more children with disabilities in school and achieving similar grades to non-disabled children; or more women with disabilities in full-time employment on equivalent remuneration to non-disabled employees) to substantiate whether predetermined assumptions of the change process have been achieved. Rights holders can ultimately report to the Committee on the CRPD and hold their government to account; with the CRPD Committee requiring governments to make changes to implement the convention and improve the quality of life (impact) of people with disabilities.

As we move from left to right in the ToC, 'outside' agencies (such as the UN) have progressively less influence, and government and civil society progressively more, as they institute the structural changes deemed necessary. Ultimately the ToC charts a process of persuasion to change structural barriers: where multiple levels are used, multiple levers adopted; where networks, personal influencers, incentives, public accountability, and many other tactics are used to push forth the strategy of change. Wescott et al. (2021a) presented a Preliminary Analysis of the United Nations Partnership on the Rights of Persons with Disabilities programme within the context of the CRPD and the Sustainable Development Goals.

Case Study 2: A Country Level Example of the Work of the UNPRPD: Deinstitutionalization and promotion of assisted decision-making in Moldova.

The ratification of the UN CRPD by the Republic of Moldova in 2010 marked important changes in the field of disability. In relation to deinstitutionalization, the Republic of Moldova approved the National Program on the Deinstitutionalization of Persons with Intellectual and Psychosocial Disabilities and the Action Plan for 2018–2026 (Government of the Republic of Moldova, Ministry of Health, Labour, and Social Protection, 2018). In the three years prior to the programme there were over 12,000 complaints from 3,665 people who used (many involuntarily) institutionalized mental health or intellectual disability services in Moldova (UNPRPD, 2018). Throughout implementation, the four partner agencies had quarterly meetings to assess progress and discuss challenges and potential threats to the successful implementation and strategize further steps (UNPRPD, 2018). In addition, UN implementing partners used, on a quarterly basis, the already existing governmental platforms, such as the National Council on Disability and the National Council on Child Protection, to bridge and consolidate partnerships across different partner ministries and other state entities directly responsible for the outcomes of the intervention (UNPRPD,

2018). As a result of the UNPRPD programme, the first Organization of Users of Psychiatry was created and empowered to participate in the promotion of disability rights (UNPRPD, 2018). Experts participated at every major event to guarantee that the voices of persons with disabilities were at the forefront of the project. As a result of UNPRPD support, this organization convened and filed a request for official registration with the Ministry of Justice (UNPRPD, 2018). The group commented on CRPD Committee Draft General Comment on Article 12: Equal recognition before the law. UNPRPD enabled work to create independent bodies that will monitor the implementation of the Convention, in line with its Article 33(2) (United Nations Development Group, 2015).

The Moldovan government also adopted a national policy on deinstitutionalization of adults with mental and intellectual disabilities and established community mental health centres in each of the country's 26 districts (UNPRPD, 2016). Two years later, the number of beds in large psychiatric institutions was reduced by 40%. In a landmark case, the Court of Justice upheld the right of an 18-year-old woman with intellectual disability to her own supported-decisions (opposed by her parents); and this led to the introduction of a programme to facilitate the legal capacity (decision-making capacity with necessary assistance) for people with intellectual disability (UNPRPD, 2016). Both the judge and legal aid lawyer in this case had participated in training on the CRPD provided by the UNPRPD project in Moldova. The project also achieved notable progress with regard to inclusive education (see UNPRPD, 2016, for more details of programmatic impact in Moldova and the other countries in the first round of the programme). According to the Ministry of Health, Labour, and Social Protection report Republic of Moldova (2020) on the UNCRPD, the National Agency for Social Assistance (NASA) reported that at the beginning of 2020 there were 1696 persons with disabilities, of them 812 women and girls, in residential institutions. In the context of deinstitutionalization and preventing new entrances of the women with disabilities in institutions: the National Program on Deinstitutionalization of Persons with Intellectual and Psychosocial Disabilities, including women in residential institutions, managed by NASA, was developed and approved, for 2018–2026. During 2017–2020, about 200 persons with disabilities were deinstitutionalized in community-based services and/or biological/extended families or independent living (Keystone Moldova, 2020, 2022). It is important to note the lack of longitudinal data to understand the impacts of deinstitutionalization (and other country interventions) beyond project timelines, particularly regarding the experiences of people with disabilities impacted by the project. Additional research is necessary to better understand how projects transition out of a country, how the next steps in service development are handled, and how these relate to meaningful outcomes for individuals. For instance, it is important to know for individuals the sort of domicile, degree of integration, and support from community they experience, as well as their opportunities for meaningful activity such as employment, volunteering, or education. Without such indicators the effects of systems and organizational change on an individual's quality of life will remain unknown.

Discussion

ToCs in international development draw on a variety of sources, including needs assessments, previous evaluations, research, and the perspectives of experts, staff, partners, and community members (Rogers, 2014). We have used this approach in our knowledge management training, and elsewhere, along with the ideas of Pierre Bourdieu (1977, 1986) who recognized the importance of power relations, symbolism, different forms of capital (beyond financial) and the general idea that the privileged often prefer to maintain things as they are (Wescott et al., 2021b; Wescott & MacLachlan, 2021). While Bourdieu's sociological scholarship was largely focused on social class, it has also been applied to other areas including disability (Byrne, 2018; Wescott et al., 2021a; Wescott & MacLachlan, 2021; Wescott, 2024) and is an important component of political economy analysis—how power and resources are distributed (Collinson, 2003). Acknowledging and finding ways to work with or around position, power, and privilege is central to the process of using a ToC approach as it is often these factors that resist change. While their role in the global theory of change presented in Case Study 1 is perhaps less apparent, it is in the implementation of these broad drivers of change at the country and local level, where power relations, contextual differences, and systems readiness to change kick in.

In Case Study 2, removing people from institutional settings and giving them more decision-making power was central to the work of the UNPRPD. Mental health and disability professionals and their representative professional bodies hold significant 'capital', in Bourdieu's terms. They also often constitute hierarchies of dominance. Thus, just as social dominance theory can be applied to societal oppression of people with disabilities, including mental health conditions (Sidanius et al, 1994), legitimizing myths can also be utilized to protect hierarchy and power differences which may exist within and between different professions. Addressing the containment and decision-making power of people/patients affects the privilege and status of different professions in different ways—some have more to lose than others. And so, it is not surprising that professions can often be a significant barrier to change which seeks to promote human rights. Of course, deinstitutionalization only works where adequate provision has been made for people who often have very significant support needs, to be so supported in community settings. In many counties, including many rich countries, this may not be the case. As such, sometimes it can be difficult to disentangle statements from professions expressing genuine concerns for service user's welfare, from the interests in those professions maintaining positions of power and privilege.

De Silva et al. (2014) suggest that the ToC approach has several distinct advantages: it makes explicit causal pathways without imposing pre-defined structure; it is more flexible than linear logic models; it allows for multiple causal pathways, along with interventions at different levels and feedback loops. This, therefore, allows ToC to represent more usefully how complex interventions happen. As De Silva et al. argue 'ToC is not a sociological or psychological theory such as Complexity Theory or the

Theory of Planned Behaviour, but a pragmatic framework which describes how the intervention effects change. The ToC can be strengthened by inserting sociological or psychological theories at key points to explain why particular links happen' (p.2). While the ToC approach has been used in a range of project contexts (see Connell & Kubisch, 1998, Breuer et al., 2014, Breuer et al., 2016), we are not aware of its previous use at the national level to address social structural change from a rights-based perspective, or for people with disabilities. As other aspects of the KnowUNPRPD project have been described elsewhere (see Wescott et al, 2021; Wescott & MacLachlan, 2021; Wescott et al, 2023; Wescott, et al., 2021a, Wescott, 2024), this paper focuses only on the ToC component of this broader programme of work.

Conclusions

Psychosocial and more general social science skills have an important role in the design, implementation, and evaluation of theories of change that seek to challenge and address social injustice at a national or regional level (MacLachlan & McVeigh, 2021). Such interventions should not replace other interventions at individual, family, group, or organizational level, but rather complement them and provide a broader planned framework in which the interactive effects of different types and levels of intervention can be collectively harnessed. An appreciation of contextual constraints and opportunities will be critical to make change happen through resources available in more local contexts. A multi-layered and contextually sensitive application of social science can contribute substantially to change at all levels, including the social structures and institutions that form an important context for how we live.

Reflective Questions

1. Big picture—little picture: sometimes the systems we work in seem just too big or too complex to change and we focus instead on what is immediately in front of us, in the hope that we will at least help some people. Do you do this and if so, what is in the big picture which discourages you from addressing it?
2. Identify a particular change that is needed in some aspect of the services in your country and identify who are the main stakeholders (potential winners or losers, influencers, gatekeepers, etc) who would need to be 'got on-board', to allow such a change to happen. How would you 'get them on-board'?
3. Draw a Venn diagram of three interlocking circles, with the titles 'What's in my own best interests?', 'What's in the best interest of my profession?', and 'What's in the best interest of people using our services?' Start in the middle of the intersecting circles and draw an arrow from that point to lower on the page, and then list those things where all three interests overlap. Do the same for the

spaces on the diagram where two of them overlap, and for where there is no overlap between them.

4. Change may be resisted because it's a bad idea. But it may also be resisted because it will impact on personal or professional standing. What sort of change can you think of which may well be a good idea, but would impact in an undesirable way on either your own or others' personal or professional standing?

5. Should governments sign up to implementing human rights legislation only once their systems are ready to respond to those rights, or before they are ready, so as to propel the obligation to change the system?

Funding

This research was funded by the Irish Research Council in Ireland [GOIPG/2019/674].

Acknowledgments

We wish to extend our gratitude to the participants in the United Nations Partnership on the Rights of Persons with Disabilities (UNPRPD).

Further Reading

1. To explore structural change, and thus their theories of how change is made as an iterative and ongoing process: Asada, Y., Gilmet, K., Welter, C., Massuda-Barnett, G., Kapadia, D., & Fagen, M. (2019). Applying theory of change to a structural change initiative: Evaluation of model communities in a diverse county. *Health, Education & Behavior, 46*(3), 377–387.

2. While this example is from a different context, this book offers an operational view into the unseen barriers and complexity of changing large organisations: Pahlka, J. (2023). Recoding America: Why government is failing in the digital age and how we can do better. Metropolitan Books.

3. To shed light on a UNPRPD country project with details of how the programmatic framework was used in practice: Wescott, H., Ferri, D., & MacLachlan, M. (2023). Participation, legal capacity and gender: Reflections from the United Nations Partnership on the Rights of Persons with Disabilities project in Serbia. *Disabilities, 3*(1), 129–146.

4. How to identify good local practices and then scale them to regional or national level in an inclusive way in this paper: Sanchez Rodriguez, A. M., MacLachlan, M., & Brus, A. (2021). The coordinates of scaling: Facilitating inclusive innovation. Systems Research and Behavioral Science, 38(6), 833–850.

References

Asada, Y., Gilmet, K., Welter, C., Massuda-Barnett, G., Kapadia, D., & Fagen, M. (2019). Applying theory of change to a structural change initiative: Evaluation of model communities in a diverse county. *Health, Education & Behavior, 46*(3), 377–387.

Bourdieu, P. (1977). *Outline of a theory of practice.* Cambridge University Press.

Bourdieu, P. (1986). The forms of capital. In J. Richardson (Eds.), *Handbook of Theory and Research for the Sociology of Education* (pp. 241–258). Westport, CT: Greenwood.

Breuer, E., De Silva, M. J., Fekadu, A., Luitel, N. P., Murhar, V., Nakku, J., Petersen, I., & Lund, C. (2014). Using workshops to develop theories of change in five low- and middle-income countries: lessons from the programme for improving mental health care (PRIME). *International Journal of Mental Health Systems, 8*(1), Article 15. https://link.springer.com/article/10.1186/1752-4458-8-15

Breuer, E., De Silva, M. J., Shidaye, R., Petersen, I., Nakku, J., Jordans, M. J., Fekadu, A., & Lund, C. (2016). Planning and evaluating mental health services in low-and middle-income countries using theory of change. *The British Journal of Psychiatry, 208*(s56), s55–s62. https://doi.org/10.1192/bjp.bp.114.153841

Byrne, B. (2018). Dis-equality: exploring the juxtaposition of disability and equality. *Social Inclusion, 6*(1), 9–17. https://www.ssoar.info/ssoar/handle/document/57051

Collinson, S. E. (2003). *Power, livelihoods and conflict: case studies in political economy analysis for humanitarian action*. London: Humanitarian Policy Group, Overseas Development Institute. https://odi.org/en/publications/power-livelihoods-and-conflict-case-studies-in-political-economy-analysis-for-humanitarian-action/

Connell, J. P., & Kubisch, A. C. (1998). Applying a theory of change approach to the evaluation of comprehensive community initiatives: progress, prospects, and problems. In K. Fulbright-Andersen, A. Kubisch, & J. Connell (Eds.), *New approaches to evaluating community initiatives Vol. 2: Theory, Measurement, and Analysis* (Vol. 2, pp. 1–16). The Aspen Institute of Human Studies. http://www.dmeforpeace.org/wp-content/uploads/2017/06/08071320AppllyingTheoryofChangeApproach.pdf

De Silva, M. J., Breuer, E., Lee, L., Asher, L., Chowdhary, N., Lund, C., & Patel, V. (2014). Theory of change: a theory-driven approach to enhance the Medical Research Council's framework for complex interventions. *Trials, 15*(1), 267. https://www.ncbi.nlm.nih.gov/pubmed/24996765

de Waal, A. (2003). Human rights, institutional wrongs. In D. Dijkzeul, & Y. Beigbeder (Eds.), *Rethinking international organisations: Pathology and promise* (pp. 234–260). New York: Berghahn Books.

Goodley, D., & Lawthom, R. (2006). *Disability studies and psychology: New allies*. Palgrave Macmillan.

Government of the Republic of Moldova, Ministry of Health, Labour, and Social Protection. (2018). National Program on the Deinstitutionalization of Persons with Intellectual and Psychosocial Disabilities and the Action Plan for 2018–2026. https://www.unwomen.org/sites/default/files/Headquarters/Attachments/Sections/CSW/64/National-reviews/Republic_of_Moldova.pdf

Grenfell, M., & Lebaron, F. (2014). *Bourdieu and data analysis: Methodological principles and practice*. Oxford: Peter Lang AG. https://doi.org/10.1002/9780470672532.wbepp253

Keystone Moldova. (2020). Deinstitutionalization of persons with disabilities in Moldova: Recommendations for 2021–2027. https://www.inclusion-europe.eu/wp-content/uploads/2020/11/Position-Paper-Deinstitutionalization-of-Persons-with-Disabilities-in-the-Republic-of-Moldova-EN.pdf

Keystone Moldova. (2022). Written submission to the UN Committee on the Rights of Persons with Disabilities on the draft guidelines on deinstitutionalization, including in emergencies.

Laing, K., & Todd, L. (2015). Theory-based methodology: Using theories of change in educational development, research and evaluation. Research Centre for Learning and Teaching, Newcastle University.

Levitt, J. (2017). Exploring how the social model of disability can be re-invigorated: in response to Mike Oliver. *Disability and Society 32*(4), 589–594. https://doi.org/10.1080/09687599.2017.1300390

MacLachlan, M. & Mannan, H. (2016). Stepping back to move forward. In UNPRPD (Ed.), *Connections: Building partnerships for disability rights* (pp. 102–104). New York: UNPRPD Secretariat. http://mptf.undp.org/document/download/16578

MacLachlan, M., & McVeigh, J. (Eds.) (2021). *Macropsychology: A population science for sustainable development goals.* Springer.

Marks D. (1997). Models of disability. *Disability and rehabilitation, 19*(3), 85–91. https://doi.org/10.3109/09638289709166831

Power, A., Lord, J., & DeFranco, A. (2013). *Active Citizenship and Disability: Implementing the Personalisation of Support* (Cambridge Disability Law and Policy Series). Cambridge University Press.

Pratto, F. & Stewart, A. (2012). Social dominance theory. In J. Daniel, & C. Christie (Eds.), *The encyclopedia of peace psychology.* Blackwell Publishing Ltd. https://doi.org/10.1002/9780470672532.wbepp253

Republic of Moldova. (2020). Implementation of the UN Convention on the rights of persons with disabilities. https://ms.gov.md/wp-content/uploads/2020/12/Report-II-and-III-Implementation-of-CRPD_EN.pdf

Rogers, P. (2014). Methodological briefs – theory of change. Florence: UNICEF Office of Research. http://www.entwicklung.at/fileadmin/user_upload/Dokumente/Evaluierung/Theory_of_Change/UNICEF_Theory_of_change.pdf

Sanchez Rodriguez, A. M., MacLachlan, M., & Brus, A. (2021). The coordinates of scaling: Facilitating inclusive innovation. *Systems Research and Behavioral Science, 38*(6), 833–850.

Sidanius, J., Liu, J., Pratto, F., & Shaw, J. (1994). Social dominance orientation, hierarchy-attenuators and hierarchy-enhancers: Social dominance theory and the criminal justice system. *Journal of Applied Social Psychology, 24,* 338–366.

Taplin, D., & Clark, H. (2012). *A primer on theory of change.* New York. ActKnowledge. http://www.theoryofchange.org/wp-content/uploads/toco_library/pdf/ToCBasics.pdf

UN General Assembly. (2006). Convention on the Rights of Persons with Disabilities, A/RES/61/106, Annex I. https://www.refworld.org/docid/4680cd212.html

United Nations Development Group. (2015). Eight case studies on integrating the United Nation' *Normative and Operational Work.* https://unsdg.un.org/sites/default/files/Normative-Operational-Study-FINAL.pdf

United Nations Development Programme (UNDP). (2020). UNPRPD strategic operational framework. https://unprpd.org/new/wp-content/uploads/2023/12/UNPRPD-SOF-2020-2025-ACC_0-737.pdf

United Nations Development Programme (UNDP). (2016). Connections: Building partnerships for disability rights. New York: UNPRPD Secretariat. https://unprpd.org/resources/

UNPRPD. (2016). Paradigm Shift: UNCT Moldova Strategic Action Supporting CRPD Implementation. https://unprpd.org/new/wp-content/uploads/2023/12/Moldova_End_of_Project_Report_Phase_I-01e.pdf

UNPRPD. (2018). Intersections: Finding common ground to advance the rights of persons with disabilities. New York: UNPRPD Secretariat.

Vogel, I. (2012). *Review of the use of 'Theory of Change' in international development.* London: UK Department of International Development. https://assets.publishing.service.gov.uk/media/57a08a5ded915d3cfd00071a/DFID_ToC_Review_VogelV7.pdf

Wescott, H. N., MacLachlan, M., & Mannan, H. (2021a). Disability inclusion and global development: A preliminary analysis of the United Nations Partnership on the Rights of Persons with Disabilities programme within the context of the Convention on the Rights of Persons with Disabilities and the Sustainable Development Goals. *Disability, CBR & Inclusive Development, 31*(4), 90–115.

Wescott, H., & MacLachlan, M. (2021). Implementing 'real' change: a Bourdieusian take on stakeholder reflections from the United Nations Partnership on the Rights of Persons with Disabilities project in Uruguay. *SN Social Sciences, 1*(12), Article 282. https://doi.org/10.1007/s43545-021-00280-w

Wescott, H., Credit, K., Tatic, D., Lorell, C., & MacLachlan, M. (2023). Full and meaningful participation: considerations for engaging persons with disabilities in development projects. In M. Meyers, M. McCloskey & G. Petri (Ed.), *Hierarchies of Disability Human Rights.* Routledge.

Wescott, H., MacLachlan, M., & Mannan, H. (2021b). The macropsychology of disability rights and structural change: Using Bourdieusian analysis to understand stakeholder power relations. In M. MacLachlan & J. McVeigh. (Eds.), *Macropsychology – A population science for Sustainable Development Goals* (pp. 175–188). Springer.

Wescott, H. (2024). *Disability inclusion and structural change: Understanding the relationship between stakeholders in the United Nations Partnership on the Rights of Persons with Disabilities (UNPRPD) programme.* [PhD thesis], Maynooth University.

Winance, M. (2016). Rethinking disability: Lessons from the past, questions for the future. Contributions and limits of the social model, the sociology of science and technology, and the ethics of care. Repenser le handicap: leçons du passé, questions pour l'avenir. Apports et limites du modèle social, de la sociologie des sciences et des techniques, de l'éthique du care. *Alter, 10*(2), 99–110.

World Health Organization & World Bank. (2011). *World report on disability.* https://www.who.int/teams/noncommunicable-diseases/sensory-functions-disability-and-rehabilitation/world-report-on-disability

13

Mental Health e-Technologies

Derek Richards

Introduction

Mental health e-technologies use available technology to deliver mental health services. These include teletherapy, telepsychiatry, self-guided mental health apps, online support groups, and guided digital interventions. These are increasingly used as treatment options in service provision. Based on the available clinical and cost-effectiveness evidence and acceptability, expert consensus recommends incorporating and utilizing these innovations within healthcare (Mohr et al., 2021). Several countries have developed virtual clinics that provide a range of mental health e-technologies in service delivery (Harty et al., 2023; Titov et al., 2018). Their inclusion in clinical guidelines has been endorsed in several jurisdictions (National Institute for Health and Care Excellence, 2023a, 2023b; Therapeutic Goods Administration, 2023). Despite the challenges with successfully implementing mental health e-technologies, the compelling assertions about their potential to enhance accessibility, eliminate disparities, and lower costs are noteworthy (Mohr et al., 2017). If these promises prove true, there is a substantial possibility that they could bring about a significant transformation in mental healthcare, offering a more accessible, equitable, and cost-effective approach to evidence-based treatment (Mohr et al., 2017). Such a promise supports the human right to access appropriate healthcare (United Nations, 1948; World Health Organization, 2008).

By providing mental health services through digital interventions, individuals who may not have otherwise been able to access care due to geographic location, transportation or financial barriers, or stigma can now receive treatment (Richards et al., 2019). Mental health e-technologies increase accessibility and convenience of care, reduce stigma, and deliver evidence-based treatments with fidelity; they are user-centred, and help address the pressing shortage of licensed professionals. Consequently, they assist in reducing the treatment gap in mental healthcare and positively impact the significant burden of mental health disorders globally. However, because of their flexibility and scalability, digital treatments should not axiomatically be identified as a panacea for the pressures on service delivery due to the shortage of trained professionals, the lack of access to evidence-based treatments, or the mental health challenges embedded in our globalized world, commonly related to the social inequities they arguably accentuate (Davies, 2021; Kelly, 2003). Additionally, the evidence demonstrates that a sizable proportion of the global population lacks access to the infrastructure, commodities, and capabilities for participation in digital life, thus propagating existing inequalities in opportunity and access to appropriate healthcare (O'Sullivan et al., 2021). This amounts to a significant global human rights challenge across healthcare.

Historically, mental health e-technologies have been standalone or point solutions for specific disorders or populations. Modern and advanced platform technologies are now overtaking point solutions with diverse capabilities, products, and services, providing an integrated system for technology-delivered services. The age of the mental health platform is upon us. The 'platformization' of industries is not new: it has developed with both positive and negative consequences across retail (e.g., Amazon), transport (e.g., Uber), banking (e.g., Revolut), and food (e.g., Deliveroo) (Lehdonvirta et al., 2020). Platforms create an ecosystem of consumers, suppliers, and services (Baldwin & Woodard, 2011); their technical infrastructure, governance, security, privacy contracts, and practices can have significant consequences for human rights protection, both in the opportunities they offer and the potential harm they can cause (Jørgensen, 2019).

Generally, platforms deliver their products and services while extracting as much data as possible to feed their precision algorithms (Zuboff, 2019). Therefore, data is viewed as capital and is very much in keeping with the neoliberal philosophy underpinning '*big tech*' (Crawford, 2021). Arguably, '*big techs*' commercial pursuit has transformed '*human subjects*' into '*data subjects*,' where all human experience is potentially the raw material of value (Crawford, 2021; DeNardis, 2020; Véliz, 2021). Modern technology platforms typically include data extraction and analytics, various applications and tools, and intelligent technologies such as artificial intelligence (AI) and the Internet of Things (IoT). Our digital world, however, is quickly moving to what DeNarids (2020) describes as the cyber-physical world. Developments in virtual reality (VR) and augmented reality (AR) technologies, and in the Internet of Bodies (Self) (biometric sensors and neurotechnology), will inevitably expand the capabilities of (mental health) platforms. In tandem, they will collect and process vast quantities of personal and sensitive data, particularly concerning aggregated, anonymized, or deidentified data, which will increasingly appropriate our personal lives. As Zuboff writes, 'the rendition of data relentlessly seeks to erode any boundaries around the self, whether physical, mental, psychological, or emotional' (Zuboff, 2019).

Advanced mobile and connected platform technologies introduce unprecedented multi-dimensional datasets of behavioural surplus rendered from our physical, mental, psychological, and emotional lives, and their computational methods provide hope for tailoring and optimizing psychological and psychiatric treatments (Insel, 2023; Tal & Torous, 2017; Zuboff, 2019) For example, machine learning could use clinical, biological, and social data to augment decisions associated with diagnosing, prognosis, and treating people with mental illness (Dwyer et al., 2018). This promise would revolutionize mental healthcare; it would reduce the uncertainty of diagnosis and prognosis and increase effectiveness (currently, psychotherapeutic and pharmaceutical treatments are effective in 30–50% of service users) by allocating service users to treatments that maximized their clinical benefit, thereby reducing overall suffering and resource consumption. Several reviews summarize the work (Aafjes-van Doorn et al., 2021; Dwyer et al., 2018; Shatte et al., 2019).

Platforms for mental health raise human rights concerns, including data breaches, bias and discrimination, and scope creep (Sun et al., 2020). Concerns exist about collecting and using personal data and sensitive health information, and about the potential for sharing this data with third parties without informed consent. For example, several entities have reported instances where service user data was shared inappropriately, without consent, or hacked, and service users were blackmailed (Federal Trade Commission, 2023; Hern, 2017; Kleinman, 2020; Lovett, 2023). There is even greater concern about the potential for machine learning to infer insights from such data. The literature is replete with examples of poorly designed machine learning algorithms, which can harm vulnerable and marginalized groups, even when they 'work' (Eubanks, 2019; O'Neil, 2016). Moreover, as we enter a more cyber-physical world, the implications of data acquisition and governance become more profound. Are we prepared to collect and derive insights from data gathered within and beyond our bodies across our physical, mental, psychological, and emotional lives?

The evolution of the mental health platform and the move to the cyber-physical world bring novel opportunities for enhanced treatments. Irrespective of the technology architecture of mental health platforms or their computational models, privacy challenges (e.g. data governance, consent, ownership) arise (Taddeo & Floridi, 2018). The human right to privacy (United Nations, 1948) has broad implications for individuals, becoming more acute for vulnerable persons who have necessarily been afforded special protections (United Nations, 1991, 2006). Therefore, regarding the moral limits of personal and sensitive data acquisition and analysis (the right to privacy), we urgently need clarification on potential human rights challenges in the 'age of the platform' for vulnerable groups such as those with mental health disorders.

Case Study

Mental health e-technologies have become commonplace in mental health services. One example is the UK NHS Talking Therapies Service, which has used various mental health e-technologies over the past 15 years. The service uses a stepped-care model to triage service users to low-intensity (e.g., guided digital interventions, bibliotherapy) or high-intensity (e.g., face-to-face therapy) interventions. Currently, mental health e-technologies are becoming even more essential, especially in light of recent funding pressures that have led to increased targets for access to care (access targets increased from 15% to 25%) (Mental Health Taskforce, 2016). Mental health platforms will likely play an increasingly important role in service delivery and treatment in the coming decade.

This is sometime in the not-too-distant future, and talking therapies continue at a pace. Most service users are provided treatment via the digital health platform.

In recent years, Bobo has had several personal setbacks, including dropping out of university, losing his job, and failing in relationships. He has been to see many medical doctors and specialists, who have offered a range of innovative interventions; individually, they have been of little consequence to him. It is time for a change, and Bobo self-referred to the Talking Therapies service via the web portal. His two-minute voice message left during intake procedures details that he is depressed. His recent neurotechnology implant details cognitive and brain dysregulation, poor concentration, and psychomotor agitation, corroborating his voice analysis findings. Not surprisingly, these findings were further illuminated by his Bluetooth biometric device embedded in his arm last year. The details highlight central features of depression symptoms, including his poor sleep and lack of exercise. The technology platform underpinning the Talking Therapies mental health service leverages its embedded precision treatment algorithm (built from 2 million previous service users) to deliver a personalized treatment package. Treatment includes a low dose of Bluetooth-enabled intelligent antidepressants, which regulate the release and uptake of the active ingredient, alongside a course of cognitive behavioural therapy guided by his chatbot that has already consumed his total medical and personal history, including his social media and work history. A licensed 'low-intensity' professional monitors the treatment, and clinical decisions are based on insights inferred from ongoing weekly data acquisition (via voice recordings, neuroanalysis, biometric feeds, passive data from his phone, and social media usage) and their analysis. After three months of treatment, the various data show that his cognition, emotions, and behaviours are better regulated; his symptom profile has altered; he has increased concentration and less psychomotor agitation; his circadian rhythms are regulated; he is beginning to exercise and has engaged positively with his social life (at least his virtual social life). He is ready to get on with life, perhaps even to find a job!

Analysis

The case study might sound like science fiction, but it is not. Voice analysis for emotion and affect detection has already been developed (Harati et al., 2022). Likewise, various biometric identification systems are highly developed and widely used, including the ability to scan and analyse fingerprints, voice, facial features, iris patterns, palm veins, and movement (DeNardis, 2020; Farahany, 2023). Similarly, neurotechnology is developing fast, and our brain data may be more unique than our fingerprints (De Ville et al., 2021). Inferential insights using machine learning and 'precision' algorithms in mental health treatment are increasingly practised (Topol, 2019). The intelligent pill has already been devised and regulated (Litvinova et al., 2022). Chatbots for mental health are increasingly deployed in treatment (Denecke Kerstin & Abd-Alrazaq, 2021). These various developments are considered part of the Internet of Self. The evidence for using these technologies, individually and collectively, in clinical practice is only beginning to emerge. The potential impact of these technologies and the insights derived from their data on the diagnosis and treatment of mental health could lead to profound epistemological shifts, perhaps evolving our current approaches. As noted earlier, platforms have transformed other industries in unimaginable ways, and we can thus be optimistic that these innovations will potentially alter our current mental healthcare models.

As illustrated in the case study, such technological developments relegate the traditional online and offline divide; cyber-physical firmly embeds the internet into the material world, which has profound implications for security, privacy, and democracy (DeNardis, 2020). These developments raise significant human rights questions, which become more pronounced with vulnerable groups who, at times, already experience a lack of agency, reduced autonomy, invasions of privacy, curtailment of expressions, and a lack of ability to participate in social life. In this present but future case scenario, the difficulty is the significant potential risk to our right to privacy concerning personal and sensitive data acquisition and analysis, including freedom from interference in personal information and the ability to be left alone and forgotten (Latanero, 2018). Gathering our concerns about the move to a data-centric world, as described in the case study, we can consider a meta-category: the 'datafication of life'. Digitalization is the rendering of, for instance, books or music into digital content; 'datafication', on the other hand, renders previously unquantified aspects of the world (physical, mental, psychological, or emotional) into digital formats for tabulation and analysis (Renieris, 2023).

Consider the Talking Therapies treatment and monitoring algorithm mentioned earlier. The data gathered and analysed in surveillance may become an authority beyond its merits, invested with credibility that outstrips its achievements (Hong, 2020). A related concern is that as AI becomes increasingly embedded in all aspects of our lives, we may become nonchalant about its presence, almost as if it were a natural force like gravity (Roose, 2021). In particular, these databases and algorithms are ripe with biases and heuristics that rely on arbitrary classifications, messy data, and many other concealed uncertainties (Hong, 2020). Data used in algorithm development are generally not representative and, therefore, not generalizable. They risk flattening complexity and can lead to essentialist understandings, promoting bias and discrimination (Crawford, 2021). The 'black box' (explainability) is not necessarily new to psychology and psychiatry (e.g., parsing the relative contributions of specific vs non-specific factors in treatment success). However, many argue that such black boxes in healthcare should be 100% explainable (Topol, 2019). Otherwise, we risk allowing big data's 'rationality' to extend across boundaries, social, political, and personal, with the likely result of privileging technocratic automation over individual experience: our lived experience, our interpersonal and intrapersonal lives, our fantasy, transference, our emotional life (joy, fears, likes, and loves), behavioural adaption, ambiguity, uncertainty and cognitive biases, all of which is the 'stuff' of psychology and psychiatry.

Intervention

Privacy and confidentiality have been ethical cornerstones in psychology and psychiatry practice, first, because the information is sensitive; it details our most personalized nature, our mental and emotional states; and second, for reasons to do with the well-documented prejudice and discrimination that so often accompanies the stigma of a mental health disorder. Without consideration and respect for the vulnerable position of individuals seeking mental health treatments, we introduce a level of risk to people's privacy that can have dire consequences across many areas of life: employment, insurance, education, relationships, and other opportunities (Gates & Arons, 2000). Personal health data is already a refined commodity in the healthcare marketplace, especially in the United States (Tanner, 2017); it seems that now, in the age of platforms for mental health and the increased rendering of our lives as data, these risks have become more pronounced (Crawford, 2021; DeNardis, 2020; Véliz, 2021).

Clinicians subscribe to the Hippocratic oath and practice in the context of a code of ethics based on beneficence (doing good), non-maleficence (not causing harm), autonomy (the right of service users to make their own decisions), and justice (to distribute resources equitably). How can these deontological principles protect vulnerable people in the datafication of life that so typifies mental health platforms? The risk of amplifying existing power asymmetries between vulnerable people seeking mental health treatment and the providers that collect voluminous data on their delivery requires clarification. The privacy of individuals' health data and clinical records is generally limited by informed consent, laws, medical ethics, and state and national policies that protect consumers (Gates & Arons, 2000). In summary, how can we assuage the potential asymmetries in data collected and analysed from vulnerable groups, such as those with mental health problems, to prevent breaches, biases, and discrimination?

Theory

Drawing on empirical research, Tomasello (2016) describes the 'Interdependence Hypothesis' to specify the evolution of morality for human cooperation. It is precisely here that we can set the stage for the evolution of human rights as a set of values determining the 'good society'. His two-stage theory focuses on dyadic cooperation in early hunter-gatherers and on group-minded cooperation in early cultural groups. He argues that morality based on these stages emerged due to (a) changes in ecology over time (environmental changes, food availability, increases in population, and group competition), (b) obligations to forage collaboratively and initial cultural organization for group survival, and (c) moving from dyadic to collective cognitive, cultural, and self-regulation abilities. He writes that 'each mode of social engagement represents a distinct set of biological adaptations for coping with distinct forms of social life (Tomasello, 2016)'. This empirically supported evolution of morality lays the foundational scripts for the development of sociality, group cooperation, and self-regulated and self-governed culture and society. In this evolutionary account, the literature suggests that humans have innate psychological capacities for morality (akin to those for language), which animate our collective adaptation and survival. It underpins the social contract upon which we evolve a good society (Ramen & Schulz, 2020). It is the basis of our human rights, advocacy, campaigning, regulation, laws, and institutions.

Evolutionary theory can help us understand human rights in establishing a good society that can adapt and survive. The good society is supported by contemporary empirical work in human rights research, including, for example, the number of countries that have abolished capital punishment, trends in genocide and politicide, reductions in violence, famine, infant mortality, and undernourishment, and access to education and sex and gender equality (Sikkink, 2019). Sikkink (2019) demonstrates the progress and regress of human rights across many areas over time and shows how evolution is neither linear nor perfect. Sikkink (2019) distinguishes between ideal and non-ideal theory, where empirical work evaluating the success of human rights advances held to the 'ideal' standard is unforgiving and can lead to pessimism about human rights outcomes. Commensurate with an evolutionary approach, it is more appropriate to understand progress against evolving, contextualized, and historical contexts. The evolutionary approach can be further specified to demonstrate how individual rights require 'contextual integrity' (Nissenbaum, 2010). For instance, privacy must be appropriate to a given context, in this case, treating service users' mental health disorders in the age of mental health platform technologies and their capabilities.

Rights Reflection

From a human rights perspective, current articulations of rights to privacy need to evolve, as rights that fail to adapt to new realities are likely to be eroded by indifference, irrelevance, and defiance (Ramen & Schulz, 2020). Digital technologies have transformed the economy and society. Data is at the centre of this transformation, resulting in the increasing datafication of life and a data-centric view of privacy (Renieris, 2023). According to Renieris, we have repeatedly centred data over people in our regulations and laws to govern technology platforms. She argues that by framing data governance as our challenge, we lean on data as abstract and neutral, arguably easier than speaking about asymmetries of power, inequality, bias, exploitation, racism, and other mounting challenges posed by digital technologies. The right to privacy predates the digital age (Diggelmann & Cleis, 2014), and we need a return to an understanding of privacy that prioritizes the protection and safety of *people*. According to Renieris, if we continue on the current path, 'our data will end up with more rights and protections than we do,' which will not facilitate the building of consensual norms about how we wish to interact with each other in a technology-mediated world. In summary, we must move from a data-driven to a human rights-centred notion of privacy.

To offset the pervasive use of data and to guard against data breaches, bias and discrimination, and scope creep (Sun et al., 2020), the original rights-based conceptualization of privacy and data protection needs to resurface, focusing on protecting people rather than merely data security and protection. To that end, some argue for establishing normative limits (or indeed a complete ban) on the rendition and datafication of aspects of our lives and experience, especially domains of our inner life and experience, our unexpressed thoughts, feelings, inclinations, and emotions (Renieris, 2023; Véliz, 2021). Indeed, this is especially important with deanonymized, deidentified data used in machine learning and the development of AI-driven algorithms that seek to infer our mental or emotional states' physiological or psychological properties; indeed, whether this is deemed personal data and therefore covered by existing laws and governance standards is debatable (Renieris, 2023; Zuiderveen Borgesius, 2020).

However, the proposal to limit data rendition and analysis may unduly compromise innovation and the promise of tailoring, developing, and optimizing psychological and psychiatric treatments. There are, however, developments that could aid in a path forward. More specifically, the technology architecture of platforms and the computational models they employ can be considered, as well as the principle of privacy by design (Hartzog, 2018), which aims to embed privacy into the creation, processing, and operations of technology. After that, privacy-enhancing technologies (PETs) may offer more confidence. PETs aim to integrate data from diverse sources securely and efficiently, guarantee data is used only for intended purposes, and disseminate outputs while preventing reverse engineering. Among the available technical solutions are multiparty computation and homomorphic encryption, along with the creation of secure enclaves to support data input privacy. Output privacy can be enhanced via methods such as statistical disclosure controls, differential privacy, the creation of synthetic data, and federated learning; for more details, see Royal Society (2023). Different input and output PET methods arrangements may be appropriate for various contexts. As with PETS, machine learning algorithms are not immune to interference attacks, and work to develop systematic, quantitative privacy risk auditing methods is underway (Hunt et al., 2018; Shokri et al., 2017; Ye et al., 2022).

However, PETs will no doubt be subject to the criticism of seeking technocentric solutions for human confidentiality, privacy, and security (Renieris, 2023). Therefore, we can also bolster traditional approaches based on policy, regulation, and jurisprudence. For instance, the American Data Privacy and Protection Act, introduced to the US Congress in 2022, would be the first federal legislation on privacy protection in the digital world since 1970. The EU has the General Data Protection Regulation (GDPR), which imposes data protection requirements on any entity, regardless of location. It gathers fundamental principles (lawfulness, fairness, transparency, purpose, minimization, accuracy, storage limitation, integrity, confidentiality, and accountability; for more detail, see https://gdpr.eu/) and significant penalties for non-compliance. The EU has also published its AI Act and established the European AI office to implement the world's first comprehensive AI law (see https://tinyurl.com/5as9dsbd). The literature also includes strengthening cybersecurity, stopping the trade in healthcare data, stopping default personal data collection, creating digital regulatory agencies, and updating antitrust, freedom of information, and criminal and administrative laws (DeNardis, 2020; Véliz, 2021; Zuiderveen Borgesius, 2020).

Finally, traditional human rights promotion activities can be important, including, for example, service user empowerment, advocacy, and updating professional training on new technologies. Also necessary are professional practice updates to guidelines and regulations, continuing professional training and development, and ongoing research. Collectively, these reflections help us to think about protecting the privacy of vulnerable individuals in the age of the platform for mental health. Our efforts may allow us to realize the potential for innovative technologies and novel computational techniques to enhance psychological treatments while protecting human rights: this would indeed amount to a public good.

Questions and Thought Experiments

How might you describe to clients the current and future use of their data in AI-driven e-technologies?

Are there circumstances to deny some individuals access to and use e-technologies for mental health treatment? And what are the reasons?

How might you accurately present the benefits of mental health e-technologies for users?

How should professional bodies seek to update current standards for ethical practice to cover mental health e-technologies?

How might you present potential opportunities and challenges for using mental health e-technologies with peer professionals?

What potential concerns or misgivings might arise for people about mental health e-technologies?

Further Reading

DeNardis, L. (2020). *The Internet in everything*. Yale University Press.
Renieris, Elizabeth. M. (2023). *Beyond data*. MIT Press.
Ramen, S., & Schulz, W. F. (2020). *The coming good society*. Harvard University Press.
Tomasello, M. (2016). *A natural history of human morality*. Harvard University Press.

References

Aafjes-van Doorn, K., Kamsteeg, C., Bate, J., & Aafjes, M. (2021). A scoping review of machine learning in psychotherapy research. *Psychotherapy Research*, *31*(1), 92–116. https://doi.org/10.1080/10503307.2020.1808729

Baldwin, C. Y., & Woodard, J. C. (2011). The architecture of platforms: a unified view. In A. Gawer (Ed.), *Platforms, Markets and Innovation* (pp. 19–44). Edward Elgar Publishing Ltd. https://doi.org/10.4337/9781849803311

Crawford, K. (2021). *Atlas of AI: Power, politics, and the planetary costs of artificial intelligence.* Yale University Press.

Davies, J. (2021). *Sedated: How modern capitalism created our mental health crisis.* Atlantic Books.

De Ville, D. Van, Farouj, Y., Preti, M. G., Liégeois, R., & Amico, E. (2021). When makes you unique: Temporality of the human brain fingerprint. *Science Advances 7*(42), eabj0751. doi: 10.1126/sciadv.abj0751

DeNardis, L. (2020). *The Internet in everything: Freedom and security in a world with no off switch.* Yale University Press.

Denecke, K., Abd-Alrazaq, A., & Househ, M. (2021). Artificial intelligence for chatbots in mental health: Opportunities and challenges. In M. Househ, E. Borycki, & A. Kushniruk (Eds.), *Multiple perspectives on artificial intelligence in healthcare: Opportunities and challenges* (pp. 115–128). Springer. https://doi.org/10.1007/978-3-030-67303-1_10

Diggelmann, O., & Cleis, M. N. (2014). How the right to privacy became a human right. *Human Rights Law Review, 14*(3), 441–458. https://doi.org/10.1093/hrlr/ngu014

Dwyer, D. B., Falkai, P., & Koutsouleris, N. (2018). Machine learning approaches for clinical psychology and psychiatry. *Annual Review of Clinical Psychology, 14,* 91–118. https://doi.org/10.1146/annurev-clinpsy-032816-045037

Eubanks, V. (2019). *Automating inequality: How high-tech tools profile, police, and punish the poor.* St. Martin's Press.

Farahany, N. A. (2023). *The battle for your brain.* St. Martin's Press.

Federal Trade Commission. (2023, July 14). *FTC Gives Final Approval to Order Banning BetterHelp from Sharing Sensitive Health Data for Advertising, Requiring It to Pay $7.8 Million.* Federal Trade Commission. https://tinyurl.com/3a5j3srz

Gates, J. G., & Arons, Bernard. S. (2000). *Privacy and confidentiality in mental health care.* Brooks Publishing.

Harati, A., Rutowski, T., Lu, Y., Chlebek, P., Oliveira, R., Shriberg, E., & Lin, D. (2022). Generalization of deep acoustic and NLP models for large-scale depression screening. In I. Obeid, J. Picone & I. Selesnick (Eds.), *Biomedical Sensing and Analysis* (pp. 99–132). Springer. https://doi.org/10.1007/978-3-030-99383-2_3

Harty, S., Enrique, A., Akkol-Solakoglu, S., Adegoke, A., Farrell, H., Connon, G., Ward, F., Kennedy, C., Chambers, D., & Richards, D. (2023). Implementing digital mental health interventions at scale: One-year evaluation of a national digital CBT service in Ireland. *International Journal of Mental Health Systems, 17*(1), 1–11.

Hartzog, W. (2018). *Privacy's blueprint: The battle to control the design of new technologies.* Harvard University Press.

Hern, A. (2017, July 3). Royal Free breached UK data law in 1.6m patient deal with Google's DeepMind. *The Guardian.* https://www.theguardian.com/technology/2017/jul/03/google-deepmind-16m-patient-royal-free-deal-data-protection-act?CMP=share_btn_url

Hong, S. (2020). *Technologies of speculation: The limits of knowledge in a data-driven society.* NYU Press.

Hunt, T., Song, C., Shokri, R., Shmatikov, V., & Witchel, E. (2018). *Chiron: Privacy-preserving machine learning as a service.* http://arxiv.org/abs/1803.05961

Insel, T. (2023). Digital mental health care: five lessons from Act 1 and a preview of Acts 2–5. *NPJ Digital Medicine, 6*(1), Article 9. https://doi.org/10.1038/s41746-023-00760-8

Jørgensen, R. F. (2019). Rights talk: In the kingdom of online giants. In R. F. Jørgensen (Ed.), *Human Rights in the Age of Platforms* (pp. 163–187). MIT Press.

Kelly, B. D. (2003). Globalisation and psychiatry. *Advances in Psychiatric Treatment, 9*(6), 464–470. https://doi.org/10.1192/apt.9.6.464

Kleinman, Z. (2020, October 26). *Therapy service user blackmailed for cash after clinic data breach*. BBC News Website. https://bbc.com/news/technology-54692120

Latanero, M. (2018). Big data analytics and human rights. In M. K. Land & J. D. Aronson (Eds.), *New technologies for human rights law and practice* (pp. 149–161). Cambridge University Press. https://doi.org/10.1017/9781316838952

Lehdonvirta, V., Park, S., Krell, T., & Friederici. (2020). *Platformization in Europe*. https://tiny url.com/bdfca6ta

Litvinova, O., Klager, E., Tzvetkov, N. T., Kimberger, O., Kletecka-Pulker, M., Willschke, H., & Atanasov, A. G. (2022). Digital pills with ingestible sensors: Patent landscape analysis. In *Pharmaceuticals, 15*(8), Article 1025. https://doi.org/10.3390/ph15081025

Lovett, L. (2023, March 13). Cerebral reveals it shared patient health information with third-party advertisers, social media companies. *Behavioural Health Business*. https://tinyurl.com/34drmjxj

Mental Health Taskforce. (2016). *The five-year forward view for mental health*. https://www.engl and.nhs.uk/mental-health/adults/nhs-talking-therapies/

Mohr, D. C., Azocar, F., Bertagnolli, A., Choudhury, T., Chrisp, P., Frank, R., Harbin, H., Histon, T., Kaysen, D., Nebeker, C., Richards, D., Schueller, S. M., Titov, N., Torous, J., & Areán, P. A. (2021). Banbury Forum consensus statement on the path forward for digital mental health treatment. *Psychiatric Services, 72*(6), 677–683. https://doi.org/10.1176/appi.ps.202000561

Mohr, D. C., Weingardt, K. R., Reddy, M., & Schueller, S. M. (2017). Three problems with current digital mental health research and three things we can do about them. *Psychiatric Services, 68*(5), 427–429. https://doi.org/10.1176/appi.ps.201600541

National Institute for Health and Care Excellence. (2023a). *Digitally enabled therapies for adults with anxiety disorders: early value assessment (HTE9)*. www.nice.org.uk/guidance/hte9

National Institute for Health and Care Excellence. (2023b). *Digitally enabled therapies for adults with depression: early value assessment (HTE8)*.www.nice.org.uk/guidance/hte8

Nissenbaum, H. (2010). *Privacy in context: Technology, policy, and the integrity of social life*. Stanford University Press.

O'Neil, C. (2016). *Weapons of math destruction: How big data increases inequality and threatens democracy*. Crown.

O'Sullivan, K., Clark, S., Marshall, K., & MacLachlan, M. (2021). A Just Digital framework to en-sure equitable achievement of the Sustainable Development Goals. *Nature Communications, 12*(1), 1–4, Article 6345. https://doi.org/10.1038/s41467-021-26217-8

Ramen, S., & Schulz, W. F. (2020). *The coming good society: Why new realities demand new rights*. Harvard University Press.

Renieris, E. M. (2023). *Beyond data: Reclaiming human rights at the dawn of the metaverse*. MIT Press.

Richards, D., Enrique, A., & Palacios, J. (2019). Internet-delivered cognitive behaviour therapy. In S. Parry (Ed.), *The handbook of brief therapies: A practical guide* (pp. 173–187). Sage.

Roose, K. (2021). *Futureproof*. John Murray.

Royal Society. (2023). *From privacy to partnership*. The Royal Society.

Shatte, A. B. R., Hutchinson, D. M., & Teague, S. J. (2019). Machine learning in mental health: A scoping review of methods and applications. *Psychological Medicine, 49*(9), 1426–1448. https://doi.org/10.1017/S0033291719000151

Shokri, R., Tech, C., Stronati, M., & Shmatikov, V. (2017). Membership inference attacks against machine learning models [Conference Session]. *IEEE Symposium on Security and Privacy*, California, United States. https://doi.org/10.48550/arXiv.1610.05820

Sikkink, K. (2019). *Evidence for hope: Making human rights work in the 21st century*. Princeton University Press.

Sun, N., Esom, K., Dhaliwal, M., & Amon, J. J. (2020). Human rights and digital health technologies. *Health and Human Rights Journal, 22*(2), 21–32.

Taddeo, M., & Floridi, L. (2018). How AI can be a force for good. *Science, 361*(6404), 751–752. https://doi.org/10.1126/science.aat5991

Tal, A., & Torous, J. (2017). The digital mental health revolution: Opportunities and risks. *Psychiatric Rehabilitation Journal, 40*(3), 263–265. https://doi.org/10.1037/prj0000285

Tanner, A. (2017). *Our bodies, our data: How companies make billions selling our medical records*. Beacon Press.

Therapeutic Goods Administration. (2023). *Digital tools and medical devices: Guidance for the mental health sector*. Australian Government Department of Health and Aged Care.

Titov, N., Dear, B., Nielssen, O., Staples, L., Hadjistavropoulos, H., Nugent, M., Adlam, K., Nordgreen, T., Bruvik, K. H., Hovland, A., Repål, A., Mathiasen, K., Kraepelien, M., Blom, K., Svanborg, C., Lindefors, N., & Kaldo, V. (2018). ICBT in routine care: A descriptive analysis of successful clinics in five countries. *Internet Interventions, 13*, 108–115. https://doi.org/10.1016/j.invent.2018.07.006

Tomasello, M. (2016). *A natural history of human morality*. Harvard University Press.

Topol, E. (2019). *Deep medicine: How artificial intelligence can make healthcare human again*. Basic Books.

United Nations. (1948). *Universal Declaration of Human Rights*. https://tinyurl.com/3v2snad3

United Nations. (1991). *Principles for the protection of persons with mental illness and the improvement of mental health care*.

United Nations. (2006). *Convention on the Rights of Persons with Disabilities*.

Véliz, C. (2021). *Privacy is power: Why and how you should take back control of your data*. Melville House Publishing.

World Health Organization. (2008). *The Right to Health*. https://tinyurl.com/2p8867sp

Ye, J., Maddi, A., Murakonda, S. K., Bindschaedler, V., & Shokri, R. (2022). Enhanced membership inference attacks against machine learning models [Conference session]. *ACM Conference on Computer and Communications Security,* Los Angeles, United States. https://doi.org/10.1145/3548606.3560675

Zuboff, S. (2019). *The age of surveillance capitalism: The fight for a human future at the new frontier of power*. Profile Books.

Zuiderveen Borgesius, F. J. (2020). Strengthening legal protection against discrimination by algorithms and artificial intelligence. *International Journal of Human Rights, 24*(10), 1572–1593. https://doi.org/10.1080/13642987.2020.1743976

14

Emerging Ethical Issues on Different Mental Health Conditions/Personality

Edmund G. Howe III

Introduction: Treating One Patient For Longer or Helping More Patients?

Psychiatrists in the United States working within institutions must regularly decide how long they will treat a patient. These psychiatric 'sessions' are one resource discussed here, but other countries might have scarcities of different resources, and so this chapter's overall reflections are generalizable. The duration of the care they give may be based on findings empirically established. Even here, however, they may have to make subjective ethical judgments. Guidelines, even for short-term treatments, provide a range of recommended sessions. Thus, providers may have to choose between more sessions or fewer (Erekson, 2022). A question more ethically taxing arises when they know that other patients also need their help, but they want to treat a patient longer despite the fact that this will deprive these other patients of treatments these psychiatrists could otherwise offer them (Gaskell et al., 2023). Whose need then should prevail?

This micro-allocation question may in some cases be decided for providers by their organization's policy. Patients may, for example, have only limited numbers of visits available to them (Bailey et al., 2021). This piece will not address the public policy question as to who should have access to psychiatric treatments. It rather will discuss how psychiatrists should decide this when this is within their discretion (Campbell and English, 2011; McAleavey et al., 2017). It will focus then on how, ethically, mental health workers of all sorts may best go about making the above micro-allocation decision that may confront them when they see that patients need longer require further care (Kent et al., 2020). A case paradigmatic of this problem will be presented and the ethical questions such cases raise analysed. The extent to which therapists can resolve this and other ethical conflicts by rational argumentation and what they should do when they can't will also be addressed. Finally, suggestions will be made regarding core concerns that providers may want to consider how providers when the confront the ethical decisions considered here.

The overall aim of this inquiry will be to suggest an outcome possibly different from what psychiatrists may now believe they should do. This piece is intended to provide therapists ethical grounds for pursuing some patients' long-term needs so that they can have increased quality in their lives, though providers may reasonably anticipate that if they do this, other patients who could benefit from their treating them instead will not.

Initial Case Example: What of Patients Who Mostly Just Talk?

An example illustrating the ethical conflict between treating a patient longer and treating more patients is offered by a patient I saw who had been homeless (Meja-Lancheros et al., 2020). He would speak over and over about his past trauma from the moment he first would enter my office until after he left (Lallier et al., 2023). I could hardly get a word in to comment or ask questions and when I did, he would usually respond in a few words, only then to continue saying whatever he was sharing. There was little I could do other than listen. He took medications but these lowered his pressured speech only to a limited extent. He had a full-time care giver who brought him to and from the clinic.

I wondered after having seen him for some time whether I should decrease the frequency of our sessions since I seemed to be helping him only a little, so allowing me time to see other patients whom hopefully, I could help much more. In some contexts, it may be possible and optimal to suggest other alternatives, e.g. a referral for a different type of support such as talk therapy with another provider or group work. In this instance, however, since he had indicated how his meeting with me was so exceptionally important to him, it seemed to me that my raising this possibility of him seeing others, he most likely might take as a deeply disturbing felt rejection and thus or regardless an option he wouldn't follow. To me, the line was paper thin between his continuing to cope reasonable well, notwithstanding his emotional deficits, and his having nothing in his life that he could look forward to.

Analysis: Deontological vs Utilitarian Approaches

How mental health providers should allocate their limited time is a question often common to all. Patients we have been seeing may continue to get better if we continue to see them. We may benefit these patients more especially because we have already gotten to know them. Ethically by continuing to see them longer, we may be fulfilling an implicit promise to them that we will give them the care that they need. Providing benefit is a utilitarian value. It is based on a factual consequence. Fulfilling a promise is a deontological value. It is not based on consequences such as the benefits patients may gain, but on respecting them and what is referred to most often as respecting their dignity as persons (Chochinov, 2007). Some ethicists believe that deontological values should always prevail over values involving utility (Robertson, 2007). In any case, when deontological values are present, they cannot be weighed and contrasted directly against utilitarian values. When deontological values are not present, on the other hand, competing utilitarian values can be weighed against each other and net utilitarian results can be determined. This net result cannot be determined when the key value on one side is treating patients longer to fulfil a promise to them and respect them. Thus, these two moral frameworks, respecting patients and maximizing their gains may be mutually exclusive and not subject to rational argumentation and therefore resolution. A deontological argument can also be extended to a collective group, e.g., people with mental health conditions and respect the dignity of members of that group, independent of utility. An example may be providers contacting loved ones of a seriously mentally ill person to gain more information about them. This may positively influence their ability to treat them, but at this same time may violate their dignity by violating their confidentiality. The goals for both individual patients and these larger groups may, too, differ. The goal of habituation (living with illness) or rehabilitation (recovering from illness) may also be different outcomes that providers may want to consider when deciding which patients they should treat for longer times. This answer may depend, of course, on the effect of patients' illness on their quality of life and may be a question they can and should optimally share with their patients. Ethical analysis may offer then no clear method for resolving the conflict posed by these two competing moral values (Feister, 2007).

Using a paradigmatic example to further illustrate this limitation, we can consider the early months when patients in the United States had COVID (Gaffney, 2022). Multiple approaches then were put forth as to how care providers should best allocate limited resources such as ventilators. Where, for example, ventilators were scarce in supply, agonizing questions existed as to who should be placed on a ventilator when not all patients needing this could be placed on one. A particularly excruciating question was whether providers should ever remove a patient from a ventilator who could survive if kept on it so that this ventilator could save more patients' lives. This dilemma involves providers implicit promise to continue a ventilator once it is started and the stakes here are as high as they can be since this question involves such a patient's life.

Here, too, age was considered as a plausibly valid ground for treating, let us imagine, a person 30-years-old over a patient of 80. The former patient statistically would be expected with the same treatment to live 50 more years. This same net calculation cannot be applied when a deontological value is chiefly at stake. The deontological ethical principle here is justice. This principle applies when this decision between treating the 30-year-old and 80-year- old patient arises (Nielsen, 2022). One means of resolving this could, at least in theory, could be to flip a coin. There are, however, other ways in which this same moral principle, justice, could be applied. The criterion of opportunity to live a full life could be used instead of the value only of life itself. By this criterion, this deontological principle of justice, the ventilator access should be given to the 30-year-old.

Another application of justice is to give most to people worst off (Kneiss, 2021). Providing equitable access to services may mean, for example, allocating proportionately more resources to those who have more barriers to accessing services. This critical consideration may be relevant to all people with disabilities. Applying this criterion of justice to psychotherapy patients then, we might reasonably ask what patients, due to their symptoms or lack of access to psychotherapeutic interventions are worst off and thus on this ground alone these patients might be those that providers should treat longer. More generally, providers assessing justice should initially then consider then which meaning of justice they should use: a life equals a life, access to a full life, or giving priority to those worst off. As we shall see with other examples that follow, there may be several different kinds of patients with mental health needs whose symptoms might place them in this worst-off category.

Conventional Approaches: Doing First or Even Exclusively What Is Evidence-Based

A conventional approach to treating many patients is to use evidence-based approaches at least first, when these approaches are proven, and then to tailor these interventions to patients' individual and even idiosyncratic emotional needs (Hill & Norcross, 2023). Short-term manualized treatment protocols may be an example of this. This limitation may be particularly justified because once patients are helped initially to progress to a certain degree, they may be able to continue then to progress further on their own. This possibility is hoped for and expected, for example, with cognitive therapies. After patients learn to question their own thinking, they hopefully can then go ahead and do this on their own. Some patients, however, may not be able to do this (Goldberg et al., 2018). They may need longer term therapies and only do better with them (Mayotte-Blum et al., 2012). If, in fact, their therapy is stopped, they may go back downhill and regress. These patients may need a long-term relationship with a trusted provider regardless of the specific type of therapy initially used (Birkhäuer et al., 2017). This rationale may be harder to support with empirical data (Kline et al., 2018). Patients' long-term benefits are, for example, more difficult to match against those of a control group. Gains from longer therapy, too, may be subtle. Patients who initially hardly respond to therapists' initial interventions may, over time, for instance, come to respond more. Their progress may not be linear.

If standard treatments do not work, less evidence-based approaches may be successful (Schulz & Hede, 2018). Providers pursuing these additional treatments may though, as a result, again, because of this, not be able to give other patients treatments that they too need. An example illustrating these additional treatments involves patients who have a post traumatic stress disorder that fails to respond to standard interventions. Newer therapies are accelerated resolution therapy (ART) and treatment with psychedelics (Howe et al., 2018). Both may have efficacy, but both also may involve providers treating these patients longer, thus further denying to other patients what these providers could otherwise offer them.

There is a panoply of other treatment interventions that could take additional time. I here will give two additional, more radical examples to especially illustrate the extent to which this same micro-allocation problem can exist. The first example involves an intervention carried out by a psychiatrist, David Mee-Lee, who presented this at a course he gave at an annual American Psychiatric Association meeting, decades ago. He spoke of how he might intervene when a patient with schizophrenia refuses to take psychotropic medicines. Mee-Lee might say, 'Maybe you are right. Maybe these meds won't help you. Would you be open to us together conducting an experiment?' Mee-Lee would then suggest that if the patient answered, 'Yes,' the patient might first go without meds for a time, and then, depending on how this patient did, go on for this same amount of time with meds. They would then both see which approach had the best results and decide this together.

This approach was likely to further two outcomes. First, these patients would be more likely in time to accept taking meds, though they might have a psychotic event due in part to not taking meds before this occurred. Second, the patient's relationship with Mee-Lee would likely be strengthened because they had pursued this experiment together. 'Patients' needs should be served as they present, rather than requiring patients to meet the needs or expectations of treatment' (Gastfriend & Mee-Lee 2022, p. 604). This plan would be shared, that is, not imposed. Mee-Lee informed, of course, other staff in advance, what he was doing and why.

A second example of a perhaps still more radical treatment was one often most associated with Jay Haley and Cloe Madanes. They and others founded Strategic Psychotherapy (Madanes, 1991; Peluso & Freund, 2023; Madanes & Haley, 1977). This therapy may involve working with patients who have not responded to prior therapies, possibly because they tended, reactively, to not respond to pressures from others but rather to oppose such pressures. All of us at some times have such oppositional responses. We do not want to do what another tells us we should do.

Haley shared, as an example, how a patient in his early teens had continued to masturbate in front of guests in his living room whenever his parents entertained. Other psychiatrists' attempts to break him of this behaviour hadn't succeeded. Haley then took another tack. As opposed to his even implicitly encouraging this boy to change, Haley encouraged him to continue doing what he was doing but more so. When at the next session, this boy reported that he failed to do what Haley had instructed to the extent that Haley had urged this, Haley expressed his disappointment. He then upped-this-ante, instructing this boy to masturbate even more and on a fixed schedule. This boy again didn't meet Haley's requirements, Haley responded in the same way, with disappointment. This continued. In a short time, this boy stopped masturbating in the living room altogether (Haley, 1973) This act had become Haley's preference so that this boy, if continuing to do what he had done before, would now be meeting Haley's prescribed agenda, not his own If then this boy's agenda was to oppose or even shock, Haley's tack had deprived him of these underlying, secondary gains. The boy's continuing to do what he had been doing would now be his complying with what Haley had prescribed and not then his alone. While he could still choose not to go along with

Haley's request, he was now in a new position of opposing Haley's request, but he then would be doing what his parent wanted. He was no longer free to make this decision wholly on his own.

I have tried this approach to a full extent only once. I was asked to see a patient whom internists informed me was dying because she had diarrhoea that they couldn't control. She had tried, she said, all standard medications and were even considering the use of 'gold therapy', a treatment sometimes used at this time primarily to treat rheumatoid arthritis, because she saw this as a potentially life-threatening emergency. Gold therapy involves the use of gold salts which are anti-inflammatory component of the metal. It is not in common use at this time. She, I found out, felt guilty because her husband had just died from a long-standing illness. He, too, had had profound diarrhoea. It is tempting to imagine that her diarrhoea stemmed from her identifying with her husband (Corradi, 2011).

She had in any case only once during all this time, which consisted of many months, left his side. She did this over a weekend. She visited relatives a plane flight away. 'I should not have done this,' she cried, when I first saw her. 'I feel so guilty.' I sought to work with her; initially by helping her reframe how she viewed her taking this trip. She might have needed this respite, I suggested, both for herself, and particularly, perhaps, for him. If she was in less pain herself as a result of this trip, it seemed reasonable, I suggested, that she would then be better able to offer him the love and support that he needed and that she wanted to give him. She would have none of this.

Meanwhile, her physical condition and risk of dying, her doctors told me, continued to get worse. I, then, wholly at loose ends, adopted a Haley-inspired, paradoxical intervention. I said finally to her, 'Well, perhaps you are right. Maybe you shouldn't have gone away, and thus maybe you should feel guilty.' She reversed herself then and for the very first time immediately defended herself. 'What are you talking about?' she retorted. 'You know nothing. I needed that time away.' The next day I repeated what I had said. She got angrier and after a few days, when she saw me poking my head in her door, would yell at me to get away. Yet, through these days, as she got angrier and angrier at me, her health got better. Her diarrhoea soon stopped, and she left the hospital just two weeks' later. Such paradoxical interventions carry risk and have ethical issues in and of themselves.

Such paradoxical interventions carry risk and have ethical issues in and of themselves. In this instance, for example, this patient may have simply not improved and only acquired, as a result of my interventions, greater distrust.

Moral Theory: How Far Can It Take Us?

The above examples raise the question how far we should go to continue to try to help one patient at the expense of a greater number of others. An analogous question arises for many health providers concerned with limiting one patient's extensive use of resources in short supply so that they can use these same resources to treat greater numbers of other patients. This common dilemma is worth our looking at in more detail to best understand how different moral theories may or may not apply. For instance, staff may want to stop treating a patient in part because they think that this treatment is futile. In many countries, laws allow them to stop, and some hospitals have specific rules that allow this also. These providers' stopping treatment may be supported also by these decisions saving resources. These providers, in addition, may view their continuing treatment in these instances as death-prolonging, as opposed to life-prolonging. Patients and families may, though, want a new treatment such as dialysis started even though this will prolong their loved one's life for no more than a week or so. The patient and family may both find even at this time seven more days or so as most meaningful. Their providers may though overrule them (Grassi et al., 2017).

All providers may feel moral distress (Vig, 2022). All may balk at the thought of acting against what they believe is right. These families may feel bitter about the patient's providers going against them for the rest of their lives. How, using moral theory, might this impasse be assessed resolved?

Providers should be aware that while both they and patients and families opposing them have power, theirs may be greater (Cassell, 2005). They may fear that patients may sue, but while this is true, this risk may not be close to the ease with which they may deny patients treatments that they see as futile. Providers risk then more imposing their view, not because they have this ethical justification, but because they have greater power to impose their view (Croskerry, 2015; Saposnik et al., 2016; Featherstone et al., 2020; Thirsk et al., 2022). Further, they may see reasons that support their view more than they see other equally valid reasons that oppose it. Then, they may additionally see their view as more justified than that of these others, but not know this Veatch, 1973; Hirsch et al., 2016).

The critical awareness regarding moral theory then may not be to know how to apply it but to know that ethical analysis may be limited. It may not allow a sound resolution in many cases (Fiester, 2007). In many contexts, a sound ethical analysis may provide a likely best answer, but in other instances, it cannot. Providers knowing this can at least then not be in as much risk of imposing their moral view and by doing this unjustifiably harm (Gibson, 2005). They can instead, then, seek other means of resolution such as changing the question from what they should do to who should decide. Here there may be mutual agreement. When a child is profoundly ill and there is no unequivocal reason that this child should be kept alive or allowed to die, all may agree to leave this decision to the parents since they are closest to their child and will live more than others with whatever they decide.

There is, of course, also, good reason to allow the parents to avoid this decision, by giving them the option of letting healthcare providers decide. This might diminish future regret or self-questioning. The value of 'You decide, doctor' is greatly underappreciated in an academic literature that values autonomy far more than most patients do, and implicitly denigrates many patients' desire to hand that autonomy to others.

On this other hand, if parent do defer this decision to their child's providers, they may later regret not having made this decision on their own. The value of 'You decide, doctor' is may be underappreciated in an academic literature since, especially in the United States, providers may value autonomy more than most patients do, in part to offset the excessive paternalism to which providers have been prone and much criticized for in the past. This bias in favour of autonomy may implicitly denigrate many patients' desire to hand over that autonomy to their providers others. Providers, patients, and families might alternatively decide to seek to resolve their differences of opinion through a medical mediator who will seek to see if there is some compromise with which all can agree.

Rights: Should They Prevail over the Care Perspective?

There is a limitation of ethics in practice that goes beyond this, beyond the limits of what ethical analysis can offer (Carson & Lepping, 2009). This is that patients and families, to respond to ethics maximally, must need to feel safe and sufficient trust (Fett et al., 2022). Practically then providers may need to seek to establish this trust more than they need to determine answers to more abstract questions as those establishing their own or their patients' rights (Veatch,1998).

This proposition is in fact embodied in an additional approach to ethical conflicts known as the Care Perspective (van Dijke et al, 2023). This framework may conflict with principle-based reasoning (Tronto, 2009; Jager & Perron, 2018). This approach highlights patients' and their families' relationships with each other and with their providers. It also gives more priority to feelings. Some advocates of this perspective assert that words alone can't adequately capture the nuances of people's relationships and emotions. The practical implication of this additional framework is then that providers may in some cases do ethically better by attending to patients' and families' feelings as opposed to what they believe, rightly or otherwise, to be right (Floresco, 2015). This might mean, then, using the prior example involving dialysis, that accepting the patient's and family's heartfelt desire so that they may have for one more week together may be warranted. Providers may see this goal as superseding the question who should prevail. Their retaining a mutually felt alliance may result in these parties wanting to walk out of the hospital hand-in-hand and together.

How might this emphasis on feelings occur? I recall when five siblings' mother had been in an ICU for weeks, remaining unresponsive. Her providers had done all they could to no avail. Thus, they wanted to meet with this family to tell them that they thought it was time to discontinue her treatment. They called me in as an ethics consultant. The staff wanted to withdraw her treatment because they believed it was futile. They shared this, and this family felt enraged. The five family members sat on my left, and the five staff members to my right. Each sat across from each other. These numbers suggest incidentally an important consideration: providers arranging such meetings should ensure that patients and their families—having less power—have enough persons with them to feel safe and supported (Little et al., 2018; Pluhar et al., 2019). The number of people necessary to achieve this is subjective. This number depends on what these people feel. A still possibly better seating arrangement—in similar circumstances might be to try to avoid 'them and us' seating, by mixing participants up. This may, though leave patient and their families feeling less secure. What they want and how they feel safest may be, then, the optimal criteria for making this seating arrangement.

The staff presented their case. One member, the family's informal leader, then said, 'But, you haven't yet come up with a diagnosis for our mother. Thus, isn't it more likely that she could recover and even get well?' The staff then reiterated why they thought she would not. I then spoke out, 'Is the family not right? There is no diagnosis and thus it would be more likely that she could get better' (Linton et al., 2017). The staff looked at me then, it seemed to me, angrily. And understandably. I had, I imagined they thought, betrayed them. I was one of them, also a staff member, at their same hospital. In the role of an ethics consultant, I had an especially absolute ethical obligation to ensure that all valid considerations were adequately fleshed out and evident to all on their decision-making table, though each 'side' would inevitably be more prone to favour the side that they were on. This obligation exists for all ethics consultants, and, patients getting well despite providers' best prognosis—that maybe they could not—is a perhaps rare, but not so uncommon occurrence. Then, however, this family leader spoke. 'Maybe the staff is right,' she said, reversing her own and her family's view. 'Maybe it is time that we should just let our mother go.' Her four other siblings then too, along with her, reversed themselves and agreed with her, their leader. This patient then ironically did do well and went home after all her treatments were withdrawn.

Patients may and do, of course, sometimes, albeit perhaps not commonly, respond in ways that providers haven't predicted. Patients with illness they and their providers believe is surely fatal may, for example, ask their providers how long they believe they have to live and providers maybe reluctant to answer for this reason.

The change in this loved one's response and the other loved ones with her too may occur not so uncommonly. One way of understanding this response or reaction is that once a provider also support an opposing person's view, they may feel less need to rigidly adhere to their position wholly on their own. With their entire focus and emotional energy not then wholly tied up in this way; they may be able to think newly about other, even opposite possibilities. This may be what happened with all in this case.

To ascertain when there may be injustice, providers may do best by asking themselves with every patient they see what they might want if they had with them a specialist on their medical disorder, an ethicist, and lawyer, and if they were rich. If using this hypothetical, they would want some other medical treatment, the principle of justice would suggest that, at least at this first cut, they should have it. What would be the result of this question if applied to my patient who had been homeless (Mezzich et al., 2017)?

Another approach is to consider this dilemma using the philosopher John Rawl's veil of ignorance thought experiment. He suggested that the best approach we could use to decide who should receive limited resources would be for us to all imagine that we were under a veil such that we don't know anything about others or ourselves. We could then be born or have become, for instance, blind, deaf, and without arms or legs, just to use these examples to illustrate his point. We would generally want to adopt then he posits, a social policy that would give us all, notwithstanding our deficits a meaningful quality of life. He favours then our giving at least limited priority to people worst off and our doing this even if this increases the gap between persons rich and poor. He does not though extend this framework to people throughout the globe. This important extension, of course, requires, then further initiative (Rawls, 1971) ().

Here, even this question, clarifying justice, wouldn't, though, help us. The Care Perspective, however, might (Carse, 1991). Returning to the considered patient in the 'Initial Case Example' section, it would suggest that based on the relationship we already had, which was like that of a family member, my continuing to see him at the frequency we had been seeing each other might more be the right thing for me to do.

Questions: Who, If Anyone, Should We Continue to See?

One unanswered question posed always is when providers should not seek ethics consultation first, but should seek medical mediation. This same question may arise, as well, in other contexts such as the law. Medical mediators undergo specific training in mediation and as a result have supreme skills, non-verbally as well as verbally, to convey that they are not judging. This training may be provided, for example, in courses or much longer educational opportunities that include practical application with experienced mentors over time. They also are especially skilled in eliciting deeper values within stake holders who initially differ. They seek then to help others, though initially diametrically opposed, to arrive at some compromise position that all can agree on and then not leave the hospital bitter.

I recall as an example of such an outcome a case in which a young man was dying of cancer. His staff believed he had six months to live. He was unconscious due to a bodily infection caused by an abscess. This abscess could be relieved by surgery his doctors believed. This would leave him conscious for these six months. They asked should they do this surgery? He might rather they did not. They asked his wife. She was his legally designated surrogate decision-maker (Kaebnick, 2017). His wife said he would not. His parents and adult siblings said he would. He is 'a fighter', they said. Ethics and the law prescribed that the doctors go forth based on whatever his wife would say that she thought he would have wanted. The task posed to the family then would be for them to forgive. All did not go this way. They agreed on a compromise solution like that they might have reached through mediation (Bergman & Fiester,

2015). He would have the surgery and have a do not resuscitate (DNR) order. This would have required his providers to not try to restart his heart in case he had a cardiac arrest. He had the surgery, recovered consciousness, and said what his wife had said he would want—not to have had the surgery.

This case raises a related question. Suppose that in a similar case a patient is unconscious or lacks capacity and surrogate decision-makers again are called in. Their task would be again to say what they think the patient would want—not, though, what they would want. There is, though, this likelihood—the patient may most likely want whatever it is they would want, if the patient had been asked. Should, then, the patient's provider tell these surrogate decision-makers how the law works initially and before they express themselves? Then they could say that what they think the patient would want was whatever they would want (Howe, 2020). This may seem only a way to skirt the law. This is, at the same time though, informing these surrogates of public information they should be enabled to know.

A key over-arching question posed in this piece is when, if ever, a psychiatrist should continue to treat patients even knowing that this would leave other patients wanting. We have seen in some detail one patient posing this question. I will say still later what I did. But there are numerous other examples. Considering these extends the application of this question.

An additional example is any patient who hurts greatly as one who feels even suicidal when stressed. These patients may endure this pain between appointments but hang on through these times because they know that they will see their therapist soon. This group includes those whose spirit is similarly sapped by a medical condition that leaves them suffering throughout every day (Strojan et al., 2017) These patients too may be able to carry on with a sense of meaning in their life in part because they look forward to therapy sessions because they can then share their pain with someone who will hopefully not so much respond by becoming depressed.

Suggestions: Choosing What We Can't Know

Many clinical outcomes lack answers. Patients may, for example, undergo trauma to their head or undergo a stroke and then be unconscious. It may not be knowable then whether they have or do not have inner awareness or will later regain this (Murtaugh et al., 2023). Whether or not these patients have awareness may be inferred by providers asking them questions and then seeing how their brain responds, using technologies such as an electroencephalogram (Wang, 2023). If these patients respond consistently, providers can infer that they have some awareness. When these patients show no evidence of awareness, their families may want these patients kept alive and their providers to regularly check for their awareness in case they develop this. If they are aware, families may want to tell them what they believe might be meaningful to these patients. There is no way to predict though whether this awareness will later occur.

Psychiatrists may have some ethical justification in continuing to keep these patients alive if this occurs, though, as a result of their doing this, they again would not be able to treat other patients who also would benefit from their care. This may fulfil a deontological value and an Ethics of Care by again giving exceptional weight to relationships and these families' and possibly, as well, these patients' feelings (Norcross & Wampold, 2018; Wampold, 2015).

More generally, providers may often, justifiably give priority to how patients will respond emotionally. If patients feel greater trust, they may respond better to all interventions. (Baier, 2020; Norberg, et al. 2017). Psychiatrists should seek then to increase this trust (Birkhäuer et al., 2017; Norcross & Lambert, 2011). A most illustrative paradigmatic example of this opportunity is when patients' individual providers first imagine that an ethical conflict could be brewing and thus forthcoming. They could then inform patients and families of this and tell them that if this conflict does arise, they will support what these patients and families want and will do this regardless of what they themselves believe. This is, of course, the opposite of providers putting first their own moral views or conscience (Churchill, 2019). Though legally they can put their own moral views first, this too may wholly erode patients' and families' trust.

Another paradigmatic example illustrates this still further. Patients commonly ask their doctors what they would do in their shoes. We need to respect patients' desire for this information, along with all the objective pros and cons of whatever in the end patients decide. To presume that they will be disproportionately influenced by our answer is disrespectful of their autonomy and of their decision to ask in the first place.

Providers sometimes say, 'No, I can't tell you, because I'm not you.' This response risks, however, leaving these patients feeling emotionally abandoned. Rather, providers might say that they will answer, but ask if they might share first with them the pros and cons of their doing this and then they can decide together whether to proceed with their responding to the patient's request. The main positive benefit from the provider's sharing this is to provide new thoughts to the patient (Pelto-Piri et al., 2013) Two cons are, however, also possible. Both may occur if the outcome for the patient is a bad one. If the patient decides what to do on the basis of what the provider has said or to not go with this this, they may blame themselves more in either case.

This sharing departs from some providers' view that they should at all cost remain neutral. They may reason, 'I should be neutral and only share information, leaving decision-making wholly up to my patients.' This view misses, however, ways in which they can benefit their patients (Cohen, 2020). An ethically preferable view may be to share with patients whatever they may have overlooked that might be important to them (Halpern, 2001). A patient wanting all-out care if later permanently unconscious may, for example, not have considered that this ongoing treatment could use up money, this patient had carefully saved to be able to fund a grandchild's college education.

How, then, might all these considerations bear on how long psychiatrists should continue to treat patients like the patient who spoke continually with whom I began this discussion. I thought I was doing him little good. Just as I was about to reduce the frequency of our sessions, he told me as if out-of-the-blue that the only moments he looked forward to and found meaningful in his life were his sessions with me (Frankl, 2006; Mulahalilović et al., 2021).

This is not uncommon. Patients' knowing that they can look forward to a future session, as I've said above, can alone sometimes sustain them through close-to-unbearable times. I feel some shame now that I failed to even imagine this with the above patient. That this may be possible is a chief underlying theme of this chapter. Psychiatrists are most often rightly wedded to empirical, evidence-based findings. These may not exist, but patients can find meaning from longer care that they could not gain in any other way (Hemberg et al., 2022). Our continuing to see some patients who want this may alone keep them from becoming worse (Knapp, et al. 2021). The regression this may prevent may, however, not be detectable. We don't see what doesn't occur. Outcomes prevented include, of course, patients being hospitalized and even their taking their lives (Li et al., 2020). This patient I've discussed? I continued to see him at the same frequency.

Questions

Numerous or at least difficult questions come up in regard to truth telling, especially when patients have fatal conditions.

1. What should providers, including those only doing psychotherapy, do when they know or suspect that a patient has a fatal disease but hasn't yet been told that this is possible or probable?
2. What, if anything, should a provider or therapist say if a family contacts them, prior to the diagnosis of a possibly lethal condition asking that if this is the case? Should the provider tell the family, not this patient? (This is the practice and preference in many cultures and even between neighbours in cultures absolutely committed to respecting individual patients' autonomy.)
3. What, if anything, should a provider or therapist do when a child has a fatal illness but this child's parents and providers won't tell this to the child? (Children may in these circumstances already know or be quite sure, but feel painfully isolated as a result of having no one with whom they can discuss their fears.). Does the age of the child matter, here? If so, how so?
4. What, if anything, again, should a provider or therapist do when parents have given birth to their stillborn infant or an infant who is alive but will shortly die and they are filled with grief and may not want to see or touch this infant? Some parents, here, having just experienced these terribly sad circumstances may fare profoundly better, later on, if they can and do see and hold these infants. They may even want then to later try to have children, though without this seeing and touching they may remain traumatized so that they do not want to ever

have children and more importantly perhaps still may grieve and always re-member and be preoccupied with this sad memory for the remainder of their lives. The core problem here is that if these parents' providers or therapists sug-gest that for these reasons they see and hold these infants, these parents experi-encing wracking grief and disappointment at this time may see them as almost incomprehensively insensitive and lose their trust in them and all desire to con-tinue to see them.

5. When, if ever, should therapists, on their own initiative suggest to their patients that they reconsider or consider mire deeply decisions they have made? (Prime examples are those that can occur at the end of life. The patient may for example want to undergo an experimental therapy for lethal cancer highly unlikely to succeed and that will require the patient to most likely live out his her or their final days alone and away from family. And, on the other extreme they may want assistance in dying when they have undergone physical losses and find no more meaning in life but plausibly, possibly or even probably could. See *Albert Camus, A Happy Death* (Penguin Modern Classics).

Disclaimers

Suggestions for further reading

Kelly, R. E. Jr, Ahmed, A. O., Hoptman, M. J., Alix, A. F., & Alexopoulos, G. S. (2021). The quest for psychiatric advancement through theory, beyond serendipity. Brain Science *12*(1), 72. doi: 10.3390/brainsci12010072

Kane, N. B., Ruck Keene, A., Owen, G. S., & Kim, S. Y. H. (2022). Difficult capacity cases-the experience of liaison psychiatrists. An interview study across three jurisdictions. *Frontiers in Psychiatry, 13*, Article 946234. doi: 10.3389/fpsyt.946234

Shadbolt, C. (2020). Psychotherapy in the time of COVID-19 (psychotherapy changes shape and steps forward). *Psychotherapy and Politics International, 18*(3), Article e1552. doi: 10.1002/ppi.1552

Avasthi, A., Grover, S., & Nischal, A. (2022). Ethical and legal issues in psychotherapy. *Indian Journal of Psychiatry, 64*(Suppl 1), S47–S61. doi: 10.4103/indianjpsychiatry. indianjpsychiatry_50_21

References

Baier, A. L., Kline, A. C., & Feeny, N. C. (2020). Therapeutic alliance as a mediator of change: a systematic review and evaluation of research. *Clinical Psychology Review, 82*, Article 101921. doi: 10.1016/j.cpr.(2020).101921

Bailey, R. J., et al. (2021). Busy therapists: examining caseload as a potential factor in outcome. *Psychological Services, 18*(4), 574–583.

Bergman, E. J., & Fiester, A. (2015). Teaching and learning the techniques of conflict resolution for challenging ethics consultations. *The Journal of Clinical Ethics, 26*(4), 312–314.

Birkhäuer, J., et al. (2017). Trust in the health care professional and health outcome: A meta-analysis. *PLoS One, 12*(2), Article e0170988. doi: 10.1371/journal.pone.0170988

Campbell, A. T., & English, A. (2011). Law, ethics, and clinical discretion: Recurring and emerging issues in adolescent health care. *Adolescent Medicine State of the Art Reviews, 22*(2), 321–334.

Carse, A. L. (1991). The 'voice of care': Implications for bioethical education. *The Journal of Medicine and Philosophy, 16*(1), 5–28.

Carson, A. M., & Lepping, P. (2009). Ethical psychiatry in an uncertain world: Conversations and parallel truths. *Philosophy, Ethics, and Humanities in Medicine, 4*, Article 7. doi: 10.1186/1747-5341-4-7

Cassell, E. J. (2005). Consent of obedience? Power and authority in medicine. *New England Journal of Medicine, 352*(4), 328–330.

Chochinov, H. M. (2007). Dignity and the essence of medicine: The A, B, C, and D of dignity conserving care. *British Medical Journal, 335*, 184–187.

Churchill, L. R. (2019). Conscience, moral reasoning, and skepticism. *Perspectives in Biology and Medicine, 62*(3), 519–526.

Cohen, S., et al. (2020). Paternalism and certitude. *Bioethics, 34*(5), 478–482.

Corradi, R. B. (2011). The role of identification in dynamic psychiatry and psychotherapy. *Journal of the American Academy of Psychoanalytic Dynamic Psychiatry, 39*(3), 539–561.

Croskerry, P. (2015). When I Say… cognitive debiasing. *Medical Education, 49*(7), 656–657.

Erekson, D. M., et al. (2022). Psychotherapy session frequency: A naturalistic examination in a university counseling center. *Journal of Counseling Psychology, 69*(4), 531–540.

Featherston, R., et al. (2020). Decision making biases in the allied health professions: A systematic scoping review. *PLoS One, 15*(10), Article e0240716. doi: 10.1371/journal.pone.0240716

Feister, A. (2007). Why the clinical ethics we teach fails patients. *Academic Medicine, 2*(7), 684–689.

Fett, A. K., et al. (2022). Learning to trust: Trust and attachment in early psychosis. *Psychological Medicine, 46*(7), 1437–1447.

Frankl, V. (2006). *Man's search for meaning*. Beacon Press.

Gaffney, A. W. (2022). Intensive care unit equity and regionalization in the COVID-19 era. *Annals of the American Thoracic Society, 19*(5), 717–719.

Gaskell, C., et al. (2023). Long-Term psychotherapy in tertiary care: A practice-based bench-marking study. *British Journal of Clinical Psychology, 62*(2), 483–500.

Gastfriend, D. R., & Mee-Lee, D. (2022). Thirty years of the ASAM criteria: A report card. *Psychiatry Clinics of North America, 45*(3), 593–609.

Gibson, S. (2005). On judgment and judgmentalism: How counselling can make people better. *Journal of Medical Ethics, 31*(10), 575–577.

Goldberg, S.B., et al. (2018). Unpacking the therapist effect: impact of treatment length differs for high- and low-performing therapists. *Psychotherapy Research, 28*(4), 532–544.

Grassi, L, et al. (2017). A person-centered approach in medicine to reduce the psychosocial and existential burden of chronic and life-threatening medical Illness. *International Review of Psychiatry, 29*(5), 377–388.

Haley, J. (1973). Strategic therapy when a child is presented as the problem. *Journal of the American Academy of Child and Adolescent Psychiatry, 12*, 641–659.

Halpern, J. (2001). *From detached concern to empathy*. Oxford University Press.

Hemberg, J., et al. (2022). Meaningfulness among frail older adults receiving home-based care in Finland. *Health Promotion International, 37*(2), Article daab087. doi: 10.1093/heapro/daab087

Hill, C. E., & Norcross, J. C. (2023). Skills and methods that work in psychotherapy: observations and conclusions from the Special Issue. *Psychotherapy (Chic), 60*(3), 407–416.

Hirsch, C. R, et al. (2016). Resolving ambiguity in emotional disorders: The nature and role of interpretation biases. *Annual Review of Clinical Psychology, 12*, 281–305.

Howe, E. G., et al. (2018). Ethical reflections on offering patients accelerated resolution therapy (ART). *Innovations in Clinical Neuroscience, 15*(7–8), 32–34.

Howe, E. G. (2020). Beyond shared decision making. *The Journal of Clinical Ethics, 31*(4), 293–302.

Jager, F. & Perron, A. (2018). Caring as coercion: Exploring the Nurse's role in mandated treatment. *Journal of Forensic Nursing, 14*(3), 148–153.

Kaebnick, G. E. (2017). Decisions and authority. *Hastings Center Report, 47*(1), 2. doi: 10.1002/hast.663

Kent, D. M., et al. (2020). When predictions are used to allocate scarce health care resources: Three considerations for models in the era of Covid-19. *Diagnostic and Prognostic Research, 4*, 11. doi: 10.1186/s41512-020-00079-y

Kline, A. C., et al. (2018). Long-term efficacy of psychotherapy for posttraumatic stress disorder: A meta-analysis of randomized controlled trials. *Clinical Psychology Review, 59*, 30–40.

Knapp, K.S., et al. (2021). Daily meaningfulness among patients with opioid use disorder: examining the role of social experiences during residential treatment and links with post-treatment relapse. *Addictive Behaviors, 119*, Article 106914. doi: 10.1016/j.addbeh.(2021).106914

Kniess, J. (2021). Health justice and Rawls's theory at fifty: Will new thinking about health and inequality influence the most influential account of justice? *Hastings Center Report, 51*(6), 44–50.

Lallier, S., et al. (2023). General practitioners' perceptions of dealing with patients with pressured speech: a qualitative study. *Family Practice, 40*(4), 575–581. doi: 10.1093/fampra/cmad088

Li, S. B, et al. (2020). The mediator effect of meaningfulness on the relationship between schizotypy traits and suicidality. *Frontiers of Psychology, 11*, Article 493. doi: 10.3389/fpsyg.(2020).00493

Linton, S. J., et al. (2017). Can training in empathetic validation improve medical students' communication with patients suffering pain? A test of concept. *Pain Reports, 2*(3), Article e600. doi: 10.1097/PR9.0000000000000600

Little, V., et al. (2018). Integrating safety plans for suicidal patients into patient portals: Challenges and Opportunities. *Psychiatric Services, 69*, 618–619

Madanes, C. (1991). *Strategic family therapy*. Jossey-Bass Publishers.

Madanes, C., & Haley, J. (1977). Dimensions of family therapy. *The Journal of Nervous and Mental Disease, 165*(2), 88–98.

Mayotte-Blum, J., et al. (2012). Therapeutic immediacy across long-term psychodynamic psychotherapy: An evidence-based case study. *Journal of Counseling Psychology, 59*(1):27–40.

Mejia-Lancheros, C., et al. (2020). Trajectories and mental health-related predictors of perceived discrimination and stigma among homeless adults with mental illness. *PLoS One, 15*(2), Article e0229385. doi: 10.1371/journal.pone.0229385

Mezzich, J., et al. (2017). A person-centered approach in medicine to reduce the psychosocial and existential burden of chronic and life-threatening medical illness. *International Review of Psychiatry, 29*(5), 377–388.

McAleavey, A. A., et al. (2019). Effectiveness of routine psychotherapy: Method matters. *Psychotherapy Research, 29*(2), 139–156.

Mulahalilović, A., et al. (2021). Meaning and the sense of meaning in life from a health perspective. *Psychiatria Danubina, 33*(Suppl 4), 1025–1031.

Murtaugh, B., et al. (2023). Clinical application of recommendations for neurobehavioral assessment in disorders of consciousness: An interdisciplinary approach. *Frontiers in Human Neuroscience, 17*, Article 1129466. doi: 10.3389/fnhum.(2023).1129466

Nielsen, L. (2022). Pandemic prioritarianism. *Journal of Medical Ethics, 48*(4), 236–239.

Norberg, B. G., et al. (2017). Trust in the early chain of healthcare: Lifeworld hermeneutics from the patient's perspective. *International Journal of Qualitative Studies on Health and Well-being, 12*(1), Article 1356674. doi: 10.1080/17482631.2017.1356674

Norcross, J. C., & Lambert, M. J. (2011). Psychotherapy relationships that work. *Psychotherapy (Chic), 48*(1), 4–8.

Norcross, J. C., & Wampold, B. E. (2018). A new therapy for each patient: Evidence-based relationships and responsiveness. *Journal of Clinical Psychology, 74*(11), 1889–1906.

Peluso, P. R., & Freund, R. (2023). Paradoxical interventions: A meta analysis. *Psychotherapy, 60*(3), 283–294.

Pelto-Piri, V., et al. (2013). Paternalism, autonomy and reciprocity: ethical perspectives in encounters with patients in psychiatric in-patient care. *BMC Medical Ethics, 14*, Article 49. doi: 10.1186/1472-6939-14-49

Pluhar, E., et al. (2019). Medical education: Guidelines for effective teaching of managing challenging patient encounters. *Medical Science Educator, 29*(3), 855–861.

Rawls, J. (1971). *A theory of justice*, Harvard University Press.

Robertson, M., et al. (2007). Overview of psychiatric ethics V: Utilitarianism and the ethics of duty. *Australasian Psychiatry, 15*(5), 402–410.

Saposnik, G., et al. (2016). Cognitive biases associated with medical decisions: A systematic review. *BMC Medical Informatics and Decision Making, 16*(1), 138. doi: 10.1186/s12911-016-0377-1

Schulz, P., & Hede, V. (2018). Alternative and complementary approaches in psychiatry: beliefs versus evidence. *Dialogues in Clinical Neuroscience, 20*(3), 207–214.

Strojan, P., et al. (2017). Treatment of late sequelae after radiotherapy for head and neck cancer. *Cancer Treatment Reviews, 59*, 79–92.

Thirsk, L. M., et al. (2022). Cognitive and implicit biases in nurses' judgment and decision-making: A scoping review. *International Journal of Nursing Studies, 133*, Article 104284. doi: 10.1016/j.ijnurstu.(2022)

Tronto, J. C. (2009). *Moral boundaries: A political argument for an ethic of care*. Routledge.

van Dijke J., et al. (2023). Engaging otherness: Care ethics radical perspectives on empathy. *Medicine, Health Care and Philosophy, 26*(3), 385–399.

Veatch, R. M. (1973). Generalization of expertise. *Hastings Center Studies, 1*(2), 29–40.

Veatch, R. M. (1998). The place of care in ethical theory. *The Journal of Medicine and Philosophy, 23*(2), 210–224.

Vig, E. K. (2022). As the pandemic recedes, will moral distress continue to surge? *American Journal of Hospice and Palliative Care, 39*(4), 401–405.

Wampold, B. E. (2015). How important are the common factors in psychotherapy? An update. *World Psychiatry, 14*, 270–277.

Wang, J., et al. (2023). Evaluation of consciousness rehabilitation via neuroimaging methods. *Frontiers of Human Neuroscience, 17*, Article 1233499. doi: 10.3389/fnhum.(2023).1233499

15
Ethical Issues in Dementia

Julian C. Hughes

Introduction

According to the Convention on the Rights of Persons with Disabilities (CRPD), dementia is a disability because 'Persons with disabilities include those who have long-term physical, mental, intellectual or sensory impairments which in interaction with various barriers may hinder their full and effective participation in society on an equal basis with others' (United Nations, 2006). Indeed, dementia can cause impairments that are physical (e.g. movement disorders), mental (e.g. hallucinations), intellectual (cognitive impairment), and sensory (e.g. visual misperceptions). In addition, there is stigma. And we need to recall that dementia is not one thing; it is many. So different dementias will present different sorts of disability. Episodic or recall memory problems in Alzheimer's disease, speech problems in vascular dementia, visual hallucinations in Lewy body dementia, sexual disinhibition in the behavioural variant of frontotemporal dementia, and so forth: people living with dementia are disabled in a variety of ways (see Dening et al., 2021; Hughes 2011a).

No one can deny that the intent and effect of the CRPD is essentially good. But there are some clauses which cause controversy. In this chapter, I shall focus on Article 12 which concerns equal recognition before the law. I shall interrogate the concept of legal capacity (paragraph 2 of Article 12). But I also wish to focus on the idea of supported decision-making, in relation to paragraph 4 of Article 12. Article 12 is discussed in some detail in the General Comment Number 1 (United Nations, 2014).

The question I wish to pose is whether these aspects of the CRPD can be regarded as wholly relevant to people living with *severe* dementia. My aim is to suggest that there are deeper, more philosophical, and more important issues at stake—which stem from the reality of dementia—than the semantic, legalistic arguments that surround these clauses of the CRPD.

Mrs Jenkins: a Hypothetical Case Study

After 12 years of worsening Alzheimer's dementia, Mr Jenkins found he could no longer cope with his wife and, with great reluctance, he arranged for her to be admitted to a care home. Sadly, her condition continued to deteriorate. Eventually, she became bed-bound. At the same time, her ability to feed herself deteriorated and eventually it was obvious that she had difficulty swallowing (dysphagia), even when she was fed very carefully. A series of chest infections seemed to result from her dysphagia, each worse than the previous one. Advice was sought from the speech and language team, who advised the use of thickened food and fluids. She did not seem to like the thickener, so getting food and drink into her became a struggle. Her son read on the internet about the use of percutaneous endoscopic gastrostomy (PEG) tubes to feed people with dementia and he suggested that this might be appropriate for his mother. His sister did not agree and preferred that she should continue to be fed by hand as this provided her with at least a little regular human contact. She felt that the risk of her mother choking was outweighed by her enjoyment when being fed. Staff were divided about what to recommend. Mr Jenkins was left in a bewildered and anxious state when he was asked for his opinion. He was told to consider what his wife might have wished for when she was able to make such decisions. He had to admit that they had never discussed such issues and he felt unable to say what she would have wanted.

Analysis of the Background Issues

The CRPD is laudable: it establishes an important framework for thinking about disabilities, including dementia, and aims to make the lives of those who live with disabilities better. But it is problematic when it comes to thinking about people with severe dementia like Mrs Jenkins. It does a good job inasmuch as it forces us to think harder about how we support decision-making around severe dementia. But in the end severe dementia poses a problem that seems to have no solution. For we cannot be sure, under these circumstances, what Mrs Jenkins would wish.

I am leaving mild to moderate dementia out of this analysis. But it is tangentially relevant to notice that even in the case of someone living with mild to moderate dementia there should at least be some concern about the possibility of coercion or of a lack of the ability to see the whole picture. Some people living with dementia might object to this suggestion. In many, perhaps most, cases they would be right to object. People living with dementia should certainly make decisions for themselves if able, even if those decisions seem unwise. Why? Well, because we should all be free to make even unwise decisions. The CRPD, in its championing of the notion of legal capacity, hammers home this point. Nevertheless, the possibility of coercion and the worry that subtle cognitive impairment might be an issue even in mild or moderate dementia needs to be kept in mind. In severe dementia, however, the point is that there is no obvious way of knowing what the person now wants.

Of course, if Mrs Jenkins has created an advance directive when able to do so, then we would know her wishes. An advance directive might take a variety of forms—verbal, written, witnessed or not, specific or general, and so forth—according to the laws and customs of the relevant country. But even with an advance directive in the correct form, doubts can still be raised. Are we sure that the person, when the advance directive was created, was fully able to weigh up the pros and cons of the decision (perhaps even a mild degree of dementia might have made this difficult) and that there was no coercion? Furthermore, are we sure that the person would still feel the same about the advance directive now she is in the position of it needing to be enacted. Perhaps she would say, if able, that she now wishes for everything possible to be done to keep her alive, despite having presumed previously that she would have wanted only palliative care. In short, some of the problems I am pointing to might yet be present in mild to moderate dementia: the reality is that our categorical classifications do not represent the true nature of states that lie on complex continua, and in severe dementia the problems are not fully obviated by an advance directive.

However, it may be that we are looking at this the wrong way round. Rather than look for a legal solution, or for a solution that is based on rules or regulations, or for a solution that can be pinned down by a pathway, it may be better to accept that there's something about the human condition that cannot be codified. Clinicians may get things wrong, but there is such a thing as good judgement which gets things right (Hughes & Ramplin, 2012). The law can provide frameworks to encourage good judgements, but at root—I want to argue—such judgements are based on something intangible embedded in a way of being in the world. This is a synopsis of my argument.

How the Convention on the Rights of Persons with Disabilities and the Mental Capacity Act 2005 Would Have Us Intervene

So, let's look at what the CRPD tells us to do. Paragraph 2 of Article 12 says that: 'States Parties shall recognize that persons with disabilities enjoy legal capacity on an equal basis with others in all aspects of life'; and paragraph 4, talks about safeguards that will 'respect the rights, will and preferences of the person' (United Nations, 2006). In the General Comment Number 1 it is made clear that 'Legal capacity is an inherent right accorded to all people'; it 'means that all people, including persons with disabilities, have legal standing and legal agency simply by virtue of being human' (paragraph 14).

Hence, for Mrs Jenkins, having recognized her legal standing and her legal agency, we should act in such a way as to respect her 'rights, will and preferences'. The question is, how do we do this given that there is no advance directive of any sort and no certain knowledge of what she would have wanted?

In England and Wales, where decision-making is governed by the Mental Capacity Act 2005 (MCA), given the inevitable finding that Mrs Jenkins lacks the requisite capacity, according to the MCA we should act in her best interests (HMSO 2005). (I say 'inevitable' partly because tests of capacity tend to be highly cognitive. Actually, however, decision-making is more complex and involves emotions, values, relationships, environments, and so forth. See Hughes, 2014, pp. 92–108; and Hughes, 2023, pp. 74–80.) Section 4 of the MCA spells out in some detail what acting in the person's best interests entails (and see Emmett & Hughes, 2019). For instance, it involves considering 'all the relevant circumstances', the person's past and present wishes, feelings, beliefs, and values, as well as other factors the person would be likely to consider; and the person must be encouraged to participate as fully as possible in decision-making, whilst the views of 'anyone engaged in caring for the person or interested in his [or her] welfare' must be taken into account; and so forth. If we are to take the idea of Mrs Jenkins's best interests seriously, we must—insofar as it is possible—do all of these things.

Theoretical Approaches

The framers of the CRPD would not, however, be happy with the description I have given of how we should act in connection with Mrs Jenkins. They would object strongly to my talk of the 'inevitable' finding of her lack of mental (decision-making) capacity. They suggest, for instance, that mental and legal capacity have been conflated. In paragraph 14 of General Comment Number 1 the philosophical position is made clear: 'The concept of mental capacity is highly controversial in and of itself. Mental capacity is not, as is commonly presented, an objective, scientific and naturally occurring phenomenon. Mental capacity is contingent on social and political contexts, as are the disciplines, professions and practices which play a dominant role in assessing mental capacity.' Thus, decision-making 'mental capacity' is firmly portrayed as socially and politically constructed.

In paragraph 15 of the General Comment Number 1, the functional approach to the assessment of capacity, used in the MCA, where the person must demonstrate the functional ability to make decisions by showing that he or she can recall the relevant information, understand it, use or weigh it up and express a choice (MCA section 3), is condemned for two key reasons. First, 'it is discriminatorily applied to people with disabilities', and secondly, 'it presumes to be able to accurately assess the inner-workings of the human mind and, when the person does not pass the assessment, it then denies him or her a core human right—the right to equal recognition before the law' (United Nations, 2014).

Now, there is something to be said in favour of the first reason. If I were to go to my lawyer and ask that my last will and testament should be changed, the lawyer would discuss the changes with me but then make them. If I were to go to the lawyer with the label of dementia and ask for changes to be made, I would almost certainly be subjected to a test of my mental (decision-making) capacity, in this case my testamentary capacity. I might then not be allowed to make the changes. The label of dementia is discriminatory. Such discrimination might be wholly unfair. Perhaps I fail the testamentary capacity assessment, but still know for sure why it is that I now wish to leave some money to my favourite charity. On the other hand, the discrimination is intended to protect me and my interests, and it might well do so. What is required here, in my view, is a dose of virtue ethics, mostly in the shape of practical wisdom. What is being aimed at and how do we achieve that end?

But let us consider the second reason for condemning the functional approach. Here, I think, it is easier to argue that the condemnation is wrong or confused. For instance, say I tell you that the tablet I am prescribing for you has three side effects, which I spell out and then repeat. If I ask you to confirm for me that you know what the possible side effects are, but you cannot recall them, am I not entitled to say that I have accurately assessed, at least to a degree, that you have poor recall of the relevant information? This is very definitely to say something about 'the inner workings of [your] human mind'. In which case, am I not entitled to say that you are lacking—at least to this degree—in this particular mental (decision-making) capacity (whatever your mental capacity in other regards)? The suggestion in the General Comment is that in saying these things I am denying you 'the right to equal recognition before the law'. A simple retort to this would be to say that of course all humans are equal, but we are not the same. In a slightly more complicated manner, I might say that recognizing your standing as a person is the reason why in this case you must be treated differently, because we have duties to care for and to protect each other.

Paragraph 15 of General Comment Number 1 highlights the requirement that people be supported in 'the exercise of [their] legal capacity'. The contrast here is with substituted judgements, as in the MCA's advocacy of best interests. In supported decision-making, I support you to make whatever decision you wish to make. In substitute decision-making, given that I have assessed you cannot make the required decision yourself (because of your lack of mental capacity), I substitute a decision on your behalf based on what I and others see as being in your best interests.

The clash between these two approaches focuses on the CRPD's talk of 'will and preferences' (Martin et al., 2014). Here is a clear-cut case. Mr Smith, who has dementia, is in hospital because of a fall. He is ready to be discharged and he wishes to go back to live in his own home. His will and preference is so to do. But the assessment of his best interests is that henceforth he requires institutional care. His 'subjective' preferences are cast aside in favour of his 'objective' best interests (Alghrani et al, 2016). It is certainly true that issues around the assessment of capacity and best interests in connection with place of residence are complex because of the evaluative judgements that come into play (Greener et al., 2012). On the one hand, it seems clear that Mr Smith's legal standing and legal agency have been undermined and ignored by the process of the best interests assessment. On the other, however paradoxical it might seem, the very things that we seek to preserve through talk of legal standing and legal agency—dignity, autonomy, authenticity, integrity, personal values, and so forth—might be under threat if Mr Smith's will and preference hold sway. The old adage about dying with your rights on comes to mind (Treffert, 1973). For example, he might live in terrible conditions and be unable to care for himself in any way, whereas in a care home with practical support he may be able to live in a manner that is true to his values. In the case of Mrs Jenkins, however, things are not so clear-cut precisely because we do not know her will and preferences *at all*.

Reflection on Rights

To summarize what I wish to say about supported decision-making, as McGettrick & Williamson (2015) said: '... the CRPD requires a totally supported decision-making legal regime which poses significant challenges in terms of operationalising this for people with very severe dementia .... This purist legal stance of supported decision-making ... is a real issue for disability activists to address and needs further debate to address the nuances'. Donnelly (2016) has also called for 'a stronger legislative endorsement of will and preferences', but she rejected the contention that substituted decision-making should be entirely abolished. She also suggested an important challenge to the wholesale adoption of a social constructionist view of the world, since 'the social model has been criticised for failing to recognise and address the lived impact of impairment (as opposed to disability)'. Thus, she argued, 'the model fails to take account of the realities of embodiment—ie people exist as bodies and experience disability both socially and corporeally' (Donnelly, 2016).

Scholten and Gather (2018) similarly pointed to problems in realizing the ideal of supported decision-making in the comatose patient or in people with severe dementia or psychosis. They argued that supported decision-making 'does not make competence assessment and substitute decision-making 'superfluous'. Sensibly they suggested that 'reasonable accommodation' requires health professionals to exhaust the available resources of [supported decision-making] before they take recourse to substitute decision-making'. They advocated a combined competence and supported decision-making model, where decision support might incorporate three aims: 'It must be provided (1) to enhance a person's [decision-making capacity], (2) to improve advance care planning and (3) to improve substitute decision-making'.

Such a strategy makes great sense when faced by the realities of Mrs Jenkins in her state of advanced dementia. All that can be done should be done to support her in making her own decisions, which is in keeping with both the MCA and the CRPD. This would include supporting her at the right time to set out her views in an advance directive in the appropriate format. Those who might yet be in the position of having to make a substituted decision for her must also be supported to make the best possible decision, one that—all things considered and as far as we know—most truly reflects what she would have wanted under the circumstances that obtain.

This laudable strategy does not, however, actually tell us what to do for Mrs Jenkins. Much of the argument has been generated by a concern for rights: the CRPD talks, after all, about 'rights, will and preferences'. Indeed, the direction of travel in theorizing about dementia care has been from person-centred care (Kitwood, 1997, 2019) via a citizenship model (Bartlett & O'Connor, 2010) to a rights-based approach (Cahill, 2018). My concern has been that, if we are not careful, talk of rights can start to seem like flag waving (Hughes, 2023, pp. 234–237). So instead, we need to see 'that citizenship is a function of personhood and that rights reflect the ethical standing of persons' (Hughes, 2023, p. 234).

Whenever there is talk of the rights of people living with dementia these need to be specified at least to some degree and the problems of such rights, how they are made enforceable, must be faced. Otherwise, it can seem like flag waving. Sometimes it is good to wave flags, but not if it is a way to limit further conversation. Saying 'People living with dementia have rights' is fine and dandy, but does not tell us very much. When someone says, 'People living with dementia have a right to be cared for in their own homes', much more conversation is required. Who, for instance, has the co-relative duty to ensure that this occurs? And do not some rights trump others? It becomes immensely complex partly because the notion of rights is itself complex: one person's rights must be limited at some point by the pressure they put on the rights of others. In the end 'rights' are hollow claims until they are made more specific and shown to be enforceable.

With these comments in mind, if we return to Mrs Jenkins, we can see that talk of her rights does not get us very far. She has all sorts of important rights that can be specified and are enforceable: a right to life, a right not to be tortured, a right to respect for her private life and for her religious beliefs, and so on. But here we are: should she be hand-fed or given a PEG tube? Of course, there is room for some discussion of rights. Will one or other route threaten her right to life? The answer is that either could shorten her life, although saying this does not mean that someone has the intention of compromising her right to life. Enforcing a PEG tube on her might be seen as torture (although this would seem to be an extreme position to take about a properly indicated and performed medical treatment), but so too might hand-feeding if this leads to choking. We could also note the rights of staff who might (but might not) consider it an infringement of their own rights to be told that they have to feed someone in a way that they consider to be causing suffering and, potentially, death. Arguing about rights does not seem to be very profitable.

Alternatively, we have recourse to empirical research which tends to argue against the use of PEG tubes or, at least, not in their favour (Davies et al., 2021). But even this does not end the dilemma around Mrs Jenkins. For facts must be aligned with values; so we need facts plus values, as well as rights (Hughes & Williamson, 2019).

What Mrs Jenkins requires is good judgement: judgement that takes everything possible and relevant into account, more or less as stipulated in the MCA but with a greater emphasis on anything that might gesture at her will and preference as suggested by the CRPD. Of course, all of this must occur within a framework that supports her legal and moral rights. In this concrete case, the law on its own does not and cannot tell us precisely what to do, and there is no relevant right specific enough to tell us how to act.

The point runs deeper than simply saying that whoever in the end must make the decision, which itself can be contentious, must do it by following the prescriptions of the CRPD and the MCA. Nor is it simply a matter of sticking to the appropriate protocol or care pathway. There is something deeper going on. Thornton (2007) put it thus: 'Even when a form of judgement can be codified as the application of a principle or rule, the application of the rule still depends on an element of uncodified skill'

(p. 222). The skill, I wish to say, is to do with genuine human engagement with Mrs Jenkins and with all those concerned with her welfare. At root, she requires the sort of solicitude that marks us out as human beings. One might call it love.

Conclusion

Interestingly, when the CRPD was drafted, there was no involvement of people living with dementia (Flynn, 2018). People with other forms of disability were involved but negotiations and compromises were required. The reality of people living with advanced, severe dementia was not, it seems, represented. In any case, my contention is that it is not a particular legal approach that will count in these circumstances. It is whether those involved in making the required judgements are thoughtful, sound, attentive, thorough, careful, open, honest, and so on. It is these sorts of virtues that are required. The law, rights, conventions, it seems to me, shape good judgements, but do not in the end specify them.

This is what Martin Luther King said when he was awarded his honorary doctorate in civil law by Newcastle University, UK, in 1967: 'And so while the law may not change the hearts of men, it does change the habits of men if vigorously enforced, and through changes in habits, pretty soon attitudinal changes will take place and even the heart may be changed in the process' (King, 1967).

The CRPD is a good thing. It pushes us in the direction of seeing people with disabilities as they should be seen. The law clearly has a role to play, as Dr King suggested, but it only takes us so far. The specification of practice will in the end rely on people making uncertain decisions as best they can. People being with other people in the world in a good way is what really counts. And I wonder if this is, after all, what 'legal capacity' might truly mean.

In a recent study in a care home a member of staff said this: 'I think sometimes, we just forget and need to be stripped back down to basics and you don't need anything apart from two people and two chairs' (Hughes et al., 2022). She was pointing to the fundamental importance of basic human communication and encounters. At the heart of the care of people living with severe dementia, such as Mrs Jenkins, is not legally specified action but a type of attention and commitment. It is not solely nor mainly a matter of rights, but a matter of human regard and the virtues (amongst others) of compassion, charity, honesty, integrity, and practical wisdom.

Questions

1. What is it like to live with advanced dementia? We cannot know for certain, but what do we imagine?
2. If people with advanced dementia were able to say after a decision had been taken whether or not they approved of the decision made for them, what would they say? (See Scholten & Gather (2018) for some indication.)

3. Can we have a right simply to live well? How would it be enforced?
4. A convention like the CRPD always requires negotiation and possibly some compromise. Does this make such conventions stronger or weaker?

Further Reading

Cahill, S. (2018). *Dementia and human rights*. Policy Press.

This is the book that sets out most fully the rights-based approach to living with dementia. It contains the essay by Flynn (2018), which explains the CRPD and legal capacity in a way more sympathetic than I have treated it here.

Foster, C., Herring, J., & Doron, I. (2014). *The law and ethics of dementia*. Hart Publishing.

This edited volume covers broad territory and is an important book to consult for anyone interested in law and ethics in relation to dementia.

Hughes, J. C. (2011b). *Thinking through dementia*. Oxford University Press.

In this book I have said a lot more about the philosophical underpinnings touched upon in this chapter. The notion of solicitude for instance, derived from the writings of the philosopher Martin Heidegger, is covered in much more detail.

Hughes, J. C. (2023). *Dementia and ethics reconsidered*. Open University Press.

This recent volume presents a raft of ethical issues and notions in connection with dementia. The topic of rights is discussed at numerous points, as is the topic of artificial feeding.

References

Alghrani, A., Case, P., & Fanning, J. (2016). The Mental Capacity Act 2005—ten years on. *Medical Law Review, 24*(3), 311–317. https://doi.org/10.1093/medlaw/fww032

Bartlett, R., & O'Connor, D. (2010). *Broadening the dementia debate*. Policy Press.

Cahill, S. (2018). *Dementia and human rights*. Policy Press.

Davies, N., Barrado-Martín, Y., Vickerstaff, V., Rait, G., Fukui, A., Candy, B., Smith, C. H., Manthorpe, J., Moore, K. J., & Sampson, E. L. (2021). Enteral tube feeding for people with severe dementia. *Cochrane Database of Systematic Reviews 2021* (8), CD013503. https://doi.org/10.1002/14651858.CD013503.pub2

Dening, T., Thomas, A., Stewart, R., & Taylor, J.-P. (Eds.) (2021). *Oxford textbook of old age psychiatry* (3rd ed.). Oxford University Press.

Donnelly, M. (2016). Best interests in the Mental Capacity Act: Time to say goodbye?' *Medical Law Review, 24*(3), 318–332. https://doi.org/10.1093/medlaw/fww030

Emmett, C., & Hughes, J. C. (2019). Best interests. In R. Jacob, M. Gunn & A. Holland (Eds.), *Mental capacity legislation: principles and practice* (2nd ed., pp. 34–55). Cambridge University Press.

Flynn, E. (2018). Legal capacity for people with dementia: a human rights approach. In S. Cahill (Ed.), *Dementia and human rights* (pp. 157–174). Policy Press.

Greener, H., Poole, M., Emmett, C., Bond, J., Louw, S. J., & Hughes, J. C. (2012). Value judgements and conceptual tensions: decision-making in relation to hospital discharge for people with dementia. *Clinical Ethics, 7*(4), 166–174. https://doi.org/10.1258/ce.2012.012028

Her Majesty's Stationery Office (HMSO). (2005). *The Mental Capacity Act 2005*. HMSO. https://www.legislation.gov.uk/ukpga/2005/9/pdfs/ukpga_20050009_en.pdf

Hughes, J. C. (2011a). *Alzheimer's and other dementias: The facts*. Oxford University Press.

Hughes, J. C. (2014). *How we think about dementia: personhood, rights, ethics, the arts and what they mean for care*. Jessica Kingsley Publishers.

Hughes, J. C. (2023). *Dementia and ethics reconsidered.* Open University Press.

Hughes, J. C., & Ramplin, S. (2012). Clinical and ethical judgement. In C. Cowley (Ed.), *Reconceiving medical ethics* (pp. 220–234). Continuum.

Hughes, J. C., & Williamson, T. (2019). *The Dementia Manifesto: Putting values-based practice to work.* Cambridge University Press.

Hughes, J. C., Baseman, J., Hearne, C., Lie, M., Smith, D., & Woods, S. (2022). Art, authenticity and citizenship for people living with dementia in a care home. *Ageing & Society, 42*(12), 2784–2804. https://www.doi.org/10.1017/S0144686X21000271

King, Jr. M. L. (1967). *Speech on receipt of Honorary Doctorate in Civil Law,* University of Newcastle upon Tyne. https://www.ncl.ac.uk/mediav8/congregations/files/Transcript%20of%20Dr%20Martin%20Luther%20King%20Jr%20speech%2013th%20November%201967_compressed.pdf

Kitwood, T. (1997). *Dementia reconsidered: The person comes first.* Open University Press.

Kitwood, T. (2019). *Dementia reconsidered, revisited: The person still comes first* (2nd ed., edited by D. Brooker). Open University Press.

Martin, W., Michalowski, S., Jütten, T., & Burch, M. (2014). *Achieving CRPD compliance: Is the Mental Capacity Act of England and Wales compatible with the UN Convention on the Rights of Persons with Disabilities? If not, what next? An Essex Autonomy Project position paper.* University of Essex. https://autonomy.essex.ac.uk/wp-content/uploads/2021/01/EAP-Position-Paper-FINAL.pdf

McGettrick, G., & Williamson, T. (2015). *Dementia, rights, and the social model of disability. A new direction for policy and practice?* Mental Health Foundation. https://www.mentalhealth.org.uk/explore-mental-health/publications/dementia-rights-and-social-model-disability

Scholten, M., & Gather, J. (2018). Adverse consequences of article 12 of the UN Convention on the Rights of Persons with Disabilities for persons with mental disabilities and an alternative way forward. *Journal of Medical Ethics, 44*(4), 226–233. https://doi.org/10.1136/medethics-2017-104414

Thornton, T. (2007). *Essential philosophy of psychiatry.* Oxford University Press.

Treffert, D. A. (1973). Dying with their rights on. *American Journal of Psychiatry, 130*(9), 1041. https://doi.org/10.1176/ajp.130.9.1041

United Nations General Assembly. (2006). *Convention on the Rights of Persons with Disabilities,* 13 December 2006, A/RES/61/106, Annex I. https://legal.un.org/avl/ha/crpd/crpd.html

United Nations General Assembly. (2014). *Convention on the Rights of Persons with Disabilities: General comment no. 1 (19th May 2014), Article 12: Equal recognition before the law.* https://www.ohchr.org/en/hrbodies/crpd/pages/gc.aspx

16

Moral Stress and Involuntary Treatment

Working in the Chasm between Idealism and Reality

Brendan D. Kelly

Introduction

While most mental healthcare occurs on a voluntary basis, admission and treatment without consent are long-standing features of mental health systems around the world (Kelly, 2022). These practices are controversial, with some commentators suggesting that the people involved should be criminalized and reparations sought (Minkowitz, 2007). Involuntary admission and treatment are, however, governed by national legislation and permitted by, for example, the European Convention on Human Rights (ECHR) (which was written in the language of the 1950s and requires updating to reflect the concepts of the 21st century):

> Everyone has the right to liberty and security of person. No one shall be deprived of his liberty save in the following cases and in accordance with a procedure prescribed by law [including] the lawful detention of persons for the prevention of the spreading of infectious diseases, of persons of unsound mind, alcoholics or drug addicts or vagrants (Council of Europe, 1950; Article 5(1)).

In 2006, the United Nations' (UN) Convention on the Rights of Persons with Disabilities (CRPD) did not provide a precise definition of 'disability', but stated that 'persons with disabilities include those who have long-term physical, mental, intellectual or sensory impairments which in interaction with various barriers may hinder their full and effective participation in society on an equal basis with others' (United Nations, 2006; Article 1). It added 'that the existence of a disability shall in no case justify a deprivation of liberty' (Article 14(1)(b)). In 2014, the UN Committee on the Rights of Persons with Disabilities interpreted the CRPD as inconsistent with involuntary mental healthcare:

> Forced treatment is a particular problem for persons with psychosocial, intellectual and other cognitive disabilities. States parties must abolish policies and legislative provisions that allow or perpetrate forced treatment, as it is an ongoing violation found in mental health laws across the globe, despite empirical evidence indicating its lack of effectiveness and the views of people using mental health

systems who have experienced deep pain and trauma as a result of forced treatment (United Nations Committee on the Rights of Persons with Disabilities, 2014; Paragraph 42).

This opinion is inconsistent with the UN Human Rights Committee and the UN Subcommittee on Prevention of Torture and Other Cruel, Inhuman or Degrading Treatment or Punishment which endorse admission and treatment without consent under specific circumstances (United Nations Human Rights Committee, 2014; paragraph 19; United Nations Subcommittee on Prevention of Torture and Other Cruel, Inhuman or Degrading Treatment or Punishment, 2016; Paragraph 14). The latter adds that, in certain circumstances, 'the withholding of medical treatment would constitute inappropriate practice and could amount to a form of cruel, inhuman or degrading treatment or punishment. It may also constitute a form of discrimination' (Paragraph 15).

Notwithstanding this view, draft Guidance on Mental Health, Human Rights, and Legislation published by the World Health Organization (WHO) and Office of the United Nations High Commissioner for Human Rights (OHCHR) in 2022 expressed the view that 'the CRPD Committee and other human rights mechanisms have asserted that all coercive practices in mental health services are prohibited under the CRPD' (World Health Organization/Office of the United Nations High Commissioner for Human Rights, 2022; p. 61). While the WHO/OHCHR document was a draft for consultation and was not their final position, it is still interesting that they stated that 'legislation should clearly prohibit all involuntary measures', while also noting that 'no country has yet eliminated all forms of coercion in mental health systems' (despite many having ratified the CRPD).

International bodies therefore present conflicting advice, with at least some of this advice not aligning with national legislation, models of practice, or professional ethical codes. This can leave practitioners unsure of exactly what international best practice is and the extent to which the system in which they work expects this of them. This diversity of views in statements of human rights and related commentaries creates a difficult situation for mental health practitioners who are commonly faced with complex situations and mental health crises that are attributable, at least in part, to failures of health and social care upstream, but which now present as acute crises involving deep human suffering and distress. Most practitioners agree with the need for radical reform of health and social care to reduce the likelihood of such situations developing in the first place and finding new ways of dealing with them when they do. But, in parallel with advocating for reform, practitioners must also navigate the world as it is, not as we wish it to be. All too frequently, this involves using imperfect services and imperfect legislation to provide imperfect solutions in situations of urgent mental distress, acute suicidality, and, on occasion, violence.

This situation can result in not only difficult dilemmas and complex decision-making, but also 'moral stress' which is a psychological state of anxiety and unrest owing to constant and routine dilemmas and tensions which are generated by professional role occupancy in specific contexts (Cribb, 2011). Moral stress can be a consequence of 'moral injury', the misalignment of moral values with actions, and the tensions which flow from that. These tensions can be acute, as in the 'moral injury' or 'moral distress' surrounding specific actions or decisions (Litz et al., 2009), but can also become routine or chronic over time, when such challenges and misalignments are part of everyday working life, resulting in sustained 'moral stress'.

To illustrate some of these issues and dilemmas, this chapter uses a hypothetical but not unusual example of involuntary admission and treatment under mental health legislation. This vignette is based in one country (the Republic of Ireland), but many of the issues are applicable across jurisdictions. In certain jurisdictions, mental health professionals other than doctors or psychiatrists play key roles in decisions about involuntary admission and treatment: approved social workers, clinical psychologists, etc. For all decision-makers, however, key moral and ethical issues will be similar, although professional backgrounds will differ, and effective teamwork can address some of the moral stress.

Brief Case Study

CJ has a long-standing diagnosis of schizophrenia with multiple hospital admissions and a generally good response to treatment including antipsychotic medication when they accept it. For the past number of years, CJ has been homeless, spending short periods in various hostels and shelters in the city centre, but CJ is usually asked to leave after a week or two owing to disruptive behaviour, especially singing at night. CJ is offered support and treatment by a community mental health team, including a psychiatrist, social worker, community nurse, and clinical psychologist, but mostly declines all interventions and support.

On this occasion, staff at a hostel contact CJ's community nurse to say that CJ is shouting and singing all night in the hostel and other residents are complaining. The nurse goes to see CJ at the hostel to offer support, but CJ declines to see the nurse, as is CJ's right. The nurse speaks with hostel staff and advises them about management.

Two days later, hostel staff phone dCJ's social worker to say that they can no longer accommodate CJ at the hostel owing to CJ's increasingly bizarre behaviour: CJ set a newspaper on fire and went out onto the hostel roof, singing loudly through the night.

CJ's social worker goes to the hostel to meet CJ and offer support, but CJ declines to see them. The social worker speaks to hostel staff who insist that CJ can no longer stay there. No other hostels will accept CJ owing to CJ's past behaviour, so CJ ends up sleeping on the street. The social worker leaves their phone number with hostel staff to pass onto CJ, in case CJ wants assistance and support. Again, CJ declines.

Three days later, police officers contact CJ's psychiatrist to say that CJ is in police custody and to request a psychiatric assessment. CJ was standing in the middle of a busy road at midnight, singing at passing cars. CJ was posing a risk to motorists and appeared to require care and support, according to police, so they took CJ into custody.

The police bring CJ to the hospital emergency department, where the psychiatrist assesses CJ, with a nurse. The psychiatrist and nurse decide that CJ is psychotic and offer outpatient treatment and support: antipsychotic medication, renewed support finding accommodation, and follow-up in the community by the community nurse and clinical psychologist. Follow-up will be challenging because CJ is sleeping on the street, but CJ declines all interventions. The psychiatrist and nurse both feel that CJ does not meet criteria for involuntary admission under mental health legislation. The police decide not to press charges. CJ is discharged, walks out of hospital, and cannot be located for follow-up support.

Two weeks later, police officers contact the psychiatrist again, to say CJ is in custody again. CJ boarded a tour bus full of tourists and went down the bus singing and shouting about 'the devil, and the gods, and everyone in between'. CJ refused to leave the bus and was again taken into custody. Once again, the psychiatrist assesses CJ in the emergency department and decides that CJ is psychotic. On this occasion, CJ is deeply distressed, saying: 'The devil and the gods know what is happening. They are coming for me. They are coming for you. You must let me go. You know what I mean. You all know. I must be killed. I must be killed.' When the psychiatrist asks if CJ intends dying by suicide, CJ responds: 'No. That won't be necessary. They will kill me. They have already started. Soon, I will be killed.'

Again, the psychiatrist offers outpatient treatment and support: antipsychotic medication, assistance finding accommodation, and follow-up by the team. Once again, CJ refuses all forms of outpatient support and treatment. CJ also declines voluntary inpatient admission. On this occasion, however, the psychiatrist feels that CJ's condition has worsened to the degree that CJ meets criteria for involuntary admission and treatment under mental health legislation, especially if CJ declines all other forms of care and support.

Despite the relative clarity of this case, involuntary admission and treatment always pose several dilemmas for mental health professionals, as perhaps they always should, given the gravity of the issues involved. Some of these dilemmas are explored next.

Analysis

CJ's case is common and complex. People often present to mental health services in acute crises that involve combinations of mental health need, social problems, and involvement with law enforcement. This frequently follows lengthy efforts by community teams to offer support and treatment on a voluntary basis in the least restrictive fashion possible. When this is declined or proves insufficient, the issue of involuntary admission and treatment can arise.

In CJ's case, the psychiatrist is aware that efforts at community treatment have failed, CJ is increasingly distressed, and treatment is likely to help with the mental health dimension of their problems, although not necessarily the social issues (based on the psychiatrist's prior knowledge of CJ's case). On the other hand, the psychiatrist knows that involuntary admission and treatment involve temporary limitations on CJ's rights to liberty and bodily integrity, and CJ has tears in their eyes as they implore the psychiatrist to let them leave the emergency department to 'meet my inevitable fate and be killed'.

The psychiatrist is acutely conscious that CJ's position is attributable in part to mental health problems, but also social circumstances. CJ achieved stability for several years when they had a room in a hostel that was run by a former psychiatric nurse who could better manage CJ's behaviours. At that time, CJ took a small amount of medication, attended a training course, and was neither admitted to hospital nor arrested for many years. When that hostel closed, CJ did not do well in standard homeless hostels, resulting in inconsistent accommodation (if any), minimal engagement with treatment, and multiple crises—such as the present one that CJ and the psychiatrist face in the emergency department.

Under most mental health legislation, it is the psychiatrist who is faced with acute decisions in these situations, especially regarding involuntary admission and treatment. The decision of the psychiatrist will, however, have implications not only for CJ, but also for other mental health team members who will be involved in CJ's care at a later point.

For instance, it is possible that, following involuntary admission, another member of the team might feel complicit in the confinement of CJ against CJ's stated wishes, might not believe this is appropriate, and might not agree with the psychiatrist's assessment of the needs and opportunities available to CJ. The staff member might feel that they are participating in an abuse of human rights, but that they do not themselves have the means to contest the case, either personally (though differences in personal power in the team), professionally (in that their profession seeks to avoid inter-professional conflict), or legally (in that the law invests power in the psychiatrist, in this case).

So, while the psychiatrist might be uncomfortable and conflicted, they do at least have opportunity to exercise agency. In many jurisdictions, other staff who have a different view to the psychiatrist might feel obliged to participate in treatment which they may personally believe is immoral, counter to the ethical principles of their discipline, and contrary to the CRPD. They might also personally believe that the proposed intervention is inappropriate, and possibly ineffective and/or harmful.

The converse also occurs: that a psychiatrist makes a decision not to involuntarily admit someone, and team members disagree with that. This disagreement is often on the basis that comprehensive community treatment has already been tried, and that a failure to admit and treat the person without consent neglects their needs and violates their rights to healthcare, health, and even life. This is a common tension in clinical practice: team members' concerns about a psychiatrist's decision not to involuntarily admit a patient with severe mental disorder, and to try voluntary community treatment once again.

While these matters can be, and often are, discussed at multidisciplinary team meetings, and are ideally resolved in this way, not all teams function to this level, and mental health legislation still invests decision-making authority in specific people, generally the psychiatrist. To compound matters, psychiatrists can feel that the retrospective views of colleagues who are not placed in these acute decision-making positions do not take sufficient account of the moral distress involved in choosing between deeply imperfect options in emergency circumstances.

Intervention

The conventional approach to the dilemma presented in CJ's case is to identify the least restrictive pathway possible, which is usually either no care, voluntary outpatient care and support, or voluntary inpatient care and support. In this case, no care has been accepted for some weeks without resolving the situation, and CJ declines another attempt at voluntary outpatient care or voluntary inpatient care. In this situation, the psychiatrist can choose to discharge CJ from the emergency department again and continue to offer outpatient support, or proceed with involuntary admission and treatment under mental health legislation. The latter option will, of course, require the involvement of other professionals and various checks and balances, and the involuntary process might not be completed for a variety of reasons. Even so, commencing it is an option in this circumstance.

Mental health legislation in most jurisdictions places the psychiatrist in the final decision-making position here. Many sources of information are relevant to such a decision: CJ, their family or friends, the police, and other health professionals who are available. In late-night, emergency settings, the latter category is often limited to nurses, but some health systems have social workers available on a 24-hours basis. Information from all sources and the views of all available stakeholders can help to shape these decisions, but most jurisdictions require that the *final* decision about involuntary admission is made by a medical practitioner, often a psychiatrist (even though other professionals often have different formal and informal roles in the process).

If the psychiatrist chooses to discharge CJ from the emergency department again, it is likely that CJ's distress and disturbance will worsen, as it did over past weeks. Nonetheless, this is an option to consider, given that, while CJ now meets legal criteria for involuntary admission and treatment, legislation permits, rather than requires, such involuntary admission and treatment. It could, however, be a breach of medical ethics not to admit CJ when such admission would be possibly clinically beneficial (even in the short term) and is legally possible. On the other hand, involuntary admission and treatment limit the observance of certain human rights for a period of time, and CJ states that they do not intend to deliberately harm themselves or others (although they are convinced that they are about to be killed).

If the psychiatrist opts for involuntary admission and treatment, they will be morally conflicted by the fact that this extreme measure, which is only ever applied to a small minority of people with a mental disorder, is necessitated by a combination of psychiatric and social factors. Also, the psychiatrist is aware that a period of involuntary admission and treatment is likely to help with symptoms in the short term and medium term, but social problems will likely persist and undermine long-term progress. This makes the psychiatrist conflicted about balancing rights; i.e. the extent to which it is reasonable to limit CJ's right to liberty and bodily integrity for a period of time in order to respect their right to healthcare and health, but with long-term prospects uncertain either way.

Standing in the loud, crowded emergency department at 3 am, the psychiatrist is fully aware that this crisis might have been prevented with health or social care that was better, different, or provided sooner. The psychiatrist is also aware that hard cases can make bad law, that balancing rights is a complex task, and that difficult crises should not form the basis for general rules in services or legislation. Nevertheless, this crisis has developed and cannot be avoided now. CJ is agitated, shouting, and weeping in the emergency department, certain of their upcoming death. Police officers shuffle impatiently, waiting for a decision. The nurse manager reminds the psychiatrist that the emergency department social worker is on sick leave and has not been replaced. They add that six critical patients from a road traffic accident are about to arrive by ambulance and 'they have rights too'. So, could the psychiatrist 'make a decision quickly, please?'

Theory

Robertson and Walter outline a range of approaches to ethical reasoning in psychiatry, including instrumental approaches (utilitarian, ethics of duty, principle-based ethics, casuistry, and common morality theory), reflective approaches (virtue ethics, ethics of care, and ethics of the other), and integrative approaches ('political' ethics and the Rawlsian approach to justice in mental health, and postmodern professional ethics) (Robertson & Walter, 2014). In the context of involuntary care, they note the obligation of the state to provide care to a reasonable standard, although this task is rendered more complex when that care is provided without consent or against the apparent wishes of the person.

'Common morality theory', which is one approach that Robertson and Walter outline, is rooted in the broad values of citizens who live in a stable democracy, as reflected, in this case, by mental health legislation and the publicly funded health system in which this vignette is located. Both options considered by the psychiatrist in this case (discharge or involuntary admission and treatment) come within the bounds of such 'common morality', with a possibly stronger argument in favour of involuntary admission and treatment in this example. This might also be supported by an 'ethics of care' approach to the dilemma, in light of CJ's suffering and previous unsuccessful efforts at treatment and support.

However, while moral reasoning in individual cases might help resolve some of these dilemmas, the role or validity of individual moral reasoning is not fully agreed, and it is inevitably difficult in practice (Coady, 2021). The issue of 'moral stress' is also engaged, and refers to the emotional and psychological stress that develops when practitioners are confronted with ethical dilemmas or conflicts between personal values and demands of work (see 'Analysis' section above). Moral stress stems from perceived misalignment between what practitioners believe to be right or morally acceptable and the situations in which they find themselves, along with the decisions and actions they are expected or required to take by the health, social, and/or legal systems within which they work. This is compounded by the operation of overstressed systems of care (Buchbinder et al., 2024), which, in CJ's case, include insufficient models of social support, poor accommodation, and resource pressures in the emergency department where the acute decision is to be made.

The issue of moral stress becomes even more highly charged in situations that involve complex combinations of care and control (Warne et al., 2011), with conflicting requirements and desires to provide care but minimize coercion. Jansen and colleagues summarize this dilemma in their qualitative study of how 'cultural and political ideals cause moral distress in acute psychiatry', and they link this with resources for mental healthcare:

> Mental health nurses working in acute psychiatric care are involved in a complex interplay between political and professional ideals to reduce the use of coercion while being responsible for the safety of both patients and staff as well as creating a therapeutic atmosphere. External constraints like inadequate resources may furthermore hinder the healthcare workers/nurses from realising the treatment ideals set before them. Caught in the middle nurses may experience moral distress that may lead to physical discomfort, uneasiness and feelings of guilt, shame, and defeat. Pressure on nurses and care providers to reduce or eliminate the use of coercion and reduction of health care spending are incompatible demands (Jansen et al., 2022).

Rights Reflection

In terms of human rights, involuntary admission and treatment in CJ's case would be consistent with positions outlined by national legislation (e.g. the Mental Health Act 2001 in Ireland), the ECHR (Council of Europe, 1950), the UN Human Rights Committee (2014), and the UN Subcommittee on Prevention of Torture and Other Cruel, Inhuman or Degrading Treatment or Punishment (2016), but inconsistent with the UN Committee on the Rights of Persons with Disabilities (2014). The CRPD itself is less clear on the matter, notwithstanding the interpretation of the UN

Committee, which was amplified in the WHO/OHCHR's draft Guidance on Mental Health, Human Rights, and Legislation (World Health Organization/Office of the United Nations High Commissioner for Human Rights, 2022). It has been (reasonably) argued that the UN Committee's interpretation does not appear to reach a fair balance between the rights of the individual and the legitimate concerns of society (Prabhu, 2021).

Large committees of experts take much time for extensive deliberation to develop UN Conventions and Declarations, European directives, and national legislation. Where inconsistencies arise between these—as is the case here—individual clinicians are placed in invidious positions of having to use their own judgement in individual cases, but knowing that they can be held open to criticism by at least some interpretations of inconsistent policy instruments. In practice, clinicians will be persuaded by the specific circumstances of the individual case, but also proximal requirements, such as the general exigencies of the emergency department or national legal obligations, rather than more distal issues, such as complying with UN conventions which might contradict national legal obligations.

In any case, even if there was an agreed interpretation of rights outlined in the CRPD, human rights approaches do not always resolve situations in which specific rights conflict with each other, as in CJ's case. This conflict between rights to liberty and bodily integrity on the one hand, and rights to healthcare and health on the other, intensifies the moral stress generated by this kind of case—stress which is often compounded by commentators who place disproportionate responsibility for involuntary admission and treatment on individual practitioners (whose options are generally very limited at the level of individual patient care) as opposed to policymakers (who are better positioned to address upstream causes) and lawmakers (who could introduce sustainable, incremental legal reforms with zero-coercion as a goal, but generally do not).

Even in situations of moral stress, however, decisions must be made, and many practitioners work hard to take into account a range of views in order to execute their clinical, ethical, and legal obligations in circumstances that are far from ideal. The resultant decisions can be based on continuing current practice (however imperfect that might be), engaging with complex ethical and moral reasoning in each individual case (which would consume considerable psychological resources), looking beyond traditional approaches in some way (to identify new solutions) (Horsfall et al., 2011), or even stepping aside from mental healthcare entirely, owing to the stresses involved. To mitigate against everyone choosing the latter option, Hem and colleagues, following a focus group study of 'ethical challenges in connection with the use of coercion', note that these 'ethical challenges deserve to be identified and handled in a systematic way' (Hem et al., 2014). To this end, 'better communication skills among healthcare professionals and improved therapeutic relationships seem to be vital'. In addition, 'systematic focus on ethics in a broad sense would be fruitful', with particular emphasis on the links between ethics and professional practice:

[...] it is sometimes difficult to view ethics and professional questions as separate from each other, in fact, they are in many cases intertwined and should be
examined together. Developing knowledge about ethics in this field is important
to better understand the differences *and* connections between ethical and professional issues, so that the focus on and contribution of ethics can be more accurate
and precise. (Hem et al., 2014)

This link between ethics on the one hand, and professional and practical issues
on the other, is essential, along with recognition that imperfect services will inevitably result in imperfect outcomes, in which 'least-worst' choices might be the best
available to distressed patients and hard-pressed practitioners. In parallel with these
difficult or impossible decisions, it is important that practitioners advocate for improved upstream services in health and social care to diminish, minimize, or eliminate some of these dilemmas. Political support and public cooperation are vital if
we are to transform the landscape of mental health and disorder in such a way as to
improve services and support, and minimize moral stress. Implementing systems of
advance healthcare directives and advance care planning could help address some
of these matters, although they are not a complete solution, and uptake is often low
(Kelly, 2016).

In the absence of comprehensive alternative solutions that will hopefully drastic-
ally reduce the need for involuntary care in the future, practitioners must continue to
respond to the suffering and distress in front of them. This means using the deeply imperfect systems that are currently available to address problems and crises that occur,
even when these situations are generated by variable mixtures of mental disorder,
substance misuse, and adverse socio-economic circumstances. Addressing these situations with knowingly imperfect tools incurs significant moral stress for practitioners
(Murray & Ehlers, 2021). This can be mitigated by commitment to radical reform
of upstream determinants of mental health, mental disorder, and service levels; advocacy for better care, to service providers, regulators, politicians, and government;
close adherence to professional and regulatory standards in clinical situations; an
awareness that alleviating suffering is a difficult but worthwhile task; and an understanding that seeking to resolve real-life dilemmas in imperfect systems brings moral
stress, but avoiding them would bring even more—and would fail to alleviate the distress of the person.

Questions and Thought Experiments

- Would you discharge CJ from the emergency department again? If so, which
  human rights, if any, would this decision protect or promote? Which human
  rights, if any, would it undermine or violate? To what extent should you reflect
  on whether CJ would opt for treatment if they had a full understanding of their
  situation now or if they were reflecting back on this episode, after recovery?

- Which human rights should most inform the decision in CJ's case: the rights to liberty and bodily integrity, or the rights to healthcare and health? Is the right to life relevant here? Are CJ's human rights the only human rights to be considered in this situation?
- How does the concept of human dignity apply in CJ's case? Would an active consideration of CJ's lived experience of dignity shift the decision towards discharge from the emergency department or towards involuntary admission and treatment?
- How would you feel if the nurse manager in the emergency department told you that the six critical patients from a road traffic accident who are about to arrive by ambulance were injured in an accident caused by CJ standing in the middle of the road, singing? Would that change your decision about CJ's management?
- If you fundamentally disagreed on principle with involuntary admission and treatment, would you avoid working in inpatient mental health services, or would you actively seek out such a position in the hope of minimizing involuntary care and its consequences?

Acknowledgements

I am very grateful to my co-editors for their comments and suggestions.

Further Reading

Robertson, M., & Walter, G. (2014). *Ethics and Mental Health: The Patient, Profession and Community.* CRC Press (especially Chapter 1: 'Methods of ethical reasoning in psychiatry').

Coady, M. M. (2021). Psychiatric ethics and the professions. In S. Bloch & S. A. Green (Eds.), *Psychiatric ethics* (5th ed., pp. 121–142). Oxford University Press.

Prabhu, M. (2021). Global mental health law and the interface with ethics. In A. R. Dyer, B. A. Kohrt & P. J. Candilis (Eds.), *Global mental health ethics* (pp. 31–45). Springer.

Jansen, T.-L., Danbolt, L. J., Hanssen, I., & Hem, M. H. (2022). How may cultural and political ideals cause moral distress in acute psychiatry? A qualitative study. *BMC Psychiatry, 22*, 212. https://doi.org/10.1186/s12888-022-03832-3

References

Buchbinder, M., Browne, A., Berlinger, N., Jenkins, T., & Buchbinder, L. (2024). Moral stress and moral distress: confronting challenges in healthcare systems under pressure. *American Journal of Bioethics, 12*, 8–22. https://doi.org/10.1080/15265161.2023.2224270

Coady, M. M. (2021). Psychiatric ethics and the professions. In S. Bloch & S. A. Green (Eds.), *Psychiatric ethics* (5th ed., pp. 121–142). Oxford University Press.

Council of Europe. (1950). *European Convention on Human Rights (Convention for the Protection of Human Rights and Fundamental Freedoms)*. Rome: Council of Europe.

Cribb, A. (2011). Integrity at work: managing routine moral stress in professional roles. *Nursing Philosophy, 12,* 119–127. https://doi.org/10.1111/j.1466-769X.2011.00484.x

Hem, M. H., Molewijk, B., & Pedersen, R. (2014). Ethical challenges in connection with the use of coercion: a focus group study of health care personnel in mental health care. *BMC Medical Ethics*; *15,* Article 82. https://doi.org/10.1186/1472-6939-15-82 (link to licence: https://crea tivecommons.org/licenses/by/4.0/)

Horsfall, J., Cleary, M., Hunt, G. E., & Walter, G. (2011). Acute care. In P. Barker (Ed.), *Mental health ethics: The human context* (pp. 197–204). Routledge.

Jansen, T.-L., Danbolt, L. J., Hanssen, I., & Hem, M. H. (2022). How may cultural and political ideals cause moral distress in acute psychiatry? A qualitative study. *BMC Psychiatry, 22,* Article 212. https://doi.org/10.1186/s12888-022-03832-3 (link to licence: https://creative commons.org/licenses/by/4.0/)

Kelly, B. D. (2016). *Mental illness, human rights and the law.* Royal College of Psychiatrists Publications.

Kelly, B. D. (2022). *In search of madness: A psychiatrist's travels through the history of mental illness.* Gill Books.

Litz, B. T, Stein, N., Delaney, E., Lebowitz, L., Nash, W. P., Silva, C., & Maguen, S. (2009). Moral injury and moral repair in war veterans: a preliminary model and intervention strategy. *Clinical Psychology Review, 29,* 695–706. https://doi.org/10.1016/j.cpr.2009.07.003

Minkowitz, T. (2007). The United Nations Convention of the Rights of Persons with Disabilities and the right to be free from nonconsensual psychiatric interventions. *Syracuse Journal of International Law and Commerce, 34,* 405–428.

Murray, H., & Ehlers, A. (2021). Cognitive therapy for moral injury in post-traumatic stress disorder. *Cognitive Behaviour Therapist, 14,* Article e8. https://doi.org/10.1017/S1754470X2 1000040

Prabhu, M. (2021). Global mental health law and the interface with ethics. In A. R. Dyer, B. A. Kohrt, & P. J. Candilis (Eds.), *Global mental health ethics* (pp. 31–45). Springer.

Robertson, M., & Walter, G. (2014). *Ethics and mental health: The patient, profession and community.* CRC Press.

United Nations. (2006). *Convention on the Rights of Persons with Disabilities.* New York: United Nations.

United Nations Committee on the Rights of Persons with Disabilities. (2014). *General Comment No. 1 (Article 12).* New York: United Nations.

United Nations Human Rights Committee. (2014). *General Comment No. 35 (Article 9).* New York: United Nations.

United Nations Subcommittee on Prevention of Torture and Other Cruel, Inhuman or Degrading Treatment or Punishment. (2016). *Approach of the Subcommittee on Prevention of Torture and Other Cruel, Inhuman or Degrading Treatment or Punishment Regarding the Rights of Persons Institutionalized and Treated Medically Without Informed Consent.* New York: United Nations.

Warne, T., McAndrew, S., & Gawthorpe, D. The mental health nurse. In P. Barker (Ed.), *Mental health ethics: The human context* (pp. 80–88). Routledge.

World Health Organization/Office of the United Nations High Commissioner for Human Rights. (2022). *Guidance on Mental Health, Human Rights, and Legislation (Draft).* Geneva: World Health Organization/Office of the United Nations High Commissioner for Human Rights.

17
Advance Directives in Mental Healthcare

Matthé Scholten and George Szmukler

Introduction

An advance directive is a document that allows a person, when well, to state treatment preferences in anticipation of a time in the future when they may not be capable of making treatment decisions according to their own deeply held values and preferences. The anticipated loss of this ability (commonly referred to as 'mental capacity' or 'competence to consent') typically occurs during a mental health crisis due to, for example, a psychotic episode, an organic confusional state, or a severe psychologically disturbing event. Treatment preferences are preferences for one treatment option (including the option of no treatment) over another and can hence involve both consent to and refusal of specific treatments. An advance directive offers the person the promise of a significant measure of control over their care and treatment during a mental health crisis, which at such a time might otherwise prove unachievable. It can support service user autonomy and offer self-protection at times when the person anticipates that serious harm may occur.

Advance directives seem highly suited to conditions characterized by recurrent episodes that temporarily impair one's decision-making abilities but with good recovery between episodes, such as bipolar affective disorder. Despite this, there is much less recognition of the value of mental health advance directives than of those for end-of-life somatic care. Mental health stigma is likely part of the explanation. The stereotype that mental disorders necessarily entail an inability to make sound judgments must be a highly significant factor. This stereotype is reflected in the almost universal absence of a capacity criterion for involuntary detention and treatment in mental health law, clearly at variance with the criteria for non-consensual treatment for all other medical or surgical conditions (Szmukler, 2018).

The extent to which advance directives are legally binding varies with the jurisdiction (Gloeckler et al., 2025). Legal binding requires a statutory basis, usually a capacity-based legal framework where a person's treatment decisions can only be overridden where there is a substantial impairment of decision-making ability. In such cases, recourse is taken to substitute decision-making (also referred to as 'proxy' or 'surrogate' decision-making) under these legal frameworks. The aim of substitute decision-making is to arrive at the treatment decision that the person would have made had they possessed the ability to make the decision according to their own deeply held values and preferences. If available, advance directives often provide the most reliable basis for such a decision and must hence be followed. In Germany, advance directives are legally binding, and involuntary mental health treatment is permissible only if it is compatible with an available advance directive (Henking & Scholten, 2023). In England and Wales, by contrast, under the Mental Capacity Act 2005, advance directives can be overridden as soon as one is detained under the Mental Health Act.

Two recent reviews have shown a range of perceived benefits of advance directives (Braun et al., 2023; Stephenson et al., 2020). The majority of service users, over 60% in 18 relevant studies, were positive about advance directives and were satisfied with their use (Braun et al., 2023). The benefits described included an increased sense of autonomy and control over treatment decisions; an increased sense of safety and prevention of harms resulting from damaging behaviour when ill; ensuring protection of rights; feeling respected; improved trust in mental health professionals and better therapeutic relationships; an improved experience of treatment; enhancing continuity of care; preventing hospitalization or making desired early intervention possible; reducing coercive interventions; increasing the engagement of family in the person's care, including improved understanding, communication, and trust in their involvement.

In this chapter, we discuss the clinical benefits of advance directives, the barriers to their use, and the legal and ethical issues surrounding them with an illustrative case study, that of Anne. The early phases of this case study appeared in a previous publication of one of us (Szmukler, 2018, 2017). In this chapter, we imagine how her story would likely continue had she drafted an advance directive, and perhaps even included a so-called 'self-binding' clause.

A Case Study: Anne

Anne is 24 years old and a student at a prestigious drama school. She has a diagnosis of bipolar disorder. She has had three episodes of mania, each resulting in admission to hospital on a compulsory order.

Anne's mother died by suicide during a depressive episode when Anne was 14. She lives with her father, a retired dentist. Her married sister, Louise, lives nearby. Anne has a close relationship with both.

Anne's education, especially during her final year at school, had been badly affected by her mental health condition, and she is determined to finish her drama course. Following recovery from the second admission, Anne made a so-called 'joint crisis plan' with the clinical team in which she expressed her preferences regarding treatment if she were to relapse again, including when she believed admission would be warranted. This was a brief document that carried no legal force.

Unfortunately, 6 months later, Anne relapsed. Unable to sleep and flimsily dressed, Anne went out wandering in the centre of the city around 2 am. She was eventually apprehended by the police. She claimed she was a great actress. The police, using a power under the Mental Health Act, escorted Anne to a 'place of safety', the local hospital. She refused any treatment and was detained on a compulsory order.

In fact, Anne had attended her local hospital the night before, accompanied by her father. She accepted the need for admission when shown her joint crisis plan. Unfortunately, the psychiatrist on-call was not impressed by the brief plan and concluded that Anne was not ill enough to be admitted, especially given the pressures on bed availability.

Analysis: Barriers to the Use of Advance Directives

Anne did not have a comprehensive advance directive. Following the events described in the case study, there was a discussion among those involved focused on challenges to drafting an advance directive. These have been recognized in the research literature (Braun et al., 2023; Stephenson et al., 2020). Creating an advance statement is a fairly complex and unfamiliar task and generally requires expert assistance. Anne had no access to an experienced facilitator in formulating her joint crisis plan. Despite the interest in advance directives among service users, their completion rates are low in the absence of expert facilitation. A facilitator could be an advocate (including a peer advocate) or a trusted mental health professional, preferably independent of the treatment team. A further role for the facilitator or independent advocate is to ensure that no undue influence is exerted. In addition, the involvement of a senior member of the treatment team is strongly recommended to enable an informed discussion of care and treatment options, to build trust, and to confirm that the service user had mental capacity when making the advance directive. In Anne's case, joint crisis plans had just been introduced in the context of a clinical trial, and there had been little experience in their application.

The complexity of drafting an advance directive is partly due to the wide scope of topics that could be addressed, and the level of detail required to describe preferences. A recent systematic review has described the range of topics and issues that may be covered in an advance directive (Gaillard et al., 2023). An overview of these issues and topics can be found in Table 17.1. The 'Preferences and Advance decisions for Crisis and Treatment' (PACT) template (Stephenson et al., 2020) illustrates how these topics and issues can be operationalized in the form of concrete prompts to draft an advance directive.

Other obstacles to making an advance directive reported in the reviews above that played a role in Anne's case included concerns that her advance directive would not be followed because health professionals may not endorse advance directives; that the advance directive would be inaccessible during a crisis; and that the advance directive can be easily overridden if it has no legal force. Successfully making an advance

Table 17.1 Possible contents of an advance directive

Topic	Subtopics and examples
Personal introduction	What kind of person am I?
Self-described mental health condition	How I understand my mental health condition and how it affects my life
Current care and treatment plan	Current medication; current talking treatments; somatic health conditions; allergies
Current care team	Treating psychiatrist; general practitioner; social worker; community nurse; others
Values statement	What do I find important? What are the things I care about? What are my convictions? What are my goals?
Signs of a mental health crisis	Early warning signs; crisis triggers; preventive strategies; what has been helpful or unhelpful in the past
Preferred general treatment approach	Preference for an emphatic and respectful approach; wish to be listened to and to be treated with dignity
Preferences (including refusals) regarding treatment setting	Preferences regarding particular hospitals or wards; preferences regarding particular healthcare professionals; preferences regarding other professionals who should be involved
Treatment preferences (including refusals)	Medication preferences; preferences regarding talking treatments; preferences around electroconvulsive therapy; other interventions that have been helpful or unhelpful
Preferences related to restrictive measures	Preferred de-escalation strategies; less restrictive alternatives; preferences around particular restrictive measures (when, if ever, such measures might be justified)
Social instructions	Persons to be notified; nominated representative; care of dependants or pets; care of property and finances

directive thus requires a substantial degree of trust in the treatment team and the mental health system on the part of the service user, as well as a high degree of commitment on the part of the treatment team.

Less important for Anne were possible concerns about an inability to foresee and decide on her preferences during a future crisis or a lack of flexibility in the advance directive. When considering making an advance directive, Anne anticipated regularly reviewing the document and updating it if required. Although she recognized a risk to privacy and a possible generation of stigma, she saw these as addressable (e.g. through adequate data security measures) or else outweighed by the perceived benefits. She did not worry about the risk of increased rather than reduced coercion, a fear reported by some as a disincentive. Anne had the advantage of a good social network supporting the idea of making an advance directive.

Intervention: Anne's Advance Directive

We can imagine Anne's story continued as follows:

Anne was discharged a month later. Following a full recovery and a detailed discussion with the clinical team and her father and sister, she decided to draft a more comprehensive advance directive, one that would be harder to dismiss. After a preparatory discussion with her family and an independent advocate, arranged by the hospital on request, Anne, her father, and the advocate met with Anne's consultant psychiatrist and her community psychiatric nurse to draft an advance directive. After 45 minutes of discussion, Anne produced the following advance directive:

---

1 Apr 2023

I am a drama student in my final year of a BA (Hons) in acting at a top drama academy. Next year I will apply for a master's degree.

I have bipolar disorder, for which I have been hospitalized three times in the last 5 years—in 2011 and 2012 during my last year in school (which I consequently had to repeat), and 2016 in my second year of my BA. On each occasion, it was for a manic episode, and I was involuntarily admitted each time.

My current medication is lithium 300 mg twice daily. I tolerate this well and don't feel it significantly blunts my acting ability.

I have no other serious health conditions.

Values statement

Since childhood I have wanted to be an actress. My mother who also had bipolar disorder, was a fine actress who died by suicide just as her career was taking off. I have been told by my tutors that I am unusually talented and can expect success as an actress. My mental health condition is potentially a huge impediment. Although the academy has been understanding, I believe that another manic episode, especially if prolonged, would seriously jeopardise my continuing studies.

I also hugely value my relationships with my father and my sister. I trust their concern for my welfare and my life goals when I am well, but not when I am in a mental health crisis. I can become seriously unpleasant then.

Signs that indicate I need treatment for a manic episode

My previous episodes have been very similar in their manifestations. I go wandering in the centre of town, on my own, after midnight, where I am likely to recite speeches from a favourite play to people in the street. And I say I am the reincarnation of Sarah Bernhardt or of another celebrated actress.

When I have reached this point, I will not be able to truly appreciate the relevance of the medical advice offered concerning my mental condition. I will deny that I am manic or say that my manic episode is life-enhancing, and I will not be able to give an account of my intentions that are in keeping with my values as noted above.

Thus far, the depressive periods have not been especially severe and there has not been a problem about my accepting treatment.

Preferences regarding treatment setting

When I am manic, the ideal would be to avoid admission. However, if my mood becomes abnormally euphoric or elated, or if I become hyperactive, or if my speech is faster than usual and my thoughts become easily derailed, or if I begin to sleep less than 4 hours, I am becoming unwell and need treatment to avoid a crisis. If possible, it should be at home, with visits by the home treatment team to supervise medication and to assess my progress.

Treatment preferences

The medication that is most likely to be helpful is the addition to my lithium of olanzapine, possibly with diazepam to help me sleep. I do not usually require more than 10 mg each. I react badly to haloperidol, which I refuse to take. At this stage of a relapse, with support from my father and the treatment team I may accept treatment. It should be stressed to me that I have myself agreed that the treatment in the circumstances described is necessary to prevent a serious crisis, and that its necessity is clearly indicated if my goals are to be given effect. Threats are likely to generate a negative reaction.

Social instructions

When I am manic, my father and sister should be contacted. I should not attend classes at the academy and should let my father hold my credit card.

Theory and Rights Reflection

As mentioned, advance directives typically work under a capacity-based legal framework. Under such a framework, advance directives are drafted at a time at which service users have the ability to make treatment decisions based on their own deeply held values and preferences; and they apply when these abilities are substantially impaired.

A specific interpretation of the United Nations (UN) Convention on the Rights of Persons with Disabilities (CRPD) poses a challenge to the implementation of advance documents and self-binding directives in mental healthcare. The CRPD is a human rights treaty adopted by the UN in 2006 and which has been ratified by 189 states parties to date. According to the interpretation advanced by the UN Committee on the Rights of Persons with Disabilities, CRPD Article 12 requires that the practices of mental capacity assessment and substitute decision-making must be abandoned. A key concept here is that of legal capacity. The CRPD Committee explains that legal capacity comprises legal standing, which is one's recognition as a person before the law, and legal agency, which is the capacity to change one's legal relationships to others (2014, par. 12–14). Importantly, a person's treatment decision within an informed consent process changes their legal relationships with the treating physician and hence involves an exercise of legal agency (Scholten & Gather 2018). The CRPD Committee now claims that 'all persons, regardless of disability or decision-making skills, inherently possess legal capacity' (2014, par. 25), and leaves little doubt about how this claim must be interpreted: 'At all times, including in crisis situations, the individual autonomy and capacity of persons with disabilities to make decisions must be respected' (2014, par 18).

Mental health advance directives, however, confront the CRPD Committee with a dilemma. On the one hand, the Committee stresses that 'all persons with disabilities have the right to engage in advance planning and should be given the opportunity to do so on an equal basis with others' (2014, par. 17). On the other hand, decision-making based on a mental health advance directive is inconsistent with the Committee's interpretation of CRPD Art. 12 that at all times, regardless of decision-making skills, the contemporaneous decisions of persons with disabilities should be respected.

There are two approaches to the dilemma. The first holds fixed the Committee's interpretation of CRPD Article 12 and hence its claim that treatment decisions must always be based on the person's contemporaneous preferences. When acknowledging that 'the ability to plan in advance is an important form of support,' the CRPD Committee at the same time restricts the use of advance directives to situations in which persons 'may not be in a position to communicate their wishes to others' (2014, par. 17). While this provides a basis for making treatment decisions based on an advance directive when a person is in a coma or in the later stages of dementia, it does not support the use of advance directives in mental healthcare. The reason is that in mental health crises, people typically have pronounced preferences and are in a position to communicate these to others. They may tell clinicians and close ones, for example, that they would prefer anything over hospital admission. The CRPD Committee's position implies that in such cases the person's contemporaneous preferences must be followed—that is, even in cases where the person has made an advance directive in which they requested such preferences to be discarded in favour of their advance care plan. While we see this as a highly undesirable implication of the Committee's position, the UN High Commissioner seems to accept it: 'Even when such instruments [advance directives] are in force, persons with psychosocial disabilities must always retain their right to modify their will' (2017, par. 28). This would in effect deprive people with mental health conditions of a full opportunity to plan their crisis care in advance (Scholten & Gather 2018; Scholten et al., 2019).

The second approach to the dilemma holds fixed the CRPD Committee's claim that 'all persons with disabilities have the right to engage in advance planning' (2014, par. 17, emphasis added). Most people with mental health conditions engage in advance care planning because they anticipate having harmful preferences during a mental health crisis and want these preferences to be overridden by the preferences described in their advance directive (Braun et al., 2023). The CRPD itself does not explicitly address the issue of whether treatment preferences described in an advance directive may be prioritized over contemporaneous preferences expressed during a mental health crisis which were directed to not be respected. This leads to a consideration of the meaning of CRPD Art. 12(4):

> States Parties shall ensure that all measures that relate to the exercise of legal capacity provide for appropriate and effective safeguards to prevent abuse in accordance with international human rights law. Such safeguards shall ensure that measures relating to the exercise of legal capacity respect the rights, will and preferences of the person [. . .].

The CRPD Committee has offered no definition of 'will and preferences'. Based on common usage of the terms 'will' and 'preference', as well as a reasonably common position in the philosophy of mind and action, we propose that these terms have quite different meanings. A person's 'will' is manifest in the person's deeply held and relatively stable beliefs and values, commitments, personal life projects, and conception of the good; a 'preference', by contrast, is a choice, in the present, between alternative courses of action: for example, whether to accept or refuse a recommended treatment (Szmukler, 2017, 2019). We suggest that if an autonomous person explicitly requests that a future 'preference', which is radically inconsistent with their 'will' and anticipated based on past experience, be overridden by their advance directive, this unwilled preference should not be respected and the advance directives should be followed.

Returning to Anne's case, this means that if after completing her advance directive Anne refuses treatment while showing the signs that she describes as indicative of the need for treatment in her advance directive (i.e. she wanders around the centre of town past midnight claiming she is the reincarnation of Sarah Bernhardt) and being unable to make decisions based on her own deeply held values and preferences, treatment decisions must be based on the instructions in her advance directive (i.e. her 'will', as defined above) rather than her contemporaneous preferences. In this case, that means that the preferred treatment would be starting olanzapine in addition to her lithium.

Note, however, that there are service users who have different preferences. For example, a service user with a psychotic disorder may use an advance directive to refuse treatment with haloperidol. We suggest that if after completing this advance directive this person is in a mental health crisis and does not object to treatment with haloperidol while being unable to make decisions according to their own deeply held values and preferences, the treatment team should base the treatment decision on the person's advance directive (i.e. their 'will') and hence refrain from starting treatment with haloperidol even if this treatment were medically indicated. This makes explicit that our proposed interpretation of the standard of 'will and preferences' is by no means biased toward consent to treatment as opposed to treatment refusal.

In this way, it can be argued that medical decision-making based on mental health advance directives (and substituted decision-making based on the 'will' of a person more generally) is compatible with the standard of 'will and preferences' expressed in CRPD Art. 12, as well as the purpose and general principles of the Convention (Szmukler, 2017, 2019; Scholten et al., 2019; Scholten et al., 2021).

Self-Binding Directives

In most jurisdictions, arranging involuntary admission and treatment according to an advance directive is possible only if the statutory criteria for this are fulfilled (Gloeckler et al., 2025). These typically include the criterion that the person should pose an acute risk of substantial harm to self or others. Anne wishes for intervention in her mental health crisis at an early stage, possibly before she fulfils all statutory criteria. One option for Anne would be to add a self-binding clause to her advance directive.

Self-binding directives are advance directives in which service users can instruct clinicians to override anticipated future treatment refusals and consent to involuntary hospital admission and treatment in advance (Gergel & Owen 2015). They are also commonly referred to as Ulysses contracts or arrangements, referring to the episode in Homer's Odyssey in which Ulysses, in order to be able to hear the enchanting song of the Sirens while preventing himself from being lured to his death, ordered his crew to plug their ears with wax, and instructed them to tie him to the mast and not to release him, however much he might plead for them to do so. In a comparable way, mental health service users can consent in advance to involuntary hospital admission and treatment in a self-binding directive to prevent themselves from engaging in anticipated self-damaging acts during a mental health crisis.

Self-binding directives are ethically and legally controversial. While some ethicists and legal scholars have argued that these documents offer substantial advantages, such as promoting service user autonomy and wellbeing, others have raised fundamental concerns (Stephenson et al., 2023). These concerns include legal issues surrounding an alleged incompatibility of self-binding directives with basic liberty rights and philosophical issues surrounding an alleged lack of personal identity between a person's well and unwell self. Such concerns may be part of the explanation for why few jurisdictions worldwide have made legal provisions for self-binding directives.

Only recently, the perspectives of key stakeholders (e.g. service users, clinicians, and family members) on the opportunities and risks of self-binding directives have been investigated systematically (Scholten et al., 2023a). Perceived benefits included making possible an early intervention in a mental health crisis based on self-defined criteria and avoiding personally defined harms (including not only health damage but also financial damage, setbacks to personal life projects, and impairments of personal relationships). Perceived risks were mostly pragmatic in nature and included lack of awareness and support, inaccessibility of the document during crisis, and the possibility of limited therapeutic flexibility due to too narrow instructions in the document. Stakeholders tended to support the implementation of self-binding directives because they felt the risks and challenges could be addressed through appropriate safeguards. We will describe possible safeguards below.

Thought Experiment: Anne's Self-Binding Directive

Let us assume that Anne added the following self-binding clause to her advance directive to ensure an early intervention in her anticipated mental health crisis.

> Based on my past episodes, I believe that I should be admitted to hospital and treated according to the instructions in my advance directive if I do or say three or more of the following:
>
> 1. I am becoming euphoric, talk faster and less coherently than usual, am hyperactive, and am irritable compared to my usual self.
> 2. I sleep less than 3 hours on two consecutive nights.
> 3. I go wandering in the centre of town, on my own, after midnight (where I am likely to recite speeches from a favourite play to people in the street).
> 4. I say I am the reincarnation of Sarah Bernhardt or of another celebrated actress.
> 5. I say that further training in drama is unnecessary and that I am totally equipped for major roles that I will be offered soon.
>
> My father and sister will be able to judge these changes in me.
>   I hope I will accept admission when I see this advance directive. If not, then I consent in advance to be admitted to hospital and treated on the basis of the instructions in my advance directive, despite my likely objections.

Analysis and Questions

A first issue is whether legislators should make legal provisions for self-binding directives. We suggest they should, provided they also put adequate safeguards in place. Potential safeguards include the close involvement of a person of trust (e.g. a close one or a personal advocate), the facilitation of the drafting process by a neutral party (e.g. a peer support worker), the specification of the content of the self-binding directive in consultation with the treating mental health team, and regular updating of the content (Scholten et al., 2023b). An implementation of self-binding directives along these lines would give people like Anne significantly more control over their lives and treatment. Research indicates that key stakeholders support self-binding directives (Scholten et al., 2023a) and that a substantial majority of people with bipolar would make use of this instrument if it were available (Hindley et al., 2019; Gergel et al., 2021).

It remains an open question whether admission and treatment based on a self-binding directive could be classed as an 'informal' (or non-compulsory) admission in the light of the person's advance consent, or whether it should be classed as a 'formal' involuntary admission. An advantage of the first approach is that it avoids the stigma attached to involuntary detention. The argument is that the person's advance consent makes it the case that admission and treatment according to the person's advance directive is not a deprivation of liberty. This is a controversial proposal. Although it offers a novel option that extends the reach of the person's autonomy, concerns about the lack of safeguards under an informal arrangement can legitimately be raised. The absence of protections such as the right of appeal and regular review is one example.

In the Netherlands, one of the few jurisdictions worldwide with explicit legal provisions for self-binding directives, the following legal arrangement is in place (Scholten et al., 2021). As long as a person does not object to admission and treatment based on their self-binding directive, the admission is classed as an informal admission (regardless of the person's capacity status); as soon as a person objects, however, the admission is classed as a 'conventional' formal admission that is subject to authorization by a judge. The underlying argument is that treating a person over their objections amounts to an encroachment of the basic right to liberty (despite advance consent), and that any intervention that encroaches on basic rights is subject to special safeguards and legal authorization. A disadvantage of this approach is that the time frame for obtaining legal authorization is often protracted, the legally defined maximum term being 4 weeks and 3 days in the Netherlands (Scholten et al., 2021). This undermines the aim of enabling early intervention. Another disadvantage is that many admissions based on a self-binding directive still have the stigma of involuntary admission and treatment attached to it.

Perhaps the risk of stigma and the lack of adequate safeguards can be avoided by allowing service users to specify their preferred arrangements in their self-binding directive itself. Anne, for example, could add the following stipulations to her self-binding directive:

The following conditions must be observed:

- If physical force, beyond taking me by my arm, is to be used to get me to hospital, then the admission should be a conventional compulsory admission with all of the safeguards that will entail.
- If physical force or seclusion is to be used when I am an inpatient, I should be placed on a compulsory order.
- My situation must be reviewed twice per week by my treating psychiatrist, my father or sister, and my independent mental health advocate to ensure that these conditions are being observed.

> - My advance consent to involuntary hospital admission and treatment is for no longer than 28 days.
> - If the indicators described above resolve before 28 days, then my advance consent ends. My father and sister will be good judges on this.

This proposal raises a least two concerns. A fundamental constitutional argument against this proposal from a civil law perspective is that any encroachment of a basic right should have a basis in statutory law and that making decisions about this is the prerogative of a judge (Henking & Scholten, 2023). A more pragmatic concern is that the task of stipulating the legal arrangements and the safeguards for one's admission is likely to be too burdensome for many—even if probably not for Anne.

A final proposal is to create a special legal basis for involuntary admission and treatment based on a self-binding directive over the person's objection, a 'self-binding authorization', which would have provisions for both suitable safeguards and an expedited procedure for obtaining legal authorization. The details of this proposal are described in Scholten et al., (2021). This proposal might avoid the disadvantages of the other approaches.

Conclusions

Advance directives offer mental health service users significantly more control over their lives and treatment and can contribute to an improved therapeutic relationship. Mental health professionals can remove barriers to the use of advance directives by raising awareness among colleagues and service users, supporting service users in drafting an advance directive, establishing an information infrastructure that secures accessibility of advance directives in a mental health crisis, and committing to following advance directives. While self-binding directives are not yet legally regulated in most jurisdictions, they can extend service user autonomy by enabling the person to specify the circumstances in which they want mental health professionals to intervene in an anticipated mental health crisis. Successful implementation of self-binding directives requires carefully constructed legal arrangements for involuntary admission and treatment based on the directive, as well as effective safeguards.

Questions and Thought Experiments

1. If you had a mental health condition with recurring mental health crises, would you want to draft an advance directive?
2. If you wanted to implement advance directives in your local mental health service, where would you start?

3. How would you ensure that the advance directives of people who use your mental health services are accessible to the relevant actors in a mental health crisis?
4. If a person used an advance directive to refuse a treatment that you as a clinician strongly believe is clearly the best therapeutic option, would you respect the treatment refusal? How would you justify your decision?
5. Would you arrange involuntary hospital admission and treatment for a person to comply with their self-binding directive, even when their clinical state would not conventionally warrant an involuntary admission and treatment?

Acknowledgements

Matthé Scholten would like to thank the German Federal Ministry of Education and Research for funding received in the context of the SALUS project (grant number 01GP1792).

Further Reading

Braun, E., Gaillard, A.-S., Vollmann, J., Gather, J., & Scholten, M. (2023). Mental health service users' perspectives on psychiatric advance directives: A systematic review. *Psychiatric Services, 74*(4), 381–392. https://doi.org/10.1176/appi.ps.202200003

Stephenson, L. A. A., Gieselmann, T., Gergel, G., Owen, J., Gather, J., & Scholten, M. (2023). Self-binding directives in psychiatric practice: A systematic review of reasons. *The Lancet Psychiatry, 10*(11), 887–895. https://doi.org/10.1016/S2215-0366(23)00221-3

Scholten, M., Efkemann, S. A., Faissner, M., Finke, M., Gather, J. Gergel, T., Gieselmann, A., van der Ham, L., Juckel, G., van Melle, L., Owen, G., Potthoff, S., Stephenson, G., Szmukler, L. A., Vellinga, A., Vollmann, J., Voskes, Y., Werning, A. & Widdershoven, G. (2023a). Opportunities and challenges of self-binding directives: A comparison of empirical research with stakeholders in three European countries. *European Psychiatry, 66*(1), e48. https://doi.org/10.1192/j.eurpsy.(2023).2421

Szmukler, G. (2019). Capacity, best interests, will and preferences and the UN Convention on the Rights of Persons with Disabilities. *World Psychiatry, 18*(1), 34–41. https://doi.org/10.1002/wps.20584

References

Braun, E., Gaillard, A.-S., Vollmann, J., Gather, J., & Scholten, M. (2023). Mental health service users' perspectives on psychiatric advance directives: A systematic review. *Psychiatric Services, 74*(4), 381–392. https://doi.org/10.1176/appi.ps.202200003

Gaillard, A.-S., Braun, E., Vollmann, J., Gather, J., & Scholten, M. (2023). The content of psychiatric advance directives: A systematic review. *Psychiatric Services, 74* (1), 44–55. https://doi.org/10.1176/appi.ps.202200002

Gergel, T., Das, P., Owen, G., Stephenson, L., Rifkin, L., Hindley, L., Dawson, J., Keene, A. R. (2021). Reasons for endorsing or rejecting self-binding directives in bipolar disorder: A qualitative study of survey responses from UK service users. *The Lancet Psychiatry, 8*(7), 599–609. https://doi.org/10.1016/S2215-0366(21)00115-2

Gloeckler, S., Scholten, M., Weller, P., Ruck Keene, A., Pathare, S., Pillutla, R., Andorno, L., & Biller-Andorno, N. (2025). An international comparison of psychiatric advance directive policy: Across eleven jurisdictions and alongside advance directive policy. *International Journal of Law and Psychiatry, 101*, 102098. https://doi.org/10.1016/j.ijlp.2025.102098

Henking, T., & Scholten, M. (2023). Respect for the will and preferences of people with mental disorders in German law. In C. Kong, J. Coggon, P. Cooper, M. Dunn & A. R. Keene (Eds.), *Capacity, Participation, and Values in Comparative Legal Perspective* (pp. 203–225). Bristol University Press.

Hindley, G., Stephenson, L. A., Keene, A. R., Rifkin, L, Gergel, T., & Owen, G. (2019). Why have I not been told about this? *Wellcome Open Research, 4*(16). https://doi.org/10.12688/wellcomeopenres.14989.2

Scholten, M., Efkemann, S. A., Faissner, M., Finke, M., Gather, J., Gergel, T., Gieselmann, A., van der Ham, L., Juckel, G., van Melle, L., Owen, G., Potthoff, S., Stephenson, L. A., Szmukler, G., Vellinga, A., Vollmann, J., Voskes, Y., Werning, A., & Widdershoven, G. (2023a). Opportunities and challenges of self-binding directives: A comparison of empirical research with stakeholders in three European countries. *European Psychiatry, 66*(1), e48. https://doi.org/10.1192/j.eurpsy.(2023).2421

Scholten, M., Efkemann, S. A., Faissner, M., Finke, M., Gather, J., Gergel, T., Gieselmann, A., van der Ham, L., Juckel, G., van Melle, L., Owen, G., Potthoff, S., Stephenson, L. A., Szmukler, G., Vellinga, A., Vollmann, J., Voskes, Y., Werning, A., & Widdershoven, G. (2023b). Implementation of self-binding directives: Recommendations based on expert consensus and input by stakeholders in three European countries. *World Psychiatry, 22*(2), 332–333. https://doi.org/10.1002/wps.21095

Scholten, M., & J. Gather. (2018). Adverse consequences of article 12 of the UN Convention on the Rights of Persons with Disabilities for persons with mental disabilities and an alternative way forward. *Journal of Medical Ethics, 44*(4), 226–233. https://doi.org/10.1136/medethics-2017-104414

Scholten, M., Gather, J., & Vollmann, J. (2021). Equality in the informed consent process: Competence to consent, substitute decision-making, and discrimination of persons with mental disorders. *The Journal of Medicine and Philosophy, 46*(1), 108–136. https://doi.org/10.1093/jmp/jhaa030

Scholten, M., Gieselmann, A., Gather, J., & Vollmann, J. (2019). Psychiatric advance directives under the Convention on the Rights of Persons with Disabilities: Why advance instructions should be able to override current preferences. *Frontiers in Psychiatry, 10*, Article 631. https://doi.org/10.3389/fpsyt.(2019).00631

Scholten, M., van Melle, L., & Widdershoven, G. (2021). Self-binding directives under the new Dutch Law on Compulsory Mental Health Care: An analysis of the legal framework and a proposal for reform. *International Journal of Law and Psychiatry, 76*, Article 101699. https://doi.org/10.1016/j.ijlp.(2021).101699

Stephenson, L. A., Gergel, T. Gieselmann, A. Scholten, M., Keene, A. R., Rifkin, L., & Owen, G. (2020). Advance decision making in bipolar: A systematic review. *Frontiers in Psychiatry, 11*, Article 538107. https://doi.org/10.3389/fpsyt.2020.538107

Stephenson, L. A., Gergel, T., Keene, A. R., Rifkin, L., & Owen, G. (2020). The PACT advance decision-making template: Preparing for Mental Health Act reforms with co-production, focus groups and consultation. *International Journal of Law and Psychiatry, 71*, Article 101563. https://doi.org/https://doi.org/10.1016/j.ijlp.2020.101563

Stephenson, L. A., Gieselmann, A., Gergel, T., Owen, G., Gather, J., & Scholten, M. (2023). Self-binding directives in psychiatric practice: A systematic review of reasons. *The Lancet Psychiatry, 10*(11), 887–895. https://doi.org/10.1016/S2215-0366(23)00221-3

Szmukler, G. (2017). The UN Convention on the Rights of Persons with Disabilities: 'Rights, will and preferences' in relation to mental health disabilities. *International Journal of Law and Psychiatry, 54*: 90–97. https://doi.org/https://doi.org/10.1016/j.ijlp.2017.06.003

Szmukler, G. (2018). *Men in white coats: Treatment under coercion.* Oxford University Press.

Szmukler, G. (2019). Capacity, best interests, will and preferences and the UN Convention on the Rights of Persons with Disabilities. *World Psychiatry, 18*(1), 34–41. https://doi.org/10.1002/wps.20584

United Nations, Committee on the Rights of Persons with Disabilities. (2014). *General comment No. 1 Article 12: Equality before the law. CRPD/C/GC/1.* https://undocs.org/en/CRPD/C/GC/1

United Nations, High Commissioner for Human Rights. (2017). *Mental health and human rights. A/HRC/34/32.* https://undocs.org/en/A/HRC/34/32

18

Mental Health Advocacy

Kristijan Grđan and Claudia Marinetti

Mental Health Europe

Introduction

Mental health advocacy regards mental health as both a personal asset and a fundamental aspect of overall health, which is a basic human right. Advocacy is essential to ensure the full respect of human rights for individuals with mental health problems (Mental Health Europe, n.d.)[1] and to promote their autonomy.

The history of mental health and human rights is complex, often marked by the persecution of those with mental health problems. In medieval times, mental health problems were believed to be caused by demonic possession, leading to brutal practices like exorcisms and executions. As leprosy declined in Europe, the established lazar houses, originally meant to isolate leprosy patients, began to be replaced with institutions for people with mental health problems, leading to their social isolation and institutionalization. By the 18th century, individuals with mental health conditions were placed in asylums, which were designed for their complete isolation from society (Foucault, 1961).

The atrocities reached a peak during World War II, when an estimated 220,000 to 269,500 individuals with schizophrenia were sterilized or killed by the Nazis, which some authors refer to as a 'psychiatric genocide' (Torrey & Yolken, 2010). These numbers do not include similar treatment received by people with other mental health problems or intellectual disabilities. Such atrocities were upheld, among others, by physicians who targeted patients and residents in institutions and who, after reviewing their medical records decided on murdering them. Non-consensual medical experimentation on psychiatric patients, including children, was rampant, resulting in mutilation and death (Weindling et al., 2016). The Nuremberg Trials, particularly the United States v. Karl Brandt et al. case, convicted seventeen doctors for atrocities committed by medical experimentation or euthanasia, leading to life imprisonment or death sentences. The 'Doctors' trials' resulted in the establishment of the Nuremberg Code for medical experimentation,

---

[1] Mental Health Europe prefers use of the term 'mental health problems'.

which would later significantly influence the development of international human rights law (Shuster, 1997).

The aftermath of World War II saw the creation of international organizations like the United Nations and the Council of Europe to protect human rights and prevent future atrocities. The Universal Declaration of Human Rights (1948) and the European Convention on Human Rights and Fundamental Freedoms (1950) were enacted, yet individuals with mental health problems continued to face institutionalization and non-consensual, often torturous treatments. Lobotomies continued in the United States until the late 1950s, and modified forms of surgical interventions in the brain, called psychosurgery is still practiced in some countries (Faria, 2013). Electroconvulsive therapy, though generally now administered with anaesthesia, can still be performed without consent in many countries (Leiknes et al., 2012). 'The voluntary consent of the human subject is absolutely essential' is the fundamental principle of the Nuremberg Code in relation to medical experimentation on humans, yet globally this principle was never fully implemented (Shuster, 1997). The Convention on Human Rights and Biomedicine (Oviedo Convention) allows substitute consenting for adults via guardians (Council of Europe, 1997).[2] Yet in 2015, thanks to advocacy efforts, Croatia enacted an absolute prohibition on non-consensual medical experimentation in psychiatry for both adults and children, despite strong opposition from mainstream psychiatry (Grđan, 2017).

In the second half of the 20th century, psychiatry was often politically abused, notably in the Soviet Union during the 1970s and 1980s, where a third of political prisoners were detained in psychiatric hospitals. Similar practices were widespread in other socialist countries, notably Romania, and continue in 21st-century China (van Voren, 2010).

Today, despite a growing number in the psychiatric sector supporting a human rights approach, thousands of people with mental health conditions are still denied their fundamental human rights in mental health settings and society at large. Involuntary treatment and coercive practices, including isolation and the use of restraints, are still common in Europe, justified by the misconception that individuals with mental health problems are inherently dangerous. This belief is challenged by the UN Convention on the Rights of Persons with Disabilities (UN CRPD Committee, 2015).

This chapter explores contemporary issues related to mental health as a human right and examines the response of international law in Europe. We will provide examples of how advocacy can shape laws and policies and how legal and policy tools can be used for advocacy to drive change.

In the first section, we detail the paradigm shift initiated by the adoption of the United Nations Convention on the Rights of Persons with Disabilities (CRPD).

---

[2] Article 17.

Following this, we present examples illustrating how Mental Health Europe endeavours to influence policy and international legislative processes across Europe.

The Era of the UN Convention on Rights of Persons with Disabilities

The adoption of the CRPD marked the beginning of a paradigm shift in mental health. The CRPD underpins the advocacy work of many disability organizations, including Mental Health Europe, which aligns its efforts with CRPD principles.

The CRPD was adopted by the UN General Assembly on 13 December 2006, and has since been ratified by 190 states, including all European Union (EU) member states and the EU itself. It is an enforceable international treaty, requiring the repeal of contradictory laws and the reform of practices. Some European countries operate under the monist legal system which means that international treaties automatically become part of the domestic legal system and are directly enforceable. In practice, there may be confusion about the applicability of laws and that may especially affect practitioners who are bound to implement national laws until they are changed according to the CRPD. Advocacy to reform laws in accordance with the CRPD is therefore vital. The UN Committee on the Rights of Persons with Disabilities (CRPD Committee) monitors implementation and harmonization of human rights standards.

The CRPD defines persons with disabilities as those with long-term physical, mental, intellectual, or sensory impairments that, in interaction with various barriers, hinder full and effective participation in society on an equal basis with others. Practically speaking, the CRPD transformed the way disability is determined; it is no longer enough to require the existence of a long-term, health-related functional impairment. The social barriers that hinder full participation in society are causes of disability. Disability is thus seen as a social concept rather than a biomedical issue. This paradigm shift brought about international human rights obligations, requiring societies to evolve to ensure the full and meaningful participation of persons with disabilities, rather than focusing solely on biomedical solutions to health conditions related to disability.

People with mental health problems can fall under the definition of disability as persons with psychosocial disabilities. Historically, they have faced stigma, discrimination, social isolation, and neglect, encountering barriers that impede their full participation in society. Lack of assistance, limited or no access to community-based services, inadequate employment opportunities, and social exclusion are causes of disability. The CRPD protects every person with mental health problems facing these societal barriers.

The CRPD ushered in a new approach to the human rights of people with psychosocial disabilities. Initially, international human rights laws applicable to people with psychosocial disabilities were derived from broader United Nations and Council of Europe laws.[3] These laws typically addressed incarceration in psychiatric hospitals and similar institutions, offering safeguards against non-consensual treatment and prohibiting certain practices (e.g. psychosurgery/lobotomy, unmodified electroconvulsive therapy, castration). However, the CRPD focuses not only on prohibition of practices but also on the interventions states must undertake to empower the human rights of persons with psychosocial disabilities, enabling their autonomy and full participation in society. As Professor Gerard Quinn, in his role as United Nations Special Rapporteur on Rights of Persons with Disabilities, stated: 'The surface of human rights can and should be mined to find a deeper, fuller, richer understanding of the person—of the human in human rights' (Quinn).

Historically, human rights for people with mental health problems have predominantly focused on biomedical interventions, reflecting the dominance of psychiatric care over other forms of support and care. This is evident in global government funding allocations for mental health care. According to a 2021 WHO report on mental health investment shortfalls, over 70% of government expenditure on mental health in middle-income countries was allocated to mental hospitals, compared to 35% in high-income countries. Only 25% of responding countries met all criteria for integrating mental health into primary care, highlighting the slow and challenging transition from institutional to community-based care.[4] When it comes to the financial burden of community-based services, it is important to note that recent research by WHO shows that in many cases such services have lower cost of service provision than comparable mainstream services (World Health Organization, 2021).

Since 2006, the implementation of the CRPD for people with psychosocial disabilities has been a highly debated aspect of this international law. There are different views in the global mental health community, which includes mental health professionals and service users, on this issue. Part of this community lobbies for maintaining biomedical dominance, opposing the changes demanded by the CRPD (Russo & Wooley, 2020). On the other hand, groups such as the Critical Psychiatrists Network often opposes the biomedical paradigm representing a counterbalance to the mainstream profession.[5] Although the CRPD promotes a social model of disability, requiring not only psychiatric practice reform, the most controversial issues concerning the autonomy and freedom of people with psychosocial disabilities often arise from government defences of traditional psychiatry and predominant biomedical approaches.

---

[3] For example, Universal Declaration of Human Rights, International Covenant on Political and Cultural Rights, European Convention on Human Rights and Fundamental Freedoms, Convention on Human Rights and Biomedicine, etc.

[4] https://www.who.int/news/item/08-10-2021-who-report-highlights-global-shortfall-in-investment-in-mental-health

[5] https://www.criticalpsychiatry.co.uk/

Mental Health Advocacy in Europe

The fact that the EU and all its member states have ratified the CRPD gives advocates within the EU precious tools towards the realization of rights of persons with psychosocial disabilities (European Union, 2021). However, influencing policy is a complex process that requires patience, persistence, and a multifaceted approach. Building relationships, gathering evidence, and effectively communicating messages are key to effecting change in European mental health policies.

Influencing European policy as a mental health non-governmental organization involves several strategic steps. This is what Mental Health Europe, as a network representing people with lived experience, their supporters, service and care providers, human rights experts, and mental health organizations across Europe, puts in place to influence European policies:

1. **Policy Recommendations**: Mental Health Europe develops policy recommendations based on the needs and experiences of individuals dealing with mental health problems, bringing to the table expertise from across its membership. These recommendations are presented to policymakers and government bodies in various forms, such as answers to consultations, requests of amendments to proposed legislation, individual meetings, and public events to name a few. Being concise, outlining the changes needed but also proposing how to create and implement such changes certainly increase the possibility of success of advocacy efforts. So does aligning with EU goals, existing policies, and frameworks. An example of such tools is policy developed specifically for people with disabilities. Following the European Disability Strategy, advocacy efforts let the European Strategy for the Rights of Persons with Disabilities to explicitly refer to persons with psychosocial disabilities.

2. **Engagement with Politicians and Policy-Makers**: Advocacy entails engaging directly with policymakers, politicians, decision-makers, and relevant institutions at local, national, and European levels. Opening doors to be listened to requires constant networking, good timing, political awareness, and attention to new windows of opportunity. Influencing policy discussions and decisions related to mental health is then facilitated by providing expertise, data, and insights. One example of the way in which Mental Health Europe engages with policy-makers at European level is the creation of a Coalition for Mental Health and Well-being[6] at the European Parliament active during each legislative term.

3. **Partnerships**: Creating alliances with likeminded non-governmental organizations (NGOs), advocacy groups, and relevant stakeholders helps to amplify messages and provide a unified front that adds strength to advocacy efforts. For instance, Mental Health Europe has created a Mental Health Advocacy Platform to work with

---

[6] https://mental-health-coalition.com/

European NGOs for whom mental health is not core business but a relevant element to those they represent (e.g. older people, children, LGBTQ+ communities).

Formal partnerships with international organizations also help with providing platforms for communication of issues around human rights and with cementing credibility. Mental Health Europe, for instance, is an accredited non-state actor for the World Health Organization (WHO) European Region. Regional accreditation of non-State actors is a privilege that the WHO Regional Committee for Europe may grant to regional non-governmental organizations among others; a benefit of this accreditation is that 'It includes an invitation to participate, without the right to vote, in meetings of the Regional Committee and the opportunity to submit written and/or oral statements through WHO/Europe.'[7] Mental Health Europe also enjoys participatory status with the Council of Europe.[8]

4. Public Awareness Campaigns: Public awareness can be raised through campaigns, pledges, social media, events, arts exhibitions, and media outreach, to name a few. A well-informed public can put pressure on policymakers to prioritize mental health in their agendas.

Nowadays people talk more and more about mental health. It is crucial that anti-stigma efforts do not limit themselves to the goal of attitude change but actively work to translate attitude change into societies that are conducive of good mental health for all. To achieve real positive change, awareness should be channelled towards legislative and policy change needed to address the socio-economic and environmental determinants of mental health.

Mental Health Europe runs campaigns and initiatives aimed at specific policy changes. These efforts might focus on destigmatization and end of discrimination, access to services, community mental health, or other specific aspects of mental health policy. Since 2020, Mental Health Europe hosts the European Mental Health Week.

5. Monitoring and Evaluation: Keep track of policy developments, monitor progress, and evaluate the impact of existing policies on mental health. This information is crucial for refining your strategies and advocating for necessary adjustments.

Mental Health Europe monitors the implementation of mental health policies and assesses their effectiveness. They provide feedback to policymakers based on real-world experiences, contributing to evidence-based policy-making.

6. Research and Data Collection: Gathering comprehensive data and research helps in supporting arguments. Robust evidence and statistics regarding mental health problems in Europe strengthen advocacy efforts. One of our most successful publications is Mapping Exclusion, which maps institutional and community care in the field of mental health in Europe. This tool has been praised by international organizations and successfully used to advocate for change at EU level, where action was

---

[7] https://www.who.int/europe/about-us/partnerships/partners/non-state-actors
[8] https://www.coe.int/en/web/ingo/overview

added as part of the European Semester[9] process to analyse and prioritize deinstitu-tionalization in a more comprehensive way.

Overall, Mental Health Europe's influence on European policy is driven by its dedication to representing the needs of individuals with mental health problems, conducting advocacy work, providing expertise, and fostering collaboration among stakeholders to bring about positive changes in mental health policies across Europe. Mental Health Europe is a hybrid organization comprising service users and their supporters, service providers, care professionals, human rights experts, and advo-cates. This facilitates co-creation, one of the pillars of the organization. Our advocacy activities stem from the contribution of all those who have a stake in mental health, keeping the well-being of persons with lived experience of mental health problems at the centre of our efforts.

Let's now dive into examples of how to produce tools for advocacy and how to in-fluence legislation and practices in mental health care.

Case Study 1: Producing Tools for Advocacy: Mapping Exclusion (Deinstitutionalization)

Since 2012, Mental Health Europe has published two comprehensive reports on map-ping and understanding exclusion in Europe (University of Kent-Tizard Centre and Mental Health Europe 2012). These reports aim to provide updated information on European countries' mental health laws, the use of involuntary or forced placements and treatments, the practice of seclusion and restraint, as well as emerging issues in the mental health field. They offer an overview of mental health systems across Europe, highlighting the human rights situation for individuals who use mental health serv-ices and those with psychosocial disabilities.

The reports include a set of recommendations for policymakers and legislators to empower civil society organizations in their respective countries, supporting their ad-vocacy initiatives. Notably, these recommendations urge states to adopt holistic de-institutionalization strategies in collaboration with representative organizations of persons with mental health problems and psychosocial disabilities. They also call for the reduction and eventual elimination of coercion in mental health care services.

These reports are aligned with CRPD requirements to respect legal capacity, right to freedom from coercion, and right to independent living in the community, dem-onstrating the interconnection between the fundamental rights of individuals with mental health problems and psychosocial disabilities—rights that are frequently de-nied. The reports serve as valuable resources, providing comparative information on

[9] https://commission.europa.eu/business-economy-euro/economic-and-fiscal-policy-coordination/european-semester_en

laws and practices across different countries, thereby supporting advocacy for better mental health care and human rights.

Case Study 2: Influencing Legislation: '#WithdrawOviedo Campaign'

In 1997, the Council of Europe adopted the Convention on Human Rights and Biomedicine, commonly known as the Oviedo Convention. This convention addresses various bioethical issues and patients' rights to consent to medical procedures, including biomedical research, organ donation, and medically assisted procreation. Only one provision of the Oviedo Convention refers to people with mental health problems and states that subject to protective conditions prescribed by law, 'a person who has a mental disorder of a serious nature may be subjected, without his or her consent, to an intervention aimed at treating his or her mental disorder only where, without such treatment, serious harm is likely to result to his or her health' (Council of Europe, 1997).

In 2004, the Committee of Ministers of the Council of Europe issued Recommendation Rec (2004)10 to Member States, focusing on the protection of the human rights and dignity of persons with mental health problems. Following its implementation, a significant disparity was observed in the laws and practices across Member States, particularly concerning the application of case law from the European Court of Human Rights. To address these inconsistencies, the Steering Committee on Bioethics (renamed in 2022 as the Steering Committee on Human Rights in the fields of Biomedicine and Health, or CD-BIO) was tasked in 2014 with developing a Draft Additional Protocol to the Oviedo Convention.[10] This protocol aimed to regulate involuntary placements and treatment.

Article 14 of the CRPD stipulates that a disability should never justify the deprivation of liberty, thus absolutely prohibiting the involuntary incarceration of individuals with psychosocial disabilities in mental health or similar institutions. The CRPD Committee's 2015 guidelines on Article 14 (Committee on the Rights of Persons with Disabilities, 2015) further clarified the obligation of State parties to respect, protect, and guarantee the right of persons with disabilities to liberty and security, confirming the absolute prohibition on the basis of impairment. This was linked to the right to non-discrimination and article 12 of the CRPD, which deals with legal capacity and autonomy of a person. Furthermore, the enjoyment of the right to liberty and security of a person is closely connected with implementation of article 19 of the CRPD about the right to live independently and live in the community.

The CRPD Committee argues that involuntary commitment in mental health facilities undermines a person's legal capacity to make decisions about their care,

---

[10] The additional protocol is an addendum to the international law, subject to the ratification, that has the same power as the convention itself.

treatment, and admission to a hospital or institution. This practice is repeatedly deemed contrary to both Articles 12 and 14 of the CRPD, and the Committee has called on State parties to repeal legislation permitting involuntary incarceration in mental health settings.

However, in 2011, the Steering Committee on Bioethics of the Council of Europe reviewed the relationship between Council of Europe standards and the CRPD. Despite the mandates of Article 14 of the CRPD, the Committee concluded that involuntary treatment or placement, while not based on disability, could be justified for serious mental health problems if the absence of such treatment or placement would likely result in serious harm to the person's health or to a third party (Steering Committee on Bioethics, 2011). This stance by the Council of Europe has created a divergence between its human rights protection standards and the United Nations' more progressive standards for the rights of persons with psychosocial disabilities.

From 2014 until 2022 the CD-BIO continuously worked on the *draft additional protocol to the Oviedo Convention*. The adoption of the draft additional protocol to the Oviedo Convention would establish conflicting standards of equal significance in international law, effectively cementing involuntary treatment and hindering state parties from fully implementing Article 14 of the CRPD. Russo and Wooley (2020) argue that there is evidence of both resistance and sabotage in the recognition of fundamental rights and freedoms for people with psychosocial disabilities. This includes explicit calls to revise the CRPD and exclude individuals with mental health problems from its scope entirely (Russo & Wooley, 2020). The development of the additional protocol to the Oviedo Convention exemplifies this resistance. It is difficult to imagine that multiple European states would deliberately create a conflicting system of international human rights law. Yet, this is precisely what is occurring, perpetuating the historical approach of social exclusion for persons with psychosocial disabilities.

In response, Mental Health Europe, in collaboration with the European Disability Forum, the European Network of (Ex)-Users and Survivors of Psychiatry, and other NGOs[11] created a coalition to advocate for a complete withdrawal of the draft additional protocol to the Oviedo Convention, launching the '#WithdrawOviedo Campaign.[12] The coalition argued that the draft additional protocol would perpetuate the status quo, hindering the full implementation of the CRPD. In 2019, Mental Health Europe published a report showcasing promising practices in preventing and eliminating coercion in mental health care across Europe[13] which they submitted to CD-BIO. We proposed that instead of creating additional protocol to the Oviedo Convention that contradicts CRPD, the Council of Europe should focus on creating an international framework aimed to reduce and ultimately eliminate coercion in mental health settings.

---

[11] Society of Social Psychiatry P. Sakellaropoulous, Validity, European Association of Service Providers for Persons with Disabilities, Inclusion Europe, Autism Europe and International Disability Alliance.

[12] https://www.withdrawoviedo.info/join

[13] https://mhe-sme.org/wp-content/uploads/2019/01/Coercion-Report.pdf

Both the Council of Europe's Parliamentary Assembly[14] and the Commissioner on Human Rights opposed the draft additional protocol, citing its inconsistency with the CRPD.[15] In 2021 the CRPD Committee issued an open letter to the Council of Europe expressing its concern over continuation of drafting the additional protocol to the Oviedo Convention and asking for its withdrawal.[16]

Acknowledging the advocacy efforts, the CD-BIO decided to simultaneously work on a compendium of good voluntary practices in mental health care: this was completed and published in 2021 (Goodin, 2021). However, it did not withdraw the draft additional protocol but rather chose to present the work on voluntary practices as a complementary matter.

In 2022, the Committee of Ministers suspended the work on the draft additional protocol until the end of 2024, directing CD-BIO to focus on promoting voluntary care in mental health settings. In 2023, Mental Health Europe and its partners began negotiations with CD-BIO on a draft recommendation to respect autonomy in mental health settings and prevent coercion.

Conclusion

Reforms aimed at advancing the rights and social positions of individuals with mental health problems, particularly in areas such as deinstitutionalization, respect for autonomy, and the elimination of coercion in mental health settings, often face significant challenges. These challenges are rooted in societal fears that people with mental health problems pose a danger to themselves and others. Part of the user movement also upholds such approach. Appelbaum (2019) encapsulates this sentiment, stating, 'in the name of protecting all these people from discrimination, they would be free to destroy their own lives and ruin the lives of their loved ones.' This fear is frequently used to undermine advocacy efforts aimed at progressive reforms.

We acknowledge that individuals with mental health problems can experience severe crises in the course of their lives. However, we argue that the political focus of legislators and the dominance of the biomedical model on involuntary treatment and coercion, combined with social exclusion, create mental health care systems that only respond to extreme cases. The lack of early interventions and community-based support makes people with mental health problems overly dependent on institutional mental health care, which, like other health conditions, is often reserved

---

[14] https://assembly.coe.int/nw/xml/XRef/Xref-XML2HTML-en.asp?fileid=28038&lang=en
[15] https://rm.coe.int/comments-by-dunja-mijatovic-council-of-europe-commissioner-for-human-r/16808f1111
[16] Open letter to the Secretary-General of the Council of Europe, the Committee of Ministries of the Council of Europe, the Committee on Bioethics of the Council of Europe, the Steering Committee for Human Rights, the Commissioner of Human Rights, the Parliamentary Assembly of the Council of Europe and other organizations and entities of the Council of Europe, Adopted by the Committee on the Rights of Persons with Disabilities and the Special Rapporteur on the Rights of Persons with Disabilities, June 2021.

for the most severe situations. When accessible, these institutional practices, especially those involving coercion, can be extremely stressful and damaging. This fear of coercion or abuse often deters individuals from seeking help during mental health crises.

Advocacy should bring about international laws that respect autonomy and set the highest standards, guiding states towards deinstitutionalization, developing community-based supports, and ultimately ending coercion in mental health settings. If the focus remains on coercion, states may believe that merely placing safeguards around involuntary treatment and coercive practices suffices to respect the human rights of people with mental health problems. Proponents of coercive practices often argue that coercion is used only as a last resort when other supports fail. Yet, where non-coercive supports, such as peer support services or community crisis teams or mobile unites, do not exist or are not accessible for persons with mental health problems, institutional and coercive methods might seem to be only available resort.

Evidence from Mental Health Europe and WHO can be used in advocacy to show that alternatives to coercion are both possible and more effective, respecting human rights and individual autonomy.[17] This growing body of evidence supports the view that a community-based approach to mental health care, which fully respects the autonomy of individuals with mental health problems, is the future direction for mental health systems in Europe. While these practices exist and they have been shown to be effective, they also need to be adequately resourced to be sustainable. This approach moves away from the historical paradigm of neglect and marginalization faced by these individuals.

As people with lived experience argue, people with mental health problems do not need a different psychiatry, but a different system of care that goes beyond the biomedical dominance and enables different social actors in providing support (Russo and Wooley, 2020). This is what we must advocate for.

Questions and Thought Experiments

1. In your view, are there rights that are more fundamental than others?
2. What do you think are barriers to successful advocacy by civil society?
3. What actions or tools do you feel would lead to successful advocacy in your community?
4. How do you see the future of UN CRPD implementation in mental health?

---

[17] See for example case of Kliniken Landkreis Heindenheim GmbH from Germany, which through a series of community-based supports based on respecting of autonomy of their patients, significantly reduced the use of coercion and forced treatment when compared to average of these practices in other German mental health care settings, in WHO (2021, pp. 43–48).

Further Reading

WHO. (2021). Guidance on Community Based Services: Promoting person-centred and rights-based approaches. https://www.who.int/publications/i/item/9789240025707

WHO and OHCHR. (2023). Guidance and Practice on Mental Health, Human Rights and Legislation. https://www.who.int/publications/b/70051#:~:text=The%20guidance%20p roposes%20new%20objectives,with%20current%20human%20rights%20standards.&text= Some%20rights%20reserved.,subject%20to%20permission%20from%20WHO

Mental Health Europe. (2023). Mental Health: The Power of Language. A glossary of terms and words. https://www.mentalhealtheurope.org/library/mhe-releases-

Mental Health Europe. (2023). Promoting understanding of the Psychosocial Model of Mental Health. https://www.mentalhealtheurope.org/library/mhe-releases-psychosocial-toolkit/

References

Committee on the Rights of Persons with Disabilities. (2015). Guidelines on Article 14 of the Convention on the Rights of Persons with Disabilities: The right to liberty and security of the person. Adopted during the Committee's 14th Session, held in September 2015. https:// www.ohchr.org/en/documents/legal-standards-and-guidelines/guidelines-article-14-con vention-rights-persons-disabilities

Council of Europe. (1997). *Convention on Human Rights and Biomedicine* (Oviedo Convention). https://www.coe.int/en/web/bioethics/oviedo-convention

European Union. (2021). Strategy for the rights of persons with disabilities 2021–2030. https:// ec.europa.eu/social/main.jsp?catId=1484&langId=en

Faria, M. A. Jr. (2013). Violence, mental illness and the brain – A brief history of psychosur-gery: Part 1 – From trephination to lobotomy. *Surgical Neurology International, 4*, Article 49. https://doi.org/10.4103/2152-7806.110146

Foucault, M. (1961). *Madness and civilization*. Librarie Plon.

Gooding, Piers. (2021). *Compendium report: Good practices in the Council of Europe to promote voluntary measures in mental health services*. https://rm.coe.int/compendium-final-en/168 0a45740

Grdan, K. (2017). Biomedical research in psychiatry and the right to the autonomy of partici-pants. *Almanac of the University of Rijeka Law School, 38*(3), 1133–1161. https://hrcak.srce. hr/file/288017

Leiknes, K. A., Jarosh-von Schweder, L., & Høie, B. (2012). Contemporary use and practice of electroconvulsive therapy worldwide. *Brain and Behavior, 2*(3), 283–344. https://doi.org/ 10.1002/brb3.37

Mental Health Europe. (n.d.). *A glossary of terms and words*. https://www.mentalhealtheurope. org/library/mhe-releases-glossary

Quinn, G. (2021, 21 June). *Putting the human back into human rights: Intersectional perspec-tives*. Paper presented at the Annual Conference of Netherlands Institute for Human Rights Research.

Russo, J., & Wooley, S. (2020). The implementation of the Convention on the Rights of Persons with Disabilities: More than just another reform of psychiatry. *Health and Human Rights Journal, 22*(1), 151–162. https://www.hhrjournal.org/2020/06/the-implementation-of-the-convention-on-the-rights-of-persons-with-disabilities-more-than-just-another-reform-of-psychiatry/

Shuster, E. (1997). Fifty years later: The significance of the Nuremberg Code. *The New England Journal of Medicine, 337*(20), 1436–1440. https://doi.org/10.1056/NEJM199711133372006

Steering Committee on Bioethics. (2011). *Statement on the United Nations Convention on Rights of Persons with Disabilities.* https://rm.coe.int/inf-2011-10-statement-un-conv-en/16804553b0

Torrey, E. F., & Yolken, R. H. (2010). Psychiatric genocide: Nazi attempts to eradicate schizophrenia. *Schizophrenia Bulletin, 36*(1), 26–32. https://doi.org/10.1093/schbul/sbp097

UN CRPD Committee. (2015). *Guidelines on Article 14 of the Convention on the Rights of Persons with Disabilities.* https://www.ohchr.org/en/documents/legal-standards-and-guidelines/guidelines-article-14-convention-rights-persons-disabilities

University of Kent-Tizard Centre and Mental Health Europe. (2012). *Mapping and understanding exclusion in Europe* (Report). https://kar.kent.ac.uk/64970/

van Voren, R. (2010). Political abuse of psychiatry—An historical overview. *Schizophrenia Bulletin, 36*(1), 33–35. https://doi.org/10.1093/schbul/sbp119

Weindling, P., von Villiez, A., Loewenau, A., & Farron, N. (2016). The victims of unethical human experiments and coerced research under National Socialism. *Endeavour, 40*(1), 1–6. https://doi.org/10.1016/j.endeavour.2015.10.005

World Health Organization. (2021). *Guidance on community mental health services: Promoting person-centred and rights-based approaches.* https://www.who.int/publications/i/item/9789240025707

19

Antipsychotics in Delirium and Dementia

Mediating Pressures to Treat

Shaun T. O'Keeffe

Introduction

The Nature of the Dilemma

Behavioural and psychological symptoms of dementia (BPSD) affect most people with Alzheimer's disease and other dementias at some stage and commonly precipitate admission to nursing home care. Similar symptoms are common in acutely unwell patients with delirium. (BPSD will refer to both in this chapter.) They can result in considerable suffering for patients and families and create significant management difficulties for healthcare professionals and carers. Antipsychotic agents, mainly atypical antipsychotics, have been widely used to suppress such symptoms especially when other interventions have been ineffective.

In a widely publicized report, Banerjee (2009) analysed the existing evidence and concluded that treating 1,000 people with dementia and with BPSD with an atypical antipsychotic drug for 12 weeks would result in:

- An additional 91–200 patients showing clinically significant improvement in these symptoms;
- An additional 10 deaths; and
- An additional 18 strokes, about half of them severe.

Antipsychotic drugs also increase the risk of falling and perhaps of cognitive decline (Dyer et al., 2021).

Safety concerns have also been expressed about the use of antipsychotics in delirium (Marcantonio, 2019). Multiple studies have found they do not reduce delirium duration and severity while causing potentially harmful cardiac and other effects, and adverse effects on mortality can occur even within 30 days of initiating antipsychotic therapy.

We continue to learn more about the risk profile of specific drugs; there is a better understanding of why death occurs (such as more clots, arrhythmias, and metabolic disturbances) and what subgroups of patients are at most risk. However, one core message persists—there is an unavoidable trade-off between a significant risk of serious adverse effects and a modest degree of benefit in improving unpleasant and distressing symptoms.

How to make difficult trade-offs is primarily an ethical and moral rather than an evidence-based issue. Judgement as well as statistics is required to determine where an acceptable balance of risk and benefit lies. The fact that significant behavioural problems affect not only individuals with dementia or delirium but those around them, such as family and healthcare workers, adds an additional layer of moral complexity to the decisions that must be made.

What Moral Principles and Human Rights Require Consideration?

Principlism and its Limitations

Principlism, advocated by Beachamp & Childress (2008), has been very influential as a normative ethical framework for analysing difficult healthcare decisions. It requires balancing the potentially competing principles of autonomy, beneficence, non-maleficence, and justice. It may be a parody, but one with some degree of truth, to see many ethical issues reduced to a tussle between the demands of autonomy (over-simplified as 'patient choice') and of beneficence (over-simplified as 'what is in the person's best interests'). The four principles have also been criticized as 'fatuous jargon' and as promoting a simplistic 'cook-book approach' to ethics (Lannon & O'Keeffe, 2010, p. 25).

This criticism may be too harsh, but principlism cannot tell us how to weigh the different principles, including in situations such as managing BPSD in those with cognitive impairment where promoting autonomy and self-determination is more challenging.

Relevant Human Rights Treaties

Several human rights treaties are relevant to antipsychotic use for BPSD but, again, none provides a simple guide as to what to do.

The Convention on the Rights of Persons with Disabilities (CRPD) (2006) Article 12—'Parties shall recognize that persons with disabilities enjoy legal capacity on an equal basis with others'—emphasizes the continued importance of promoting autonomy and self-determination in those with dementia or delirium despite the difficulties this may entail.

It might be argued that giving antipsychotic medications without consent and where there is significant risk of harm is contrary to the International Covenant on Civil and Political Rights Article 7: 'No one shall be subjected to torture or to cruel, inhuman or degrading treatment or punishment' (Joseph & Catan, 2013). Conversely, it could be argued that a failure to adequately control troublesome symptoms would be discriminatory against the right to health and fail to show the respect for inherent dignity required under Article 3 of the CRPD (2006).

Need to Consider Different Ethical Theories and Approaches

As Beachamp & Childress (2008, p. 408) noted regarding the misuse of their four principles: 'to assign priority to [any one] factor as the key ingredient is a dubious project, as is the attempt to dispense with ethical theory altogether'. Instead, they noted: 'in moral reasoning we often blend appeals to principles, rules, rights, virtues, analogies, paradigms, parables, and interpretations'.

Different ethical theories might of course lead to different conclusions or emphasize different aspects of choices regarding the use of antipsychotic medications by physicians. However, rather than relying solely on one ethical theory, an integrative approach would allow for a more comprehensive and nuanced assessment of the issue.

Case Studies

John: Dementia

John is 85 years old and has Alzheimer's disease and a history of transient ischaemic attacks. He is cared for by his wife of the same age. They live in a remote setting where services are limited. He has deteriorated over the last few months. He needs increased assistance with daily activities and is incontinent of urine. He has fallen a few times. He sometimes fails to recognize his wife and can often become agitated and upset at night and ask to go 'home'. Despite support and advice from professionals, his wife admits that she is exhausted and finds the situation very stressful and difficult. She is, however, very keen to maintain John at home which is where he wants to remain. There has been no benefit from non-antipsychotic medications. She asks if John can receive 'stronger medication' to help her cope.

Mary: Delirium

Mary is an 80-year-old woman with heart disease admitted with hyperactive delirium due to urosepsis. She is causing significant disruption on her ward. She sings loudly at night and shouts abuse at other patients who ask her to stop. There is no single room available. Staff also note that she is at risk of falling, and they don't have enough staff to look after her safely. Medical staff have tried giving her a benzodiazepine at night, but that didn't influence her behaviour and made her balance worse. There have been complaints from other patients and their families. Nursing staff ask doctors to start antipsychotic medications.

Issues Raised by the Case Studies

In both cases, the primary issue is whether starting an antipsychotic medication would be justified to manage significant behavioural disturbance.

An important additional complexity in both cases is the involvement of, and impact on, other people which is contributing to the pressure to use antipsychotics. John's behaviour is upsetting his wife who is struggling to maintain him at home. Mary's behaviour is disruptive for other patients on her ward and for healthcare staff. Do the other people affected matter, and to what extent, when deciding about antipsychotic use?

Both cases will require a complex balancing of the potential risks and benefits of antipsychotic use to reach a decision. There is no easy short-cut to an answer, and this will require assessing each case and the specific contextual details individually as well as considering relevant moral principles and ethical theories.

The Conventional Approach to Intervention and Treatment Dilemmas

The Conventional Approach to Intervention

Interventions Other than Antipsychotics

Medications other than antipsychotics may be helpful, such as giving analgesia for pain and managing depression with antidepressants. Treatment of any physical illness causing delirium is essential, although recovery of cognitive status can take some time and may be incomplete. Non-pharmacological measures are also essential first-line interventions. Challenging behaviours often occur as a result of unmet needs when people with cognitive impairment cannot communicate those needs and provide for themselves.

Unfortunately, not all needs can be identified or met, and notwithstanding the importance of non-pharmacological approaches, they will not always work. Staff cannot conjure up additional community supports in areas where services are lacking. Through no fault of staff, busy acute hospitals are often antitherapeutic environments for those with dementia or delirium.

Current Use of Antipsychotic Drugs in Delirium and Dementia

Although studies have shown a significant decrease in the prescribing of antipsychotics in people with dementia in recent years, inappropriately high use and long duration of use persists (Gurwitz et al., 2017). This is a particular concern in nursing home residents. Indeed, a US study found that it was common to find creation of a new, but false, diagnosis of 'psychosis' to allow continued use of antipsychotic medications (Urick et al., 2016). There have been similar findings that antipsychotic use in delirium has reduced but remains too high (Marcantonio, 2019).

Pressure to Treat

Clinicians may experience real difficulties in resisting constant pressure from family and staff that 'something must be done' if behaviour is causing a problem. Even if a clinician is strong-willed enough to resist, colleagues may not be similarly resistant. Indeed, a qualitative study of hospital decision-making noted: 'Ultimately when nurses decided an antipsychotic medication was needed to sedate a patient, nurses were able to influence decisions to get antipsychotics prescribed' (Tomlinson et al., 2021, p. 10).

Can Current Use of Antipsychotics Be Justified: The Clinical Dilemmas

Clinicians may in the past have been able to avoid the increasing number of journal articles about the hazards of antipsychotics ('I'm so busy it's hard to keep up with the literature'). The temporal distance between writing a prescription for an antipsychotic and an event such a sudden death, and the lack of an obvious cause and effect relationship ('after all he had cardiac disease—we'll never know what happened'), may have allowed an emotional distance not granted to, for example, an oncologist whose patient succumbs to neutropenic sepsis after chemotherapy. However, after the Banerjee report and multiple official guidelines on management of dementia and delirium, ignoring the issue is no longer possible: the real harms of antipsychotics, the trade-offs to be made, and the dilemma for clinicians are now concrete and 'official'.

Use Antipsychotics within the Terms of Their Licence

Most clinicians will agree that there is a role for antipsychotic drugs in some circumstances but there is no consensus on those circumstances. One response is that their use should be strictly in accordance with the evidence (and the licence) for their use and, even then, only as a last resort in the most serious situations. Corbett and colleagues (2014, p. 2), for example, advise that 'risperidone is the only recommended antipsychotic, and should be used only in people with dementia who have pre-existing psychotic disorders or severe aggression . . . and for no more than 12 weeks'.

Off-label Use of Antipsychotics

Other guidelines and commentators suggest, explicitly or implicitly, that this is too restrictive, and that judicious use of antipsychotics can be considered, for example, to manage severe agitation or distress if other approaches have failed. It is also argued by some that the limitations of the current evidence-base for antipsychotics should not deny patients a potentially helpful therapy, even accepting that this involves real risk.

For example: 'There appears to be a gap between the evidence base that informs BPSD treatment guidelines, and the reality faced by clinicians in the field ... Any clinician caring for patients with dementia knows that antipsychotic medication can rapidly calm severe agitation' (Passmore et al., 2012).

It might be seen as a comfort to those prescribing unlicensed antipsychotics that they are not alone in this practice. Off-label prescribing, where drugs are used outside of their approved terms of use, is common among all practitioners. However, this is usually reserved for when there is a reasonable presumption of efficacy based on scientific evidence and expert consensus but there have been few randomized controlled trials. This doesn't apply to the use of antipsychotics where there are explicit warnings and recommendations against their use, other than in those with severe psychosis or aggression unresponsive to other approaches, because of findings of harm or lack of benefit in trials (Ellett & Lim 2020). 'Off-piste prescribing' may be a more apt description.

Consideration of Relevant Moral Principles and Ethics Theories

Autonomy

Respecting Autonomy

Respecting the autonomy of patients—their ability to govern their lives according to their own beliefs and values—is an important moral duty for professionals in deontological and rights-based ethics. Maximizing autonomy remains important in those with dementia and delirium. However, the value of this principle in dealing with challenging behaviours can be limited when, despite genuine efforts, the unmet need triggering the behaviours cannot be identified or easily met or when the autonomy of the person comes up against the needs of others.

Informed Consent

Autonomy underpins the importance of informed consent for treatment. While unlikely to be possible for those with severe BPSD or delirium, it may be possible to obtain informed consent for antipsychotic use in some with milder cognitive impairment.

This would require providing accurate and balanced information in a comprehensible manner. What might the essential information look like? 'We wish to prescribe medication that might reduce some of the symptoms that you have been experiencing. Unfortunately, this medication also has significant side effects and increases your risk of dying or having a severe stroke within the next few months.' This is certainly a manageable amount of information, and the likelihood that many would refuse treatment is, of course, the purpose of seeking consent.

Seeking informed consent for antipsychotic treatment from, depending on the jurisdiction, a substitute or legally authorized decision-maker is recommended by some authors. The intention is often protection of the prescriber in case of an adverse outcome. There is also an argument that independent oversight of the decision is important given the stakes. However, on occasion there may be a conflict between the interests of the substitute decision-maker and the person.

Dignity

Respect for Dignity

The concepts of 'dignity' and of 'respect for dignity' offer a more egalitarian alternative to autonomy that is not linked to, and perhaps limited by, decision-making capacity (Henry, 2011). The Latin roots—'dignitus' and 'dignus', merit and worth—emphasize the broad scope of the word 'dignity', including the value of life and the need to treat everyone with respect and compassion. Respect for dignity also requires respect for the humanity of the person and is related to Kitwood's (1998) definition of personhood as 'A standing or status that is bestowed upon one human being by others, in the context of social being. It implies recognition, respect, and trust'.

Dignity and Antipsychotic Treatment

It seems clear that dignity and respect for dignity are 'good things' but less clear how they should influence antipsychotic prescribing. BPSD are often inherently 'undignified' (and many have also commented on the 'indignities of old age').

Respect for dignity seems a strong argument for adequately treating those in great distress. Can it be used more broadly? Respecting dignity requires consideration of the person's views of what is dignified. It is probably true that a person's earlier self would be horrified by many subsequent behavioural problems (Passmore et al., 2012). However, it would be easy to weaponize the concept of dignity as, effectively, an injunction to 'be dignified' and to justify antipsychotic use to make people 'more manageable' on the basis that it is to make them 'more dignified'.

Can a Palliative Care Model for Dementia Justify Antipsychotic Treatment?

Treloar and colleagues (2010) have argued that 'antipsychotics may be justified using a palliative model: by reducing severe distress in those whose life expectancy is short'. They suggest an analogy between the use of antipsychotics in people with dementia and palliative treatment in terminal cancer 'to improve quality of life in the short term even though these treatments are associated with side effects that may shorten life' and that discussions should be informed by the doctrine of double effect.

There are a number of different arguments here that are worth disentangling. While I agree that alleviation of severe distress is a justification for antipsychotic use in dementia, there are reasons to suggest that those prescribing antipsychotics cannot claim the full reassurance that they are merely adapting a palliative care model and providing psychiatric palliative care.

Dementia as a Terminal Illness

Dementia does reduce life expectancy. It also seems inarguable that those with dementia should, but often don't, receive the benefit of high-quality end-of-life palliative care. However, the fact that doctors are often poor at recognizing and responding to those entering the final stages of life in dementia does not justify treating all with dementia as though death were imminent: 'terminal illness' is not an endlessly elastic concept. While a short life expectancy can influence judgements of the balance between the burdens and benefits of interventions, this does not imply that the remaining time is not precious or important.

The Doctrine of Double Effect: An Analogy between Antipsychotic and Palliative Care Interventions

The Doctrine of Double Effect

The doctrine of double effect states that an action aimed at a good outcome is acceptable even if acting also means a foreseeable risk of a bad outcome (Quinn, 1989). Four conditions are required:

- The action itself must be morally good or neutral.
- The bad outcome must not be the means of achieving the good effect: good ends cannot justify evil means.
- The bad effect must be unintended and reasonable measures taken to prevent it.
- There must be a proportionately serious reason for risking the bad effect: the good outcome must outweigh the bad outcome.

In bioethics, the doctrine of double effect is often discussed as a justification for giving opioid medication to relieve pain even though it may lead to an unintended but foreseeable, and even sometimes inevitable, risk of hastening death by causing respiratory depression. Can a similar argument be used to support use of antipsychotics to treat BPSD?

Problems with Using the Doctrine of Double Effect to Justify Antipsychotic Use

There may be situations where this doctrine may reasonably apply to justify antipsychotic use, but there are three problems in my view with its general use as a justification.

- Although interventions such as palliative chemotherapy, palliative radiotherapy, and opioid use at the end of life can have serious side effects, palliative care physicians reject the premise that they shorten life: they are more likely to prolong life as well as provide better symptom control and quality of life. As Sykes & Thorns (2003) have noted regarding opioids:

  ' … there is no evidence that initiation of treatment, or increases in dose of opioids or sedatives, is associated with precipitation of death. Thus, we conclude that the doctrine of double effect is not essential for justification of the use of these drugs, and may act as a deterrent to the provision of good symptom control'.

- A second problem is with regard to the proportionality requirement under the doctrine of double effect. It is worth highlighting how uniquely bad the risk benefit ratio is for antipsychotics. Comments that the additional mortality due to antipsychotic use for 12 weeks is 'small' (Trifiro et al., 2007) miss the point: no other drug class used in medicine has consistently been shown to increase mortality and shorten life when used in appropriate doses in the appropriate target population. For example, high-risk medications such as chemotherapeutic drugs for treating cancer, immunomodulators for treating autoimmune conditions, and antithrombotic medications can all lead to fatal adverse events but all prolong life for most patients.

- Discussions of the doctrine of double effect often focus on whether interventions can hasten death or prolong life. Many people with chronic progressive conditions will ultimately prefer to maximize quality of life rather than duration of life. Death from a sudden and painless cardiac arrhythmia, or even from pneumonia, may well be seen as an acceptable risk to run. However, this is not true of other potential side effects of antipsychotics that may have a devastating effect on quality of life such as severe stroke.

Does Severe Distress Justify Antipsychotic Use?

Psychological distress is as real and can cause as much suffering as physical distress. (Of course, in dementia psychological distress can result from a physical cause such as pain). Unremitting severe distress can in my view get over the 'proportionality hurdle' in the doctrine of double effect. It is also arguable that respect for dignity also requires every effort to relieve severe distress even if it involves a significant risk of harm. However, a number of caveats seem necessary to justify this approach. The distress should be that of the person themselves not of others; the specific symptom or source of distress should be clearly identified and described; BPSD—a mixture of different behaviours often reflecting different needs—should not be automatically conflated with distress; and non-pharmacological interventions should have been tried and found to be ineffective.

The Role of Virtue Ethics

A virtue ethics framework focuses on the virtues, character traits, and intentions of the actor rather than the rightness of an action. The virtuous clinician would of course be competent, and resolute when necessary. While sensitive to the importance of relationships and the impact of challenging behaviours on others, one would expect him or her to be able to resist pressure to use antipsychotics where that would be the wrong option for the person.

How do we expect a clinician faced with another person's severe distress due to BPSD to think and to behave? An imperative to relieve distress and suffering is core to professional ethics. Not acting—accepting the status quo and not considering antipsychotic treatment in this situation—would also be a morally significant action with the potential for a very poor outcome for the person, including, for example, an inability to remain at home. We would expect a compassionate, empathetic clinician to be desperate to try to help the person, even if sometimes that involved providing a treatment such as an antipsychotic with some trepidation.

Can Antipsychotic Use Be Justified by Reference to Others Affected by BPSD?

Many of the approaches discussed so far emphasize the person suffering from BPSD. While this is the most important consideration, challenging behaviours can also have a major impact on, and cause distress, and even danger, to family members, carers, and healthcare staff. To what degree do their interests need to be considered?

Utilitarianism
Utilitarianism holds that the most ethical action is the one that will maximize overall happiness or well-being for all affected individuals, that is the greatest good for the greatest number. A utilitarian approach would consider the potential benefits of reducing agitation or aggression using antipsychotics not only for patients with dementia or delirium but for others involved in their care. This may be a valid approach when a person's aggressive behaviour results in a genuine danger to others, in which case there is a justification for antipsychotic use. However, utilitarianism doesn't provide any metric for balancing less tangible benefits for others against a real risk of serious harm for the person from use of antipsychotics.

Relational Ethics
Relational ethics places a strong emphasis on the importance of relationships and interconnectedness in ethical decision-making. In the context of antipsychotic use in

dementia and delirium, relational ethics highlights the significance of understanding the relationships between the person with dementia, their caregivers, and healthcare providers.

It would also require consideration of whether relationships entail obligations to others, especially to those with whom there is a close personal relationship that supports them. If a person with BPSD can't speak for themselves, it is necessary to consider whether a relationship is such that they might want or expect clinicians to take the interests of others into account and to potentially lower the threshold for antipsychotic treatment as a result.

Revisiting the Case Studies

John

Of John's symptoms, only his agitation might potentially benefit from an antipsychotic: continence and mobility may get worse and there is a risk of death and stroke. It is distressing and frightening for someone with dementia to be unaware of one's surroundings at times. Reassurance and reorientation will often be most effective (although this will usually have been advised and tried without success in such a case), and antipsychotics will not improve, and may worsen, John's cognitive status and disorientation. Also, arguably, John's symptoms, as described, don't pass a threshold to merit the term 'severe distress'.

However, there is one good reason why a conscientious clinician may often be willing to have a trial of antipsychotics in John's case, whatever their concerns about possible harm: that is his relationship with his wife, and their shared goal of maintaining John at home. A carer who is exhausted by the demands of caring has needs of his or her own. It is reasonable to say that John has obligations to his devoted wife and to presume that he would want her interests considered. Indeed, one could justify seeing them as a long-standing and mutually supportive unit or dyad. In this situation, a cautious trial of an antipsychotic, after discussing the pros and cons with his wife, could in my view be justified.

Mary

In contrast, there seems no reasonable justification for antipsychotic use in Mary's case. Singing and being verbally abusive are not symptoms that necessarily indicate distress or that, short of causing significant sedation, would respond to antipsychotics. There are no benefits to Mary herself that would justify the potential harms from even a brief trial of low-dose antipsychotics.

One would have sympathy for other patients kept awake by Mary who are themselves sick and who need their sleep, and for hard-pressed healthcare staff. However, a utilitarian argument that the greatest good for the greatest number would be achieved by giving Mary an antipsychotic is unsustainable when the benefits for others (better sleep) is of such a lower magnitude than the serious harms that Mary would risk. Similarly relational ethics would note that the other people affected are in effect strangers to Mary and that it seems impossible to argue that Mary has any moral obligation to receive treatment presenting serious hazards to herself for their benefit.

Conclusions and Suggestions

The use of antipsychotic medications in dementia and delirium raises important moral, ethical, and rights considerations due to the potential for serious complications. Several ethical theories and approaches are relevant and should be considered, including those that address the potential harms to others of not providing treatment. No single approach will provide as easy answer, and rather than relying on any one theory, an integrative approach will provide a better and nuanced assessment of the complexities of individual cases.

It is also important that the reasoning, and the trade-offs made in decision-making, are clearly documented in the notes. Knowing the ethical basis for such decisions may be helpful for other clinicians involved in the care of the person.

What if a patient does have a serious vascular event that might be attributed to use of antipsychotics, especially if that use was off-label? Knowing that one did engage in careful ethical reasoning before prescribing an antipsychotic might benefit a clinician by alleviating feelings of responsibility or guilt. (Harding & Peel (2013) have argued that a successful claim of negligence would be unlikely to succeed in such cases.

It doesn't seem enough to leave this to the conscience of the prescribing clinician. It could be argued that serious vascular events occurring within, say 3 months of initiating an antipsychotic should be identified and should trigger a careful review to ensure that there was an ethical reasoning and justification for the prescription.

A lack of resources and of appropriate facilities may lead to difficulties in implementing non-pharmacological approaches in individual cases. However, these are not one-off, unpredictable scenarios: they are predictably recurrent problems for many people with dementia. There is an ethical imperative for clinicians and their professional bodies to advocate for services that will reduce the need for antipsychotic use. Given the significant mortality and morbidity, 'shroud waving' would seem justified.

Finally, given that people experiencing BPSD may be unable at that time to consider treatment options, it could be argued that they should be encouraged, while they have decision-making capacity, in creating an advance directive or statement expressing their own wishes and the trade-offs they would feel justified.

References

Banerjee, S. (2009). The use of antipsychotic medication for people with dementia: time for action. Department of Health, London.

Beauchamp, T. L., & Childress, T. F., (2008). *Principles of biomedical ethics* (6th ed.). Oxford University Press.

Corbett, A., Burns, A., & Ballard, C. (2014). Don't use antipsychotics routinely to treat agitation and aggression in people with dementia. *British Medical Journal, 349*, g6420.

Dyer, A. H., Murphy, C., Lawlor, B., Kennelly, S. P., & NILVAD Study Group. (2021). Long-term antipsychotic use and cognitive decline in community-dwelling older adults with mild–moderate Alzheimer disease: Data from NILVAD. *International Journal of Geriatric Psychiatry, 36*(11), 1708–1721.

Ellett, L. M. K., & Lim, R. (2020). We need to do better: most people with dementia living in aged care facilities use antipsychotics for too long, for off-label indications and without documented consent. *International Psychogeriatrics, 32*(3), 299–302.

Gurwitz, J. H., Bonner, A., & Berwick, D. M. (2017). Reducing excessive use of antipsychotic agents in nursing homes. *Journal of the American Medical Association, 318*(2), 118–119.

Harding, R., & Peel, E. (2013). 'He was like a zombie': off-label prescription of antipsychotic drugs in dementia. *Medical Law Review, 21*(2), 243–277.

Henry, L. M. (2011). The jurisprudence of dignity. *University of Pennsylvania Law Review, 160*, 169.

Joseph, S., & Castan, M. (2013). *The international covenant on civil and political rights: cases, materials, and commentary*. Oxford University Press.

Kitwood, T. (1998). Toward a theory of dementia care: ethics and interaction. *The Journal of Clinical Ethics, 9*(1), 23–34.

Lannon, R., & O'Keeffe, S. T. (2010). Cardiopulmonary resuscitation in older people–a review. *Reviews in Clinical Gerontology, 20*(1), 20–29.

Marcantonio, E. R. (2019). Old habits die hard: antipsychotics for treatment of delirium. *Annals of Internal Medicine, 171*(7), 516–517.

Passmore, M. J., Ho, A., & Gallagher, R. (2012). Behavioral and psychological symptoms in moderate to severe Alzheimer's disease: a palliative care approach emphasizing recognition of personhood and preservation of dignity. *Journal of Alzheimer's Disease, 29*(1), 1–13.

Quinn, W. S. (1989). Actions, intentions, and consequences: The doctrine of double effect. *Philosophy & Public Affairs, 8*(4), 334–351.

Sykes, N., & Thorns, A. (2003). The use of opioids and sedatives at the end of life. *The Lancet Oncology, 4*(5), 312–318.

Tomlinson, E. J., Rawson, H., Manias, E., Phillips, N. N. M., Darzins, P., & Hutchinson, A.M. (2021). Factors associated with the decision to prescribe and administer antipsychotics for older people with delirium: a qualitative descriptive study. *British Medical Journal Open, 11*(7), Article e047247.

Treloar, A., Crugel, M., Prasanna, A., Solomons, L., Fox, C., Paton, C., & Katona, C. (2010). Ethical dilemmas: should antipsychotics ever be prescribed for people with dementia? *British Journal of Psychiatry, 197*(2), 88–90.

Trifirò, G., Verhamme, K. M., Ziere, G., Caputi, A. P., Ch Stricker, B. H., & Sturkenboom, M. C. (2007). All-cause mortality associated with atypical and typical antipsychotics in demented outpatients. *Pharmacoepidemiology and Drug Safety, 16*(5), 538–544.

United Nations. (2006). Convention on the Rights of Persons with Disabilities. New York: United Nations.

Urick, B. Y., Kaskie, B. P., & Carnahan, R. M. (2016). Improving antipsychotic prescribing practices in nursing facilities: The role of surveyor methods and surveying agencies in upholding the Nursing Home Reform Act. *Research in Social and Administrative Pharmacy, 12*(1), 91–103.

20
Human Rights and Wrongs in National Constitutions

A Case Study of the Irish Constitution

J. McVeigh and R. McVeigh

Introduction

When delivering judgments on issues relating to constitutional or human rights, courts make significant decisions about the principles that apply, impacting the development of case law (Whelan, 2021). This chapter discusses the interpretation by the European Court of Human Rights (ECtHR) of the European Convention on Human Rights, as the basis of the European human rights system (IHREC, 2015), incorporated into law in Ireland by the European Convention on Human Rights Act 2003. Furthermore, this chapter examines approaches to the interpretation by the Irish courts of the Constitution, as the fundamental law of the State.

Domestic constitutions establish basic principles for governing a polity, which guide and demonstrate the shared values of a State (Mazzi, 2020). As contended by Prakash (2024), the origins of constitutional government date back to the works of Greek philosophers, predominantly Aristotle; to the charter of Magna Carta (1215) in the middle ages; and subsequently to the American and French Revolutions and the works of John Locke (1632–1704) and Montesquieu (1689–1775), which gave rise to a more systematic development of constitutional government. National constitutions are deemed 'the most vital expressions of government responsibility and individual entitlements, and therefore one of the channels best suited to endorsing states' commitments to human rights' (Berro Pizzarossa & Perehudoff, 2017, p. 281).

The number of domestic constitutions globally is rapidly increasing; associated with the higher number of independent States and the transformation of countries in central Europe and across the former East European bloc in the aftermath of the Soviet Union (World Bank, 2017). The Irish Constitution was ratified by the Irish State in 1937 and has therefore had significant longevity, relative to the majority of domestic constitutions (Humphreys, 2017); with the average time span of constitutions globally being 19 years and just 8 years in Latin America and eastern Europe (World Bank, 2017). Comparable to the framing of UN human rights treaties as broad agreements (O'Brien & Gowan, 2012), constitutions are broad and abstract in nature, so that they can be used to address a wide array of unforeseen and context-specific issues

(Chandrachud, 2016). Several approaches may therefore be used by judges to interpret constitutions, including the literal approach, harmonious approach, hierarchy of rights approach, broad or purposive approach, historical approach, and the natural law approach.

Correspondingly, the ECtHR adopts various doctrines in the interpretation and advancement of rights set out in the European Convention on Human Rights, including the doctrines of autonomous concepts and the margin of appreciation (Moreno-Lax, 2021). This chapter focuses on two such doctrines, namely the living-instrument doctrine (and the associated European consensus doctrine) and the positive-obligations doctrine. The application of the living-instrument doctrine by the Strasbourg Court has been the subject of much criticism, specifically that it has damaged the Court's legitimacy and overexpanded the obligations imposed by the Convention on High Contracting Parties. As proposed by Masterman (2018), 'it has become commonplace for the European Court of Human Rights to be accused of over-reach, of utilizing the "living instrument" doctrine to develop the Convention's protections illegitimately and, as a consequence, of increasingly interfering with national sovereignty'. Similarly, some commentators have argued that positive obligations pose a risk of significantly adding to the Convention obligations that are imposed on States Parties.

This chapter first briefly examines the interpretation of international human rights law by the Irish courts. This chapter then provides a case study on the interpretation of mental health law in Ireland. Approaches to interpretation of the Irish Constitution are then examined, with particular reference to the historical approach to constitutional interpretation. Finally, this chapter examines the interpretation by the ECtHR of the European Convention on Human Rights, particularly with reference to the living-instrument and positive-obligations doctrines, which are each examined in turn with respect to their strengths, risks, and challenges as approaches to interpreting and advancing the Convention rights. In contrast with commentary that the application of these doctrines has damaged the Court's legitimacy and overexpanded the obligations of the Convention, this chapter argues in support of both doctrines as mechanisms to ensure the relevance, practicality, and longevity of the Convention and to increase human rights protection for vulnerable groups.

A goal of this edited volume is to encourage personal reflection on values that guide our judgments, and this chapter aims to examine such values in the context of those that guide legal judgments. In accordance with the approach of this book, we are not seeking to advocate *what* legal interpretations should be made, but rather to examine different approaches to legal interpretation that guide *how* such judgments are made.

Interpretation of International Human Rights Law by the Irish Courts

Ireland adopts a dualist approach to international law. Although Ireland is legally bound by the treaties that it ratifies, such treaties are therefore not directly applicable in Irish law (Houses of the Oireachtas, 2016). As set out in the Irish Constitution, in Article 29.6: 'No international agreement shall be part of the domestic law of the State save as may be determined by the Oireachtas'. To implement a convention or treaty in the Irish State, the Oireachtas must therefore pass an Act that integrates the convention or treaty or its obligations into legislation, with the exception of EU treaties that have 'direct effect' (Forde & Leonard, 2013). Both the Supreme Court and Court of Appeal have affirmed that an international agreement will not have direct effect in Irish law unless the Oireachtas determines that it does so (Hogan, 2019). For example, while Ireland ratified the European Convention on Human Rights in 1953, the Convention was not incorporated into Irish law until the European Convention on Human Rights Act 2003.

However, unincorporated international agreements may have indirect legal effect due to the *presumption of compatibility* of national legislation with international conventions (Hogan et al., 2018). For example, as the United Nations Convention on the Rights of Persons with Disabilities (CRPD) has been ratified by both the Irish State and by the EU, in accordance with Article 216(2) of the Treaty on the Functioning of the EU, a dual effect from the Convention arises in Irish law;[1] and an approach of progressive realization has been adopted with regards to the CRPD (Committee on the Rights of Persons with Disabilities, 2021). As outlined by the Irish Human Rights and Equality Commission (IHREC), although the CRPD has not been incorporated into Irish law and does not have direct effect, it is a binding international agreement and the State must fulfil its obligations.[2] It is therefore critical that domestic legislation is interpreted in accordance with the spirit and ethos of the CRPD.

For example, in a recent landmark case, *A.B. v HSE & Ors* (HSE signifies the Health Service Executive, Ireland's public health and social care service), the Irish Court of Appeal examined whether an assessment of need conducted pursuant to s.8 of the Disability Act 2005 could be considered complete without providing a diagnostic assessment of the child's disability.[3] The case related to a child who had been referred for an assessment under the Disability Act in accordance with the HSE's new Standard Operating Procedure (operating since 2020), whereby the child was identified as having a disability, but the HSE refused to diagnose the nature or severity of the disability on the grounds that the Act did not obligate it to do so; and the HSE instead referred the child for supports and services (Law Society of Ireland, 2023). The IHREC, acting as *amicus curiae*, argued that it was critical to interpret the Act's provisions in a way that was consistent with the State's obligations pursuant to the CRPD. Ms Justice Máire Whelan asserted (at paragraph 110): 'I am satisfied that this court is entitled to have regard to the fact that the CRPD was ratified by the State in 2018. It is an ancillary

---

[1] Submissions on Behalf of the Amicus Curiae, the Irish Human Rights and Equality Commission, *Nano Nagle School v Marie Daly* (Record No: SAPIE/2018/37), at [4.13].

[2] Submissions on Behalf of the Amicus Curiae, the Irish Human Rights and Equality Commission, *Nano Nagle School v Marie Daly* (Record No: SAPIE/2018/37), at [4.14].

[3] *A.B. v HSE & Ors* [2023] IECA 275.

factor to be taken into account in approaching the construction of s. 8.' In its judgment, the court held that an assessment of need conducted under s.8 of the Act could not be deemed to be complete without a diagnostic assessment of a child's disability, unless in the reasonable opinion of the assessment officer such a diagnostic evaluation was not needed.

Correspondingly, in the landmark judgment on disability discrimination, *Nano Nagle School v Daly*, the Irish Supreme Court judgment overturned a Court of Appeal judgment that was repugnant to the CRPD by limiting the employment rights of persons with disabilities and reducing the duty on employers to provide reasonable accommodation (Bruton & McVeigh, 2018). In the Supreme Court judgment, Mr Justice John MacMenamin asserted that it was necessary to advert to the CRPD to determine if unlawful discrimination had arisen under the Employment Equality Act 1998–2011. Similarly, Mr Justice Peter Charleton (dissenting) stated that 'the United Nations Convention on the Rights of Persons with Disabilities, ratified by both the State and the European Union, is part of the necessary backdrop to this appeal'.[4] It is evident, therefore, that the Irish courts are willing to take into consideration the CRPD in their interpretation of domestic legislation.

Arguably, however, the courts' interpretation of legislation in alignment with the CRPD may not be steadfast. For example, in *Reeves v Disabled Drivers Medical Board of Appeal, Lennon v Disabled Drivers Medical Board of Appeal*, the Supreme Court quashed a decision by the Disabled Drivers Medical Board of Appeal (DDMBA) to refuse medical certificates for the families of two children with disabilities.[5] The DDMBA, a statutory body for reviewing unsuccessful applications for a Primary Medical Certificate, had repeatedly expressed concern in relation to strict criteria in the Disabled Drivers Regulations for obtaining a medical certificate to access tax concessions to purchase an adapted vehicle. The Supreme Court held that the regulations excluded some people with severe disability, whose limited mobility resulted in the need for an adapted car. However, although the court's judgment was astute, it failed to consider the regulations as an inherently flawed statutory instrument that contradicts the rights enshrined in the CRPD (McVeigh, 2023).

Case study: Interpretation of Mental Health Law in Ireland

This section provides a case study in relation to interpretation by the Irish courts of the Mental Health Act 2001. While the Act introduced rights-based mental health law in Ireland, the extent to which the provisions of the Act have a de facto effect on the protection of rights is dependent on the judicial approach to the Act's implementation

---

[4] *Nano Nagle School v Daly* [2019] IESC 63, at [3].
[5] *Reeves v Disabled Drivers Medical Board of Appeal, Lennon v Disabled Drivers Medical Board of Appeal* [2020] IESC 31.

(Murray, 2010). Section 4(1) of the Act states that the best interests of the person should be the primary consideration, while also considering the interests of other persons who may be at risk of serious harm. This reference to the 'best interests' of the person as a primary consideration, in addition to the generally 'purposive interpretation' of the Act, has resulted in the Irish courts interpreting such principles in a paternalistic way, in accordance with case law before the commencement of the Act (Department of Health, 2015). As asserted by Mr Justice McMahon in *S.M. v. Mental Health Commission*: '[T]he courts in considering the Mental Health Acts should where possible adopt such a purposive or teleological approach to the legislation and should in appropriate cases do so bearing in mind the paternal nature of the legislation itself'.[6]

For example, *E.H. v. Clinical Director of St. Vincent's Hospital* concerned an appeal from the High Court, which refused to discharge the applicant from detention at St Vincent's Hospital. The court was tasked with deciding if the applicant was a voluntary patient under the meaning of the Mental Health Act 2001, and if the definition of a voluntary patient in the Act was incompatible with Article 5 of the European Convention on Human Rights. Furthermore, the court examined the statutory interpretation of the Mental Health Act 2001 and if legal challenge to detention of patients is justified unless it is in the best interests of the patient.

A declaration was sought by the applicant that she was not a 'voluntary patient' and that the definition of voluntary patient under s.2 of the Mental Health Act was incompatible with Article 5 of the European Convention. The applicant asserted that she was not a 'voluntary patient' under the meaning of the Act as she had a mental disorder that was clearly demonstrated, that she had been prohibited from leaving, and that protections provided by the Act had been denied to her. The Supreme Court held that the applicant was a voluntary patient under the meaning of the Act. If procedural protections had been denied to the applicant, she had not been removed from the protection of the Act. The first named respondent had carried out a very high level of supervision of the applicant's condition. As asserted by Mr Justice Kearns:

> The terminology adopted in s.2 of the Act of 2001 ascribes a very particular meaning to the term 'voluntary patient'. It does not describe such a person as one who freely and voluntarily gives consent to an admission order. Instead the express statutory language defines a 'voluntary patient' as a person receiving care and treatment in an approved centre who is not the subject of an admission order or a renewal order.

The appeal was deemed to be moot. The reliefs sought were therefore refused and the appeal was dismissed.[7] Accordingly, the Supreme Court held that the meaning afforded to the term 'voluntary patient' within s. 2 of the Act did not necessitate that the person 'freely and voluntarily gives consent to an admission order'; and that, using

---

[6] *S.M. v. Mental Health Commission* [2009] 2 ILRM 127.
[7] *E.H. v. Clinical Director of St. Vincent's Hospital* [2009] 2 ILRM 149.

a paternalistic approach to interpret the Act, the lack of a requirement to determine the capacity of the patient to give their consent to the admission order did not violate the right to autonomy at the level of the Convention or the Constitution (Department of Health, 2015). This meaning of s.2, whereby neither capacity nor consent are deemed relevant factors to establish the status of a patient, has implications for the State's adherence to its international human rights obligations (Irish Human Rights Commission, 2010).

As contended by Whelan (2021, p. 223), the Irish courts continue to interpret mental health law in a paternalistic way, thereby raising 'profound questions about judicial attitudes to people with mental health conditions and judicial reluctance to confer full personhood on people with disabilities'. As emphasized by the *Expert Group on the Review of the Mental Health Act 2001*, to fulfil the CRPD and the European Convention on Human Rights, a departure is needed from the frequently paternalistic interpretation of mental health legislation by the Irish courts (Department of Health, 2015). The paternalistic approach contravenes a person-centred approach, and the current interpretation by the courts of the 'best interests' of the person is antithetical to the right to autonomy (Department of Health, 2015).

When delivering judgments on issues relating to constitutional or human rights, the courts make significant decisions about the principles that apply (Whelan, 2021), as evidenced by the interpretation of mental health legislation briefly discussed above. The following sections examine principles and approaches in the interpretation of law in relation to the Irish Constitution and the European Convention on Human Rights.

Constitutional Interpretation: The Historical Approach

Comparable to the framing of UN human rights treaties as broad agreements (O'Brien & Gowan, 2012), constitutions are broad and abstract in nature, so that they can be used to address a wide array of unforeseen and context-specific issues (Chandrachud, 2016). As contended by Goldsworthy (2007, p. 1):

> The provisions of national constitutions, like other laws, are often ambiguous, vague, contradictory, insufficiently explicit, or even silent as to constitutional disputes that judges must decide. In addition, they sometimes seem inadequate to deal appropriately with developments that threaten principles the constitution was intended to safeguard, developments that its founders either failed, or were unable to anticipate.

The text of the Irish Constitution therefore requires interpretation; although notably De Valera, unfeasibly, called for an unambiguous Constitution (Ní Loinsigh, 2014). The Constitution, in Article 34.3.2, grants the High Court and Supreme Court sole authority to establish the constitutionality of legislation enacted after 1937 (Forde & Leonard, 2013).

Several approaches may be used by judges to interpret the Constitution, including the literal approach, harmonious approach, hierarchy of rights approach, broad or purposive approach, historical approach, and the natural law approach. While the 'broad' and 'harmonious interpretation' approaches are the principal methods of constitutional interpretation in Ireland, several approaches continue to be applied in the courts (Hogan et al., 2018). For some cases, the Irish courts have used a literal or grammatical approach to constitutional interpretation, while a historical approach has been used in other instances (Byrne et al., 2020).

In the seminal case of *Curtin v. Dáil Éireann*, the Irish Supreme Court considered, in some detail, criteria to apply as the correct approach to interpretation of the Constitution. It was acknowledged that 'different interpretative elements are emphasised in individual judgments according to the particular context in which questions arise and the particular types of interpretative problem'.[8] Chief Justice John Murray further contended that:

> Where words are found to be plain and unambiguous, the courts must apply them in their literal sense. Where the text is silent or the meaning of words is not totally plain, resort may be had to principles, such as the obligation to respect personal rights, derived from other parts of the Constitution. The historical context of particular language may, in certain cases, be helpful.[9]

The historical approach refers to judicial interpretation of the Constitution with regards to the proposed intentions of the 'founding fathers' and public opinion when the Constitution was drafted and enacted. In effect, it comprises the 'instrumentalisation of history' (Maggs Campbell, 2018, p. 44). The manner in which courts may avail of constitutional history, and the reasons for doing so, are varied, depending on factors such as the type of history, the pattern of usage, and the type of provision (Greene & Tew, 2018). Proponents of originalism are divided on whether the original *meaning* or the original *intentions* should be relied upon (Sunstein, 2015). Nonetheless, originalism—or historicism in the Irish context—interprets the Constitution through the lens of the original drafters (Easterbrook, 2008). There is a long-standing debate between those who believe that a constitution should be interpreted more steadily in light of its original meaning, with the exception of amendments; and those who contend that a constitution should be interpreted more flexibly as a 'living Constitution' (Stokes Paulsen & Paulsen, 2017).

Common law countries such as Ireland and the United States have comparable constitutional traditions (Tew, 2014). Nonetheless, the principle of originalism has gained significant traction in the United States, relative to Ireland where it has

---

[8] *Curtin v. Dáil Éireann* [2006] 2 IR 556.
[9] *Curtin v. Dáil Éireann* [2006] 2 IR 556.

been applied less consistently (Carolan, 2013). As proposed by Byrne et al. (2020, at section 15.126): 'While references to the historical state of the law in 1937 are likely to continue, they are unlikely to prove decisive in many instances.' It is widely acknowledged that the Irish Constitution *Bunreacht na hÉireann* is a living constitution, which should be interpreted in response to evolving conditions, values, and attitudes in Irish society (O'Mahony, 2017). As contended by Charleton et al. (2020), the Irish Constitution is a living document, which is not limited by characteristics of Irish society in the 1930s. However, as proposed by de Blacam (2017, at section 8.46):

> [I]t has the paradoxical feature that it is both fixed and changing. In any given case its requirements must of course be determined and applied; and to that extent, at least, it is fixed. On the other hand, it is also clear that the Constitution and its meaning may change over time.

Indeed, the Irish courts usually attempt to balance contemporary meanings with a historical perspective (Hogan et al., 2018). In the Supreme Court case of *Sinnott v. Minister for Education*, Mr Justice Murray asserted that, while the constitution is a living document, it cannot be separated from its historical context:

> Agreeing as I do with the view that the constitution is a living document which falls to be interpreted in accordance with contemporary circumstances including prevailing ideas and mores, this does not mean, and I do not think it has ever been so suggested, that it can be divorced from its historical *context* [emphasis in original].[10]

Advantages and Challenges of the Historical Approach

The Irish Constitution is a 'historically embedded document' that was drafted in a historically significant era, at a time of dismantling liberal democratic regimes in Europe and unstable attachment of Ireland to the British Commonwealth of Nations (Coffey, 2018, p. xi). As emphasized by Kavanagh (2012, p. 71): 'Apart from the usual legal guarantees one might find in any democratic Constitution, Bunreacht na hÉireann also gave expression to aspects of Irish life and identity in the 1930s, reflecting both the history of the struggle for independence and future aspirations of a fledgling independent State.' Indeed, the Irish Constitution is referred to as both 'law and manifesto' (Kelly, 1988, p. 208), comprising both fundamental legal principles and broad aspirations (Byrne et al., 2020).

---

[10] *Sinnott v. Minister for Education* [2001] 2 IR 545.

Proponents of the historical approach argue that it protects against judicial legislation and restrains judges from adding to the text of the Constitution. For example, in recent years, Mr Justice O'Donnell has called for 'judicial restraint' in relation to constitutional interpretation and for more critical reflection on the obligation of the courts to develop rights beyond those set out in the Constitution (Carolan, 2017). It may be argued that by abiding by the words or intentions of the drafters of the Constitution, we are abiding by an agreement that was ratified democratically (Rubenfeld, 1995). Accordingly, an important question is whether it is anti-democratic for courts to creatively interpret legal provisions to align with societal changes (Humphreys, 2017).

The legitimacy of an 'unwritten Constitution' is controversial, however (Scalia, 1989a, p. 1). Such criticisms argue that the Constitution should be treated as a living instrument, without undue influence being given to the dead hand of history. A 'living Constitution' is deemed to contain meanings that can flexibly transition and adapt across generations, without the need for formal amendments (Strauss, 2010). From this perspective, the Irish Constitution may be conceptualized 'not as a foundational moment but rather as a seminal moment in an ongoing constitutional evolution' (Doyle, 2018, p. 32).

The 'living instrument' approach has been applied in judgments where interpretations of the Constitution clearly do not reflect the original meaning, but rather reflect current societal values and attitudes (O'Mahony, 2017). In *McGee v. Attorney General*, Mr Justice O'Keeffe, for the High Court, dismissed the claim made by the plaintiff that s. 17 of the Criminal Law Amendment Act 1935, which prohibited contraceptive items from being imported into Ireland, contravened her right to marital privacy.[11] Mr Justice O'Keeffe did not agree that the right to marital privacy existed, as this would assume that voters to enact the Constitution had voted to also establish a right to marital privacy and to repeal s. 17 of the 1935 Act; which he did not believe was the intention of the polity (Byrne et al., 2020). However, the Supreme Court rejected this historical account, and affirmed that s. 17 of the 1935 Act was invalid. Walsh J declared that 'no interpretation of the Constitution is intended to be final for all time. It is given in the light of prevailing ideas and concepts.'

Several cases subsequent to *McGee* have also applied this approach (Byrne et al., 2020). For example, in the Supreme Court ruling of *State (Healy) v. Donoghue*, Chief Justice O'Higgins observed that '... rights given by the Constitution must be considered in accordance with concepts of prudence, justice and charity which may gradually change or develop as society changes and develops, and which fall to be interpreted from time to time in accordance with prevailing ideas' (p. 347).[12]

A key criticism of historicism is that it is anti-democratic, in that it 'ties the judiciary, not to deference to a present legislator and its democratic mandate but to deference to the intentions of past legislators whose democratic mandate is long gone'

---

[11] *McGee v. Attorney General* [1974] IR 284.
[12] *State (Healy) v. Donoghue* [1976] IR 325.

(Langwallner, 2008a, p. 114). Similarly, Rubenfeld (1995, p. 1121) contends that '[o]riginalism cannot explain the supremacy of the democratic voice of the past over that of the present'. Furthermore, it is not evident that it was envisaged by the framers of the 1937 Constitution that their intentions, when drafting the Constitution, would guide future generations indefinitely (Langwallner, 2008b).

It is frequently challenging to determine the intended meanings of phrasing or sections by those who drafted a Constitution; and there is seldom explicit guidance on how contradictory rights should be balanced for example (Forde & Leonard, 2013). While in-depth information on the drafting of the 1787 Constitutional Convention is available to the courts in the United States, the Irish 1937 Constitution was drafted in secret and the Dáil debates seldom clarify the drafters' intentions (Hogan et al., 2018). Accordingly, a key criticism of the historical approach to interpretation of the Irish Constitution is the challenge of deciphering the intentions and opinions of the instrument's drafters.

As judges cannot be certain of the intentions of the drafters of the Constitution, the historical approach is highly subjective. Historical analyses may be influenced by our historical pre-opinions and prejudgments, which may lead to inaccurate interpretations (Gadamer, 2013). From this perspective, our understanding of the past is shaped by our prejudices and preconceptions (Brest, 1980). Furthermore, due to historical contexts being multifaceted, it is challenging for the Supreme Court to provide accurate historical interpretations of constitutional provisions (Shaman, 2001).

Using originalism, it is also possible to selectively include some evidence, while ignoring other evidence, resulting in an inaccurate historical interpretation (Cornell, 2019). As asserted by Scalia (1989b, p. 852), judicial opinions are often 'rendered not on the basis of what the Constitution originally meant, but on the basis of what the judges currently thought it desirable for it to mean'. Similarly, Hogan et al. observe (2018, at section 1.1.12):

> [T]he courts have shown no consistency with regard to any particular approach and this gives rise to the suspicion that individual judges are willing to rely on any such approach as will offer adventitious support for a conclusion which they have already reached – a results-oriented approach, or 'ad hoc' approach.

A further criticism of the historical approach is the frequent lack of representation of marginalized groups during the drafting of a constitution. For example, regarding the United States' constitution, in relation to women's representation, Schwarzenbach (2003, p. 7) argues that ' ... in questions of interpretation to the founding fathers' "intentions" in drafting the Constitution, begs the very issue at question: why should women listen to this group of men holding a convention more than two hundred years ago in which women had no participation?'. As emphasized by the UN, inclusive constitution-making processes incorporate the perspectives and lived experiences of marginalized groups such as people living in poverty, women, and youth; with the aim of strengthening their opportunities, increasing the perceived legitimacy of the development and content of Constitutions, and strengthening buy-in from all segments of society (United Nations Development Programme, 2014).

In the Irish context, criticisms include the lack of women's representation in the formulation of the 1937 Constitution; alongside numerous discriminatory provisions, such as Article 45.4.2, which stipulates that ' … citizens shall not be forced by economic necessity to enter avocations unsuited to their sex, age or strength' (Mohr, 2006). Furthermore, Article 41.2.1 of the Constitution stipulates: 'In particular, the State recognises that by her life within the home, woman gives to the State a support without which the common good cannot be achieved'. IHREC has highlighted continued calls at the national and international levels to amend or eliminate Article 41.2 (IHREC, 2020, 2023).

Human rights have also evolved significantly since the enactment of the 1937 Constitution. This includes the evolution of the rights of children at the national and international levels (Heffernan, 2020), operationalized in Ireland's ratification of the UN Convention on the Rights of the Child in 1992, and the rights of persons with disabilities as set out by the CRPD, ratified by Ireland in 2018 (Flynn, 2020). It is argued, therefore, that the historical approach is particularly ineffective in human rights cases, which reflect current public and judicial perspectives on rights and contemporary social and political affairs.

European Convention on Human Rights: The Living-Instrument Doctrine

As outlined above, there is a long-standing debate between those who propose that a Constitution should be interpreted with respect to its original meaning, with the exception of amendments; and those who assert that a constitution should be interpreted more flexibly as a 'living Constitution' (Stokes Paulsen & Paulsen, 2017). Correspondingly, there is much debate surrounding the interpretation of international human rights treaties as living instruments (Letsas, 2013). Proponents of the living-instrument approach argue that the European Convention on Human Rights (hereafter the Convention) should be interpreted with regards to evolving and widely accepted norms, attitudes, and standards in Member States of the Council of Europe (Bychawska-Siniarska, 2017). As asserted by Heffernan (2020, at section 1.07), 'the phenomena of law and justice evolve *in tandem* with society, serving as a bedrock to support both stability and change' [emphasis in original].

The living-instrument doctrine was applied first in *Tyrer v. United Kingdom* with regards to the legality (as determined by the Convention) of corporal punishment in the criminal justice system (Mowbray, 2013). In *Tyrer*, the Convention was therefore first identified as a living instrument by the Strasbourg Court: 'As a living instrument, the Convention must be interpreted in the light of present-day conditions, and the

Court would be influenced by commonly accepted standards in the penal policy of Member States.'[13]

In determining if rights in the Convention should be developed, the Court may assess if there is a 'European consensus' or an 'emerging trend' in a particular area, denoting the evolution of common approaches amongst the legal systems of Contracting States (United Nations, 2005; Pinto de Albuquerque, 2017; European Court of Human Rights, 2020). The ECtHR therefore seeks to identify a broad consensus on a particular standard of protection across Member States when deciding if the Convention's obligations should evolve. Rather than seeking to identify identical laws or unanimity across States, the ECtHR examines if there is a general *convergence* towards a particular trend or direction amongst numerous Member States (Kleinlein, 2017).

Inherent challenges arise in the interpretation of the Convention using the living-instrument doctrine and consensus method, as the ECtHR is tasked with identifying consensus in standards of protection, abstract values, and norms across Member States. As proposed by Letsas (2013, p. 108):

> [W]hat is distinctive about human rights law is that it engages abstract values that are meant to serve as general normative standards against which to judge the soundness of a legal system as a whole. Radical changes in societal beliefs about these abstract values poses a distinctive challenge for any court, be it domestic or international, that adjudicates on issues of fundamental human rights.

The living-instrument doctrine has been the subject of much criticism in recent years. A primary concern noted by commentators is that the frequent use of the living-instrument doctrine to interpret the Convention will result in States Parties being unable to predict their obligations with respect to human rights (Byron, 2016). In further developing the interpretation of the Convention, there is also a risk of *contra legem* interpretations (Bjorge, 2017).

Although it may be contended that the living-instrument doctrine has ensured the longevity, practicality, and relevance of the Convention, there have also been widespread concerns that the ECtHR has usurped formerly domestic areas of law and policy (Masterman, 2015). Critics contend that the living-instrument doctrine threatens national sovereignty and the policy autonomy of States Parties (Masterman, 2018), limiting the margin of appreciation of States Parties (Ita & Hicks, 2021). Such arguments relate to the perceived 'invention' of new rights by the ECtHR and its interference into domestic law and policy by subverting the authority and expertise of national policymakers (Masterman, 2015). Certain commentators therefore caution of 'mission creep' by the ECtHR, namely the expansion of rights beyond the intent of the framers of the

---

[13] *Tyrer v. United Kingdom* (1979-80) 2 EHRR 1, at 1–2.

Convention and the overruling by the ECtHR of decisions made by domestic courts and democratically-elected legislators and policy-makers (UK Conservative Party, 2014).

However, interpreting the Convention as a living instrument ensures that the protection of human rights is 'not theoretical or illusory, but practical and effective' (Wildhaber, 2007, p. 223), particularly for vulnerable and marginalized groups. As suggested by Letsas (2010, p. 527):

> [T]he Court has used the living-instrument approach in order to establish the autonomy of the Convention rights, not from domestic definitions and classification this time, but from the various moralistic views that dominated member states when the Convention was drafted and may still survive in some respondent states. By 'moralistic' I mean views which propose that someone should be deprived of a liberty or an opportunity solely because others (usually the majority) think of him as less than an equal or do not care about him as they care about others.

In *Beizaras and Levickas v. Lithuania*, the applicants claimed that they had experienced discrimination on the grounds of sexual orientation, whereby the public authorities had refused to initiate an investigation of hostile comments posted on the Facebook page of the first applicant. The ECtHR held that there had been a violation of Article 8 on the 'Right to Respect for Private and Family Life', Article 13 on the 'Right to an Effective Remedy', and Article 14 on the 'Prohibition of Discrimination'. In the Strasbourg Court's assessment, it referred to the living-instrument doctrine, stating:

> [G]iven that the Convention is a living instrument, to be interpreted in the light of present-day conditions, the State, in its choice of means designed to protect the family and to secure, as required by Article 8, respect for family life, must necessarily take into account developments in society and changes in the perception of social, civil status and relational issues, including the fact that there is not just one way or one choice in the sphere of leading and living one's family or private life.[14]

European Convention on Human Rights: Positive-Obligations Doctrine

Interpreting the Convention as a living instrument has facilitated the development of positive obligations (Donald et al., 2012; Xenos, 2012). While States must not impede the exercise of human rights, they must also act positively to ensure the protection of rights, such as preventing the interference by private and non-state bodies in the rights of individuals (Bychawska-Siniarska, 2017). Positive obligations are typically relevant to economic, social, and cultural rights and often impose financial obligations on States Parties (Madden, 2016). Positive obligations are especially pertinent

---

[14] *Beizaras and Levickas v. Lithuania* (App. No. 41288/15) - [2020] ECHR 41288/15, at [48].

to the right not to be subjected to torture or to inhuman or degrading treatment or punishment, the right to life, alongside the right to respect for private and family life, where the right to private life is interpreted broadly to comprise the mental and physical integrity of a person (IHREC, 2015).

For example, a seminal case in relation to Article 2 ECHR on the right to life and the protective obligation of a State towards a potential victim is *Osman v. United Kingdom*. The second applicant incurred an injury in a shooting incident, which led to his father's death, the husband of the first applicant. The applicants invoked Articles 2, 6, 8, and 13 of the Convention and complained that the State had failed in its duty to protect the lives of both the second applicant and his father and to prevent harassment experienced by their family. The ECtHR held that there had been no violation of Articles 2 and 8 of the Convention and that it was unnecessary to assess the complaints made by the applicant pursuant to Article 13. The Court held that Article 6(1) had however been violated. The Court affirmed that Article 2 cannot be interpreted in such a way that creates an unfeasible or disproportionate burden on authorities. The court further examined the positive obligation of the right to life, as follows:

> Where there is an allegation that the authorities have violated their positive obligation to protect the right to life in the context of their abovementioned duty to prevent and suppress offences against the person, it must be established to the Court's satisfaction that the authorities knew or ought to have known at the time of the existence of a real and immediate risk to the life of an identified individual or individuals from the criminal acts of a third party and that they failed to take measures within the scope of their powers which, judged reasonably, might have been expected to avoid that risk.[15]

In determining that Article 2 'may also imply in certain well-defined circumstances a positive obligation',[16] the ECtHR exercised restraint in expanding the obligations that the Convention places on High Contracting Parties. The Convention does not therefore create an obligation on authorities to protect individuals from all claimed risks to life (European Court of Human Rights, 2021). Similarly, in *O'Keeffe v. Ireland*, in relation to Article 1 on the 'Obligation to Respect Human Rights' and Article 3 on the 'Prohibition of Torture', the ECtHR affirmed:

> This positive obligation to protect is to be interpreted in such a way as not to impose an excessive burden on the authorities, bearing in mind, in particular, the unpredictability of human conduct and operational choices which must be made in terms of priorities and resources.[17]

---

[15] *Osman v. United Kingdom* (2000) 29 EHRR 245, at 246.
[16] *Osman v. United Kingdom* (2000) 29 EHRR 245, at 305.
[17] *O'Keeffe v. Ireland* (App. No. 35810/09, 28th January 2014), at [144].

Positive obligations with regards to Article 2 were further examined in *Savage v South Essex Partnership NHS Foundation Trust*. With respect to Article 2 ECHR, the House of Lords emphasized that 'health authorities are under an over-arching obligation to protect the lives of patients in their hospitals'.[18] The court held that this obligation, depending on the particular circumstances, may necessitate the fulfilment of complementary obligations, including the need for health authorities to employ competent and highly trained staff and to put in place organizational systems that protect patients' lives. The House of Lords further held that Article 2 ECHR places an additional 'operational' obligation on health authorities and their hospital staff, when members of staff know or ought to know that a patient presents a 'real and immediate' risk of suicide. In such circumstances, Article 2 requires such staff to do all that can be reasonably expected to prevent the patient from committing suicide. If staff do not take steps to do so, they and the health authorities will be liable for negligence *in addition to* liability for infringing the operational obligation under Article 2.

Similarly, in *Rabone & Anor v Pennine Care NHS Foundation Trust*,[19] the UK Supreme Court held that the State had a special operational obligation to protect the right to life of informal psychiatric in-patients, in contrast to general medical or surgical patients (Szmukler et al., 2013). The Supreme Court emphasized that Article 2 ECHR places three separate obligations on the State:

> "The first, which does not arise here, is a negative obligation, not itself to take life except in the limited cases provided for in article 2(2). The second, which also does not arise here, is a positive obligation to conduct a proper investigation into any death for which the State might bear some degree of responsibility. And the third, with which this case is concerned, is a positive obligation to protect life ... In the health care context, this also entails having effective administrative and regulatory systems in place, designed to protect patients from professional incompetence resulting in death" (at paragraph 93).

More recently, in *Griffiths v Chief Constable of the Suffolk Police, Norfolk and Suffolk NHS Foundation Trust*, the Queen's Bench Division held that an NHS Trust was not negligent in determining that a person who had attempted suicide did not meet the criteria for compulsory admission to hospital under the Mental Health Act 1983, and therefore no breach of duty arose towards the woman that he murdered soon after. There had been no duty on the NHS Trust to give a warning to the victim or to the police.[20] Mr Justice Ouseley asserted that 'the operational duty did not arise because the NHS Trust did not know, nor ought it to have known of any real or immediate risk to Ms Griffith's life' (at paragraph 484).

---

[18] *Savage v South Essex Partnership NHS Foundation Trust* [2008] UKHL 74, at paragraph 68.

[19] *Rabone & Anor v Pennine Care NHS Foundation Trust* [2012] UKSC 2.

[20] *Griffiths v Chief Constable of the Suffolk Police, Norfolk and Suffolk NHS Foundation Trust* [2018] EWHC 2538 (QB).

Although positive obligations are therefore imposed on States to ensure the protection of rights, commentators have argued that positive obligations pose a risk of significantly adding to Convention obligations that are imposed on States Parties. As proposed by Bjorge (2017, p. 255), 'the Strasbourg Court should take to heart the classic dictum of the International Court, which can apply no less to the European Court than to the International: "It is the duty of the Court to interpret", "not to revise", the Convention'.

However, in accordance with the principle of 'attribution', the ECtHR may only protect rights that are rooted in the Convention, requiring European judges to connect each positive obligation to a particular clause set out in the Convention (Akandji-Kombe, 2007). The ECtHR imposes positive obligations on States to implement measures that are deemed necessary, reasonable, and appropriate to protect an individual's rights (Akandji-Kombe, 2007). The ECtHR has explicitly and consistently emphasized that the breadth of positive obligations must be reasonable and that positive obligations arise if State authorities had knowledge or ought to have had knowledge of a risk of harm (Stoyanova, 2020). Furthermore, the ECtHR has held consistently that when positive obligations are placed on a Contracting Party, the margin of appreciation will in principle determine the State's choice of means (European Court of Human Rights, 2021).

A primary concern that is raised regarding positive obligations is that legal human rights instruments in force in numerous States only protect against intrusions into rights by the State, but do not require the State to actively *fulfil* human rights. As such, it is contended that interpreting the Convention through the lens of positive obligations conflicts with the obligations and spirit of other international rights instruments. However, under international law, States are required to respect, protect, and fulfil rights (IHREC, 2015). For example, the right to health comprises three levels of obligations: the obligation to *respect*, whereby the State must not interfere with the enjoyment of the right to health; the obligation to *protect*, necessitating that States adopt measures to prevent third parties from interfering with the right to health; and the obligation to *fulfil*, requiring States to implement necessary legislative, administrative, budgetary, judicial, and other courses of action to realize the right to health (Office of the High Commissioner for Human Rights, 2000).

Proponents of the positive-obligations doctrine argue that the development of positive obligations has led to increased human rights protection for vulnerable cohorts in society, including victims of domestic violence, rape, and/or human trafficking (Donald et al., 2012). As emphasized by Peroni and Timmer (2013, p. 1076): 'Substantive equality does not confine itself to a duty to refrain from discrimination. Substantive equality involves more than that; it requires the state to take a proactive role and to adopt positive steps to promote equality'. In *Chapman v. United Kingdom*, the Strasbourg Court reflected on the 'consensus amongst the Member States of the Council of Europe recognizing the special needs of minorities and an obligation to protect their security, identity and lifestyle', requiring 'not only that Contracting States refrain from policies or practices which discriminate against them but that also, where necessary, they should take positive steps to improve their situation through, for example, legislation or specific programmes'.[21] The ECtHR's reasoning in *Chapman* chimes with the principle of equity, signifying the fulfilment of human rights and the distribution of resources in accordance with the needs of minority, marginalized, and vulnerable groups to provide them with equal opportunities that are enjoyed by others (Amin et al., 2011).

Conclusion

Historicism can supplement other approaches to interpretation of the Irish Constitution by shining a light on the reasoning for the structure of Articles and by enabling a more holistic reading of the Constitution (Coffey, 2018). However, as contended by Albert (2015, p. 406), 'originalism is one of several reasonable ways to give meaning to a text whose meaning may admit of a multiplicity of morally, legally and sociologically legitimate meanings'. Indeed, Hogan et al. (2018) note that compartmentalizing different approaches may be redundant, as all approaches are used to some extent when interpreting the Constitution. In *Sinnott v. Minister for Education*, Hardiman J affirmed:[22]

> Tensions are said to exist between the methods of construction summarised in the use of adjectives such as '*historical*', '*harmonious*' and '*purposive*'. In my view, much of this debate is otiose, because each of these words connotes an aspect of interpretation which legitimately forms part, but only part, of every exercise in constitutional construction [emphasis in original].

Scalia (1989a, p. 1) proposes that '[m]any, if not most, of the provisions of the Constitution do not make sense except as they are given meaning by the historical background in which they were adopted'. In the Irish context, the courts will usually attempt to balance contemporary meanings with a historical perspective (Hogan et al., 2018). Accordingly, the Irish Courts avail of both a written and an 'unwritten' Constitution. While the 1937 Constitution can provide guidance in relation to the essence and extent of rights and provisions, these must be modified and interpreted to reflect current meanings and social contexts (Langwallner, 2008a).

Correspondingly, there is much debate surrounding the interpretation of international human rights treaties as living instruments (Letsas, 2013). To support the legitimacy of the consensus method, it is imperative for the ECtHR to be clear and transparent when determining 'European consensus' in a particular area. For example, in *Tyrer*, the Strasbourg Court did not provide any detailed evidence of commonly accepted standards underpinning the policy of States Parties (Letsas, 2010).

---

[21] *Chapman v. United Kingdom* (2001) 33 E.H.R.R. 18, at 435–436.
[22] *Sinnott v. Minister for Education* [2001] 2 IR 545.

The ECtHR also requires a clear and transparent theory of 'positive obligations' to justify the Court's rationale when deviating from precedent and to support the legitimacy of its rulings (Kolliniati, 2019).

In relation to the difference between positive and negative obligations, Dickson (2010, p. 203) notes that 'the dichotomy is a false one', as positive obligations can be simply reiterated as negative obligations and vice versa and every human right has correlative positive and negative obligations. Similarly, Karp (2020, p. 86) asserts that a central aim of the 'respect, protect, and fulfil' framework is 'to reject and to move beyond a false binary divide between so-called "negative" and "positive" rights. Instead, *all* human rights, whether civil–political or socio-economic, are associated with a full spectrum of duties' [emphasis in original].

In relation to the consensus method, Kleinlein (2017, p. 873) cautions that '[p]rogressive, rights-friendly judgments that consider a mere trend in "vanguard" state parties as a European consensus will probably provoke domestic contestation in "laggard" states'. However, by affording a margin of appreciation, the Strasbourg Court can apply the consensus method, while reducing the possibility of backlash by States Parties who may otherwise be found to be in violation of a Convention right (Dothan, 2018). Similarly, with regards to positive obligations, States Parties are given a broad margin of appreciation in implementing the requirements to comply with the Convention (McGoldrick, 2016). Indeed, Protocol No. 15 has amended the Convention to explicitly refer to the principle of subsidiarity and the doctrine of the margin of appreciation (Council of Europe, 2021).

The application of the living-instrument doctrine by the Strasbourg Court, through its case law, has resulted in the expansion of the breadth of Convention rights and the development of positive obligations (McGoldrick, 2016). Case law has therefore demonstrated that public bodies must adopt positive measures to protect human rights, in addition to preventing infringements of rights (IHREC, 2015). As such, the ECtHR's broad interpretation of the Convention has led to increased promotion and protection of the rights of vulnerable groups, such as refugees, persons with disabilities, victims of domestic violence, and victims of violence against women (Gilmore, 2020).

Key Reflective Questions

1. Article 12(2) of the CRPD stipulates that 'States Parties shall recognize that persons with disabilities enjoy legal capacity on an equal basis with others in all aspects of life.' General Comment No. 1 on Article 12 (Committee on the Rights of Persons with Disabilities, 2014, p. 5) provides: 'Where, after significant efforts have been made, it is not practicable to determine the will and preferences of an individual, the 'best interpretation of will and preferences' must replace the 'best interests' determinations'. Furthermore, Article 14 CRPD requires States Parties to

ensure liberty and security of person for people with disabilities. In its interpretation of Article 14, the UN Committee on the Rights of Persons with Disabilities has called for States Parties to repeal any legislation that enables detentions based on the existence of a psychosocial disability, including in relation to perceived dangerousness or need for treatment (Doyle Guilloud, 2019). However, the legislation of many countries allows for involuntary incarceration on the grounds of a (mental health) disability, thereby conflicting with the rights set out in the CRPD. Yet clinicians who want to abide by the CRPD have a legal obligation to comply with their country's mental health law. How would you advise a group of clinicians who have approached you for advice on what they should do to promote the rights enshrined in the CRPD whilst abiding by domestic law?

2. The Office of the United Nations High Commission for Human Rights (OHCHR) (2009, p. 15) argues that '[i]n the area of criminal law, recognition of the legal capacity of persons with disabilities requires abolishing a defence based on the negation of criminal responsibility because of the existence of a mental or intellectual disability' (commonly known as the 'insanity defence'). The OHCHR advises that disability-neutral doctrines on the subjective component of the crime (*mens rea*) should instead be adopted, which take into account the particular situation of the individual defendant. From this perspective, if an individual could be deprived of their volition by virtue of a psychosocial disability alone, then laws that limit decision-making ability due to psychosocial disability could continue to operate, which Article 12 CRPD aims to prevent (Barsky & Stein, 2023). However, mental health problems can be used as a substantive defence in international criminal law, particularly at the International Criminal Court (Freckelton & Karagiannakis, 2022) and in domestic criminal courts including the Irish criminal justice system (McCutcheon, 2022). What approach would you recommend to clinicians who are invited to provide expert evidence to the courts with regards to the 'insanity defence', for example as *amicus curiae*, on how to provide such evidence while aligning with the rights enshrined in the CRPD?

3. The Indian Mental HealthCare Act 2017 was developed to 'align and harmonise the existing laws' with the CRPD (Ministry of Law and Justice of India, 2017). This obligation to 'adopt all appropriate legislative, administrative and other measures for the implementation of the rights recognized in the present Convention' is set out in Article 4(1)(a) CRPD. However, in many countries, there remain significant legislative gaps and discriminatory laws, contrary to the Convention (International Disability Alliance, 2023; Joint Committee on Disability Matters Ireland, 2024). If psychiatry is to 'lead the way in legislating for health and wellbeing' as the medical field most acquainted with the use of legislation in daily clinical health services (Duffy & Kelly, 2017), how can clinicians more effectively support reform and harmonization of domestic legislation to align with the CRPD?

Further Reading

Byrne, R., McCutcheon, P., Cahillane, L., & Roche-Cagney, E. (2020). *Byrne and McCutcheon on the Irish legal system* (7th ed.). Bloomsbury.

Hogan, G., Whyte, G., Kenny, D., & Walsh, R. (2018). *Kelly: The Irish Constitution*. Bloomsbury.

Letsas, G. (2010). Strasbourg's interpretive ethic: Lessons for the international lawyer. *European Journal of International Law, 21*(3), 509–541. https://doi.org/10.1093/ejil/chq056

Masterman, R. (2015). *Supreme, submissive or symbiotic? United Kingdom courts and the European Court of Human Rights*. The Constitution Unit, School of Public Policy, University College London.

References

Akandji-Kombe, J. F. (2007). *Positive obligations under the European Convention on Human Rights: A guide to the implementation of the European Convention on Human Rights*. Council of Europe.

Albert, R. (2015). How unwritten constitutional norms change written constitutions. *Dublin University Law Journal, 38*(2), 387–418.

Amin, M., MacLachlan, M., Mannan, H., El Tayeb, S., El Khatim, A., Swartz, L., Munthali, A., Van Rooy, G., McVeigh, J., Eide, A., & Schneider, M. (2011). EquiFrame: A framework for analysis of the inclusion of human rights and vulnerable groups in health policies. *Health and Human Rights, 13*(2), 1–20.

Barsky, B. A., & Stein, M. A. (2023). The United Nations Convention on the Rights of Persons with Disabilities, neuroscience, and criminal legal capacity. *Journal of Law and the Biosciences, 10*(1), Article lsad010. https://doi.org/10.1093/jlb/lsad010

Berro Pizzarossa, L., & Perehudoff, K. (2017). Global survey of national constitutions: Mapping constitutional commitments to sexual and reproductive health and rights. *Health and Human Rights Journal, 19*(2), 279–293.

Bjorge, E. (2017). The Convention as a living instrument: Rooted in the past, looking to the future. *Human Rights Law Journal, 36*, 243–255.

Brest, P. (1980). The misconceived quest for the original understanding. *Boston University Law Review, 60*, 209–217.

Bruton, C., & McVeigh, K. (2018). Effects of the judgment of the Court of Appeal in Nano Nagle v Daly on the duty to provide reasonable accommodation. *Irish Employment Law Journal, 15*(2), 36–47.

Bychawska-Siniarska, D. (2017). *Protecting the right to freedom of expression under the European Convention on Human Rights: A handbook for legal practitioners*. Council of Europe.

Byrne, R., McCutcheon, P., Cahillane, L., & Roche-Cagney, E. (2020). *Byrne and McCutcheon on the Irish legal system* (7th ed.). Bloomsbury.

Byron, C. (2016). The European Court of Human Rights: A living instrument as applied to homosexuality. *The Judges' Journal, 55*(3), 36–39.

Carolan, E. (2013). Originalism enabled? The role of historical records in constitutional adjudication. *Dublin University Law Journal, 36*, 311–322.

Carolan, M. (2017, 12 November). Judge advocates judicial restraint in interpreting the constitution. *The Irish Times*.

Chandrachud, C. (2016). Constitutional interpretation. In S. Choudhry, M. Khosla, & P. Bhanu Mehta (Eds.), *The Oxford handbook of the Indian constitution* (pp. 73–93). Oxford University Press.

Charleton, P., McDermott, P. A., Herlihy, C., & Byrne, S. (2020). *Charleton & McDermott's criminal law and evidence* (2nd ed.). Bloomsbury.

Coffey, D. K. (2018). *Drafting the Irish constitution, 1935–1937: Transnational influences in interwar Europe*. Palgrave Macmillan.

Committee on the Rights of Persons with Disabilities. (2014). General comment No. 1 (2014). Article 12: Equal recognition before the law. https://www.ohchr.org/en/documents/general-comments-and-recommendations/general-comment-no-1-article-12-equal-recognition-1

Committee on the Rights of Persons with Disabilities. (2021). *Initial Report of Ireland under the Convention on the Rights of Persons with Disabilities; Prepared by the Department of Children, Equality, Disability, Integration and Youth*. https://www.gov.ie/en/publication/75e45-irelands-first-report-to-the-united-nations-committee-on-the-rights-of-persons-with-disabilities/

Cornell, S. (2019). Reading the constitution, 1787–91: History, originalism, and constitutional meaning. *Law and History Review, 37*(3), 821–845.

Council of Europe. (2021). *Protocol No. 15 Amending the Convention on the Protection of Human Rights and Fundamental Freedoms*.

de Blacam, M. (2017). *Judicial review*. Bloomsbury.

Department of Health (Ireland). (2015). *Report of the Expert Group Review of the Mental Health Act, 2001*. https://www.gov.ie/en/publication/637ccf-report-of-the-expert-group-review-of-the-mental-health-act-2001/

Dickson, B. (2010). Positive obligations and the European Court of Human Rights. *Northern Ireland Legal Quarterly, 61*(3), 203–208.

Donald, A., Gordon, J., & Leach, P. (2012). *The UK and the European Court of Human Rights; Equality and Human Rights Commission research report 83*. Equality and Human Rights Commission.

Dothan, S. (2018). Judicial deference allows European consensus to emerge. *Chicago Journal of International Law, 18*(2), 393–419.

Doyle, O. (2018). *The constitution of Ireland: A contextual analysis*. Bloomsbury.

Doyle Guilloud, S. (2019). The right to liberty of persons with psychosocial disabilities at the United Nations: A tale of two interpretations. *International Journal of Law and Psychiatry, 66*, Article 101497.

Duffy, R. M., & Kelly, B. D. (2017). Can psychiatry lead the way in legislating for health and wellbeing? *Irish Medical Journal, 110*(6), 591.

Easterbrook, F. H. (2008). Originalism and pragmatism: Pragmatism's role in interpretation. *Harvard Journal of Law and Public Policy, 31*, 901–906.

European Court of Human Rights. (2020). *Judicial seminar 2020; The Convention as a living instrument at 70*.

European Court of Human Rights. (2021). *Guide on Article 2 of the European Convention on Human Rights; Right to life*. Council of Europe.

Flynn, E. (2020). The long road to ratification: Ireland and the CRPD. In E. J. Kakoullis & K. Johnson (Eds.), *Recognising human rights in different cultural contexts: The United Nations Convention on the Rights of Persons with Disabilities (CRPD)* (pp. 133–156). Palgrave Macmillan.

Forde, M., & Leonard, D. (2013). *Constitutional law of Ireland* (3rd ed.). Bloomsbury.

Freckelton, I., & Karagiannakis, M. (2022). The insanity defence under international criminal law. In R. Mackay & W. Brookbanks (Eds.), *The insanity defence: International and comparative perspectives, Oxford Monographs on Criminal Law and Justice* (pp. 334–354). Oxford. https://doi.org/10.1093/oso/9780198854944.003.0015

Gadamer, H. G. (2013). *Truth and method*. Bloomsbury.

Gilmore, E. (2020, 3 November). European Court of Human Rights has driven social change in Ireland. *The Irish Times*.

Goldsworthy, J. (2007). Introduction. In J. Goldsworthy (Ed.), *Interpreting constitutions: A comparative study* (pp. 1–6). Oxford University Press.

Greene, J., & Tew, Y. (2018). Comparative approaches to constitutional history. In E. F. Delaney & R. Dixon (Eds.), *Comparative judicial review*. Edward Elgar Publishing. Columbia Public Law Research Paper No. 14-613. https://scholarship.law.columbia.edu/faculty_scholarship/2519

Heffernan, L. (2020). *Evidence in criminal trials* (2nd ed.). Bloomsbury.

Houses of the Oireachtas (Oireachtas Library and Research Service). (2016). *International human rights law: operation and impact*.

Hogan, G., Whyte, G., Kenny, D., & Walsh, R. (2018). *Kelly: The Irish constitution*. Bloomsbury.

Hogan, G. (2019). Ireland: The Constitution of Ireland and EU law: The complex constitutional debates of a small country. In A. Albi & S. Bardutzky (Eds.), *National Constitutions in European and global governance: Democracy, rights, the rule of law; National reports* (pp. 1323–1372). Springer.

Humphreys, R. (2017). The constitution and law as living instruments for a living society. *Dublin University Law Journal, 40*(2), 45–70.

International Disability Alliance. (2023). *The CRPD Committee closed its 28th session and published its Concluding Observations on the countries under review*. https://www.internationaldisabilityalliance.org/blog/crpd-committee-closed-its-28th-session-and-published-its-concluding-observations-countries

Irish Human Rights Commission. (2010). *Policy paper concerning the definition of a "voluntary patient" under s.2 of the Mental Health Act 2001*.

Irish Human Rights and Equality Commission (IHREC). (2015). *Human rights explained: Guide to human rights law*.

Irish Human Rights and Equality Commission (IHREC). (2020). *Submission to the Citizens' Assembly on gender equality*.

Irish Human Rights and Equality Commission (IHREC). (2023). *Comments on Ireland's 20th National Report on the Implementation of the European Social Charter*.

Ita, R., & Hicks, D. (2021). Beyond expansion or restriction? Models of interaction between the living instrument and margin of appreciation doctrines and the scope of the ECHR. *International Human Rights Law Review, 10*(1), 40–74. https://doi.org/10.1163/22131035-01001004

Joint Committee on Disability Matters Ireland. (2024). *Towards harmonisation of national legislation with the United Nations Convention on the Rights of Persons with Disabilities*.

Karp, D. J. (2020). What is the responsibility to respect human rights? Reconsidering the 'respect, protect, and fulfil' framework. *International Theory, 12*(1), 83–108.

Kavanagh, A. (2012). The Irish constitution at 75 Years: Natural law, Christian values and the ideal of justice. *Irish Jurist, 48*, 71–101.

Kelly, J. (1988). The constitution: Law and manifesto. In F. Litton (Ed.), *The constitution of Ireland 1937–1987* (pp. 208–217). Institute of Public Administration.

Kleinlein, T. (2017). Consensus and contestability: The ECtHR and the combined potential of European consensus and procedural rationality control. *European Journal of International Law, 28*(3), 871–894.

Kolliniati, M. A. (2019). *Human rights and positive obligations to healthcare: Reading the European Convention on Human Rights through Joseph Raz's theory of rights*. Nomos.

Langwallner, D. (2008a). The incoherence of historicism in Irish constitutional interpretation. *The Bar Review, 13*(5), 109–114.

Langwallner, D. (2008b). The incoherence of historicism and originalism in Irish constitutional interpretation. *Independent Law Review, 4*, 17–25.

Law Society of Ireland (Law Society Gazette). (2023). *HSE's disability approach 'undermines rights'*. https://www.lawsociety.ie/gazette/top-stories/2023/november/hses-disability-appro ach-undermines-rights

Letsas, G. (2010). Strasbourg's interpretive ethic: Lessons for the international lawyer. *European Journal of International Law, 21*(3), 509–541. https://doi.org/10.1093/ejil/chq056

Letsas, G. (2013). The ECHR as a living instrument: Its meaning and legitimacy. In A. Føllesdal, B. Peters & G. Ulfstein (Eds.), *Constituting Europe: The European Court of Human Rights in a national, European and global context* (pp. 106–141). Cambridge University Press.

Madden, D. (2016). *Medicine, ethics and the law* (3rd ed.). Bloomsbury.

Maggs Campbell, C. G. (2018). The preventative potential of instrumentalising history? The 'right to truth' in Northern Ireland and Cambodia. *Hibernian Law Journal, 17*(1), 43–72.

Masterman, R. (2015). *Supreme, submissive or symbiotic? United Kingdom courts and the European Court of Human Rights*. The Constitution Unit, School of Public Policy, University College London.

Masterman, R. (2018). Federal dynamics of the UK/Strasbourg relationship. In R. Schütze & S. Tierney (Eds.), *The United Kingdom and the federal idea* (pp. 203–226). Hart Publishing.

Mazzi, D. (2020). *A discourse perspective on Bunreacht na hÉireann: A sound constitution?* Cambridge Scholars Publishing.

McCutcheon, P. (2022). The insanity defence in Irish law. In R. Mackay & W. Brookbanks (Eds.), *The insanity defence: International and comparative perspectives, Oxford Monographs on Criminal Law and Justice* (pp. 100–121). Oxford. https://doi.org/10.1093/oso/978019 8854944.003.0005

McGoldrick, D. (2016). A defence of the margin of appreciation and an argument for its application by the Human Rights Committee. *International and Comparative Law Quarterly, 65*(1), 21–60.

McVeigh, J. (2023). Transport for All: Reeves and Lennon v Disabled Drivers Medical Board of Appeal and the need for alignment with international human rights law—Part III. *Irish Law Times, 41*(5), 69–73.

Ministry of Law and Justice of India. (2017). *Mental HealthCare Act, 2017*. https://prsindia.org/ acts/parliament

Mohr, T. (2006). The rights of women under the constitution of the Irish Free State. *Irish Jurist, 41*, 20–59.

Moreno-Lax, V. (2021). Intersectionality, forced migration, and the jus-generation of the right to flee: Theorising a composite entitlement to leave to escape irreversible harm. In B. Çalı, L. Bianku & I. Motoc (Eds.), *Migration and the European Convention on Human Rights* (pp. 43–84). Oxford University Press.

Mowbray, A. (2013). Between the will of the Contracting Parties and the needs of today: Extending the scope of Convention rights and freedoms beyond what could have been foreseen by the drafters of the ECHR. In E. Brems & J. Gerards (Eds.), *Shaping rights in the ECHR: The role of the European Court of Human Rights in determining the scope of human rights* (pp. 17–37). Cambridge University Press.

Murray, C. (2010). Reinforcing paternalism within Irish mental health law – Contrasting the decisions in Eh v St. Vincents Hospital and Others and Sm v The Mental Health Commission and Others. *Dublin University Law Journal, 32*(1), 273–290.

Ní Loinsigh, N. (2014). Judicial dissent in Ireland: Theory, practice and the constraints of the Single Opinion Rule. *Irish Jurist, 51*, 123–148.

O'Brien, E., & Gowan, R. (2012). *What makes international agreements work: Defining factors for success.* Center on International Cooperation.

Office of the High Commissioner for Human Rights. (2000). *CESCR General Comment No. 14: The Right to the highest attainable standard of health (Art. 12).*

Office of the United Nations High Commission for Human Rights. (2009). *Thematic study by the Office of the United Nations High Commissioner for Human Rights on enhancing awareness and understanding of the Convention on the Rights of Persons with Disabilities.* https://digitallibrary.un.org/record/647817?ln=en

O'Mahony, C. (2017). *Marriage equality in the United States and Ireland: How history shaped the future.* University of Illinois Law Review.

Peroni, L., & Timmer, A. (2013). Vulnerable groups: The promise of an emerging concept in European Human Rights Convention law. *International Journal of Constitutional Law, 11*(4), 1056–1085.

Pinto de Albuquerque, P. (2017). *Is the ECHR facing an existential crisis?* Judge at the European Court of Human Rights; Speech delivered at the Mansfield College, Oxford.

Prakash, O. (2024). Indian constitution: Antecedents, philosophy and basic features. In M. Kumar Jha & K. Nayan Choubey (Eds.), *Indian politics and political processes: Ideas, institutions and practices* (pp. 35–52). Routledge.

Rubenfeld, J. (1995). Reading the constitution as spoken. *Yale Law Journal, 104*(5), 1119–1186.

Scalia, A. (1989a). Is there an unwritten constitution? *Harvard Journal of Law and Public Policy, 12*(1), 1–2.

Scalia, A. (1989b). Originalism: The lesser evil. *University of Cincinnati Law Review, 57*(3), 849–866.

Schwarzenbach, S. A. (2003). Women and constitutional interpretation: The forgotten value of civic friendship. In S. A. Schwarzenbach & P. Smith (Eds.), *Women and the United States constitution: History, interpretation and practice* (pp. 1–20). Columbia University Press.

Shaman, J. M. (2001). *Constitutional interpretation: Illusion and reality.* Greenwood Press.

Szmukler, G., Richardson, G., & Owen, G. (2013). 'Rabone' and four unresolved problems in mental health law. *The Psychiatrist, 37*, 297–301. doi: 10.1192/pb.bp.113.043273

Stokes Paulsen, M., & Paulsen, L. (2017). *The constitution: An introduction.* Basic Books.

Stoyanova, V. (2020). Fault, knowledge, and risk within the framework of positive obligations under the European Convention on Human Rights. *Leiden Journal of International Law, 33*(3), 601–620.

Strauss, D. A. (2010). *The living constitution.* Oxford University Press.

Sunstein, C. R. (2015). *Constitutional personae.* Oxford University Press.

Tew, Y. (2014). Originalism at home and abroad. *Columbia Journal of Transnational Law, 52,* 780–895.

UK Conservative Party. (2014). *Protecting human rights in the UK: The conservatives' proposals for changing Britain's human rights laws.*

United Nations. (2005). *Vienna Convention on the Law of Treaties 1969.*

United Nations Development Programme (UNDP). (2014). *UNDP guidance note on constitution-making support.*

Whelan, D. (2021). Application of the paternalism principle to constitutional rights: Mental health case-law in Ireland. *European Journal of Health Law, 28*(3), 223–243.

Wildhaber, L. (2007). The European Convention on Human Rights and international law. *International and Comparative Law Quarterly, 56*(2), 217–232.

World Bank. (2017). *World Development Report 2017: Governance and the Law.* World Bank.

Xenos, D. (2012). *The positive obligations of the State under the European Convention of Human Rights.* Routledge.

21
Psychologists as Community Scribes
The Case of Project Salaam

Shemana Cassim, Darrin Hodgetts, Veronica Hopner,
Jennifer Khan-Janif, and Naima Ali

Introduction

Issues of social justice are central to psychological practice and the fair treatment and rights of people with whom we work. In psychological practice many scholar activists and practitioners have strived to address issues of social injustice. Yet, we have also acted unjustly towards particular groups throughout our disciplinary history, contributing at times to their marginality in society (Hodgetts et al., 2020). These injustices are evident in real world applications of psychological science that reify Eurocentric worldviews onto and discriminate against marginalized communities. Central here are instances whereby we have failed to adequately recognize and address the different needs of persons from lower social classes, minoritized ethnicities, genders, sexualities, religions, and [dis]abilities (Fine & Asch, 1988; Guthrie, 2004; Hegarty, 2017; Hodgetts et al., 2020). This chapter contributes to efforts to pluralize and extend applications of psychological knowledge in partnership *with* societally marginalized community groups, and in ways that are led by, recognizable to, and embrace the worldviews of these communities (Decolonial Psychology Editorial Collective, 2021; Guimarães, 2020; Hodgetts et al., 2023). Central to this chapter are issues regarding how we work ethically as accomplices in partnership with communities (Li et al., 2021) to co-produce and apply knowledge *with*, rather than impose research and interventions *on* [un]suspecting locales (Cornish et al., 2023).

Concerns around our disciplinary self-positioning as objective outsiders rather than engaged advocates and accomplices are not restricted to psychologists and our internal disciplinary chatter or professional reflections. Communities on the societal margins have questioned distal or outsider-driven research and practices being imposed on them. Many communities now expect to exercise their human rights to self-determination to not be practiced *on* by outsiders in the production and application of psychological knowledge and seek proximal engagements with psychologists as accomplices in their efforts to realize social justice (Cornish et al., 2023; Rua et al. 2022). The resulting proximal relations raise issues of allyship and relational ethics in the collaborative design, conduct, and implementation of research-based praxis in community settings (Forber-Pratt et al., 2019; Hodgetts et al., 2021). Here, the notion of relational ethics refers to working alongside and co-creating knowledge in dialogue with communities, respecting and valuing their lived, experiential knowledge. This ethical orientation requires that our scholarly activities can benefit the communities with whom we work (Hodgetts et al., 2021). It is also crucial to acknowledge that such proximal relations have been a feature of community and applied social psychologies at least since the early 20th century and are growing presently in momentum (Hodgetts et al., 2020; O'Doherty & Hodgetts, 2019). For example, Dewey's (1916) approach to knowledge co-production in Hull House[1] in Chicago was anchored in a proximal and experiential form of 'experimentalism' designed to foster democratic relationships and power sharing. This approach to community praxis requires scholar activists to cultivate partnerships *within* marginalized communities that feature equity of control, meaningful associations, sustained relations, and a mutual ethos towards inclusion and social justice in shared efforts to transform situations of adversity and exclusion (Dewey, 1969/1991). Relatedly and reflecting on her seminal work from the 1930s, Jahoda (1992) also emphasized the importance of proximal relations in psychological practice whereby we immerse ourselves within equitable relations to work *with,* rather than *on* communities to identify and address their needs.

This orientation to psychological praxis is particularly pertinent to contemporary participative efforts to help improve the situations of marginalized indigenous, migrant, worker, religious, and mental health service survivor groups (Erskine & Bilimoria 2019). Such allyship is now recognized as a form of scholar activism that enacts key principles of relational ethics with the practical intention of supporting positive community-driven and controlled initiatives (Hodgetts et al., 2021; Said 1994). These immersive relationships are underpinned by ethical values of benevolence, compassion, reciprocal cooperation, human heartedness, and mutually beneficial action. These values are particularly relevant in continuing to shift our modes of practice out beyond the dominant instrumentally orientated practitioner and client relationships in psychology to more proximal and friendship like relations (Beauchamp 2019; Li et al., 2021). It centralizes a will to openness, listening to, hearing, and embracing insights from local experiential wisdom (phronetic knowledge) and combining such phronetic knowledge regarding 'how things work around here' with the resources (libraries, time, knowledge of societal and governmental systems) and skills (expertise in research, facilitation, and advocacy) that we bring to the table as scholar activists (Derickson & Routledge, 2015). Such practice work features mutually beneficial and relationally ethical partnerships between communities and scholarly activists (Li et al., 2021).

Collaborative efforts such as those discussed above, raise key considerations around human rights, inclusion, and social justice that are particularly pertinent to

---

[1] Building on insights from her visit to relief agencies in London in the early 1880s, Jane Addams established Hull House in Chicago in 1889 to facilitate processes of urbanization and poverty reduction *with* working class and new migrant groups through the provision of cutting edge educational, social, and community arts programmes.

the everyday situations and experiences of groups, such as refugees and new migrants. We use the case exemplar of Project Salaam that reminds participants that they are within the moral envelope. As psychologists we can contribute substantively here, not only when we ourselves are members of marginalized communities, but also as allied accomplices who have been invited in to share our expertise and skills (see case exemplar discussed in 'Project Salaam' section below). A central construct for our ongoing work within this tradition of community-engaged psychology is the scope of justice (Opotow, 2012), or moral envelope of inclusion in society, which determines how rights, freedoms, and liberties are distributed, and who gets to be treated fairly. This lens provides an important foundation for our relationally ethical practice (Hodgetts et al., 2021), whereby we can contribute to practical efforts to enact the moral and material inclusion of previously marginalized groups, and in ways that respect their cultures and faiths. Inclusion in the moral envelope positions groups as deserving members of society whose human rights should not be transgressed. The scope of justice is not just about personal rights. It is also a relational construct that speaks to the importance of relational ethics, group rights to inclusion and fair treatment by other groups in society and requires us all to shoulder and share obligations towards respecting each other despite our differences (Hodgetts et al., 2020). Hence, the importance of balancing the interests of different groups and the teaching of civics and skills in conflict resolution as we work towards the cultivation of more harmonious and inclusive societies of difference.

We will pick up on these issues in relation to the focal project case for this chapter on the inclusion of Muslim youth from refugee backgrounds. This focus is important given the recent history in the West whereby refugees and new migrants are often treated with suspicion and positioned outside the scope of justice as potential 'threats' to society. Recent research also suggests that respecting the various religious or faith-based beliefs of new migrant groups and ensuring fair treatment can encourage pro-social civic engagements between new and host society groups, and contribute to the cultivation of more harmonious societies (Bagasra, 2021; Vergani et al., 2015). Respecting the religious or faith-based beliefs of these groups also then means that our orientation to rights and freedoms needs to be relevant to the communities with whom we are working. For instance, our orientation on relational ethics closely aligns with, and builds on Islamic perspectives on human rights. In Islam, dignity is seen as the foundation of human rights, where rights are perceived in a collective sense, and involve a duty towards others, and ultimately seeks to bring about social justice (or *adl*) (Bagasra, 2021; Islamic Relief, 2014). This is detailed in the hadith of the Prophet Muhammad (peace be upon him) which illustrates that a Muslim fulfils their duties to God through granting the rights of others (Sahih Muslim Book 32, *hadith* no. 6232). While the Universal Declaration of Human Rights (UDHR) is premised on the notion of dignity as well, this stance appears to refer to an individual divorced from their social commitments and/or relationship with the collective.

It is important to note here that Islam is not a monolithic entity, and the settlement process for Muslim migrants and former refugee communities in the Aotearoa New

Zealand context exhibits considerable heterogeneity, with varying durations of residence among these groups. As a result of distinct resettlement procedures undertaken by the United Nations, former refugees granted entry into Aotearoa New Zealand via the Quota Refugee programme tend to possess a higher degree of awareness regarding their human rights within the framework of safety and protection. Muslim communities entering Aotearoa New Zealand as migrants or through other refugee entry permits, such as Family Reunification, have typically acquired knowledge of the Human Rights Declaration through community advocates who educate them on their entitlements in relation to housing, healthcare, education, and other human-rights-based declarations. This educational process has also encompassed the Cairo Declaration on Human Rights in Islam (CDHR), which is rooted in faith-based human rights principles (Organisation of Islamic Conference, 1990). The integration of both the UNDHR and the CDHR has enriched our advocacy endeavours and provided guidance in our work. Although differences exist between these two declarations, it is worth noting that community advocates on the ground predominantly rely on the CDHR while remaining informed about, and responsive to the UNDHR. This dual approach holds relevance for Muslims residing in Western contexts, as it draws upon faith-based rights in conjunction with the United Nations' human rights mandate. It is important to acknowledge that countries operating under Islamic Sharia law may interpret and implement these rights differently, guided by their distinct Islamic legal frameworks and legislations.

Drawing on this orientation to human rights, in the next section, we present Project Salaam, a conflict-resolution school-based programme for Muslim refugee youth that is based on Islamic values and principles that some of the authors of this chapter recently evaluated. After considering the case of Project Salaam, we will reflect conceptually on the role of community psychologists as scribes who work in allyship with, and in service to, community groups on the margins of society and in ways that support their own efforts towards inclusion within the scope of justice and the realization of a better life somewhere new.

Project Salaam

Project Salaam was conceived in 2018, in response to experiences of racism and discrimination at school for Muslim youth from refugee backgrounds in Auckland, Aotearoa New Zealand (Collins, 2001). At the time, Muslim youth were feeling significant pressure from experiences of race-based surveillance from government agencies, and wider community-based discrimination in the country (Ward et al., 2019; Yogeeswaran et al., 2019), and grappling with experiences of discrimination, trauma, and associated grief and anger at school. Building on evidence from research in Aotearoa New Zealand (e.g. Office of Ethnic Communities, 2019; Peiris-John, et al., 2021; Education Review Office, 2023), Project Salaam is designed to support Muslim youth in strengthening leadership abilities, self-confidence, academic engagement, and achievement, and developing skills in conflict resolution and re-lationship management through a series of experiential workshops. Project Salaam is underpinned by Islamic values that function to promote secure cultural and faith identities, and participation in civil society as Muslim New Zealanders. The Project was facilitated through a series of workshops in two secondary schools in Aotearoa New Zealand.

Project Salaam is a pathway to facilitate a positive sense of Islamic self, and educa-tion in civics among refugee youth shows that such efforts can facilitate the realization of youth rights, where Muslim youth can be a person of faith *and* an active citizen in-volved in pro-social civic engagements (Bagasra, 2021; Vergani et al., 2015). As such, Project Salaam positions these youth and the Islamic community within a scope of justice. Therein, this Project demonstrates that religiosity can contribute to pro-social inclusion, positions these Islamic youth within the scope of justice of Aotearoa New Zealand.

In 2022, a group of community-orientated psychologists (SC, DH, and VH) were carefully hand-picked by local community leaders and invited onto the team, pri-marily to facilitate an evaluation of Project Salaam. This invitation was a result of the cultivation of relations of trust between a key member of the main Project Salaam team and the scholars through various other projects and engagements over the pre-vious years. While SC identified as a Muslim herself from a migrant background, DH and VH were secular in orientation, and thereby supported the project as allied accomplices. SC's role involved coordinating the evaluation project that was led by JKJ, and DH and VH provided scholarly advice and research expertise to the pro-cess. While the final report writing process was led by SC, DH, and VH, it was driven by JKJ.

The evaluation highlighted that Project Salaam achieved all its key goals by helping students to grow leadership skills, self-esteem, and effective communication as a basis for applying mediation techniques in processes of conflict resolution (Cassim et al., 2023b). The report highlighted the importance of sustaining and growing Project Salaam in collaboration with key stakeholders, including teachers and schools. In particular, the evaluation highlighted how Project Salaam can create opportunities for conversations with teachers and community members regarding how teachers and students can be better supported in developing pro-social responses to intergroup tensions and which promote the inclusion of Muslim youth. Therein, as a result of this evaluation, the team worked to craft further funding applications and proposals to en-able such flow-on initiatives to take place.

Project Salaam exemplifies the value of psychologists working to support commu-nity groups who are exercising their rights to develop their own understandings and efforts to address real world problems. As we will discuss in the following section, our role can become one of the allied community scribe who gifts technical expertise in writing through collecting, assembling, and synthesizing information, but not trying to control or direct community efforts towards self-determination and inclusion. We can still use the technologies of science to produce, share, and apply knowledge, but we do so as participating scribes who document, draw upon, and highlight the wisdom of community members as we seek to support local leaders and participants.

Theoretical Analysis: Conceptualizing the Community-Engaged Psychologist as Scribe

Dating back into antiquity, scribes did much more than function as intellectual re-corders of knowledge who merely documented faiths, big events, and the mundan-ities of everyday life by copying, translating, and authoring texts. The efforts of the scribe often stretched into diplomacy, planning, advising, and the coordination of various initiatives in support of the nation state. In eras when the skill of writing and reading was not widespread, a scribe could help to connect a community, and to ensure that information was preserved in a way that could be accessed, understood, and shared. Today, as was the case in Mesopotamia, Assyria, Egypt, China, India, Israel, and so forth, prominent scribes became embedded within the politics of the day as members of the court engaged in the governance of societies (Luukko, 2007; Pioske, 2013). Many of the historical functions of the ancient scribe have evolved over time into the contemporary professions of the lawyer, accountant, journalist, public servant, and scholar. We would propose that in many respects, the ancient functions of the scribe are now evident in the everyday work of the community-engaged psychologist. In contemporary community settings, the psychologist as scribe is drawn in to become immersed in the intricacies of community life; collab-orating with local leadership in documenting the events of the day, offering advice, liaising with external stakeholders, sharing our expertise, and so forth. As commu-nity scribes, we write proposals and reports as well as corresponding with key min-istries, institutions, and stakeholders. When immersed in such praxis, psychologists work in partnership *with* communities, rather than conducting research or interven-tions *on* them.

Community scribes in contemporary psychology occupy dialectical spaces from which to interpret events, offering skills, sharing insights into developing human rights-based approaches to addressing problems. As Johnson (1991, p.820) notes in relation to the trope of the scribe in medieval literary texts, 'scribes not only left their marks upon the manuscripts they copied, they also functioned as interpreters, editing and consequently altering the meaning of texts'. We do similar things today when col-laborating to document issues faced by communities and formulating and assessing the impacts of community-driven responses. We possess the language and the skills to articulate arguments and issues important to the community in a way that translates to those operating at the structural edifices such as funders, policymakers, and gov-ernment. We employ our scholarly skills to assist communities, to write people, who are often written out of history, back into our cultural narratives and associated scope of justice, as well as advocating for their rights and interests. We are not just authors of research, but also mediators of community experiences who witness, document, and advocate for effective and just responses in partnership with the locales.

Whilst continuing to recognize the value of psychological knowledge and our own expertise within these immersive engagements, it is important that we also remain open to the phronetic wisdom of people experiencing issues such as difficult migration transitions for refugees (Cornish et al., 2023; Hodgetts et al., 2021; Rua et al., 2020). Our articulation of the practice archetype of the community scribe character personifies a broader move in some areas of psychological practice away from the orthodox physical sciences inspired training in psychologists that emphasize distal efforts to theorize, research, and control the application of research-based knowledge on others, and with minimal input from them. We have trained generations of psychologists to embrace an 'objective' subjectivity, and respect 'boundaries' that lead us to practice at a distance from 'clients' and research participants (Li et al., 2021). This is to avoid the perceived risks of bias and to protect ourselves and clients from harm. There is some legitimacy to this self-positioning. However, this self-positioning can become problematic when working with marginalized communities and can perpetuate distinctions between 'us' and 'them'. Alternatively, many on the fringes of the discipline in community, feminist, and indigenous psychologies transgress these boundaries to emphasize the importance of collaboration and partnership in addressing real world challenges that many groups face to their personal, collective, psychological, and material well-being and human rights (Cornish et al., 2023; Hodgetts et al., 2021). Therein, we recognize and value the different forms of expertise brought into projects such as these, where our communities contribute phronetic wisdom and expertise. As psychologists, we contribute theorical and cumulative academic knowledge and techniques or ways of conducting inquiries to ensure robust knowledge production (Flyvbjerg, 2001). Although, depending on the context and relationship between the background of psychologists and particular communities, we may also contribute aspects of phronesis. Ultimately, as a team engaging in such initiatives, we find points of harmony between these forms of expertise. To engage in such proximal and mutually beneficial relations, it is crucial that we consider issues of participation, collaboration, human rights, social justice, and relational ethics as key principles of psychological practice (Hodgetts et al., 2021).

In saying this, we also acknowledge that there may be points of tension that can come with this approach outlined above. We recognize that the proximal relationships we advocate for may blur boundaries between research(er) and communities in terms of identities, social obligations, duties, and expectations with/to the group. There may also be instances where scholars and community members wear multiple 'hats' or carry different roles that can be read as manifesting conflicts of interest and related pressures affecting the team and/or the successful conduct of a project. We would also note that juggling multiple 'hats' is often a reality for the members of our team (both scholars and community members), and indeed is often necessary when contributing to community initiatives. This is how relationships work in community settings, and it requires us to cultivate ethical accountabilities in our work among ourselves and within the community of interest. Nonetheless, in both instances, we contend that such tensions can be managed through clear communication, and the cultivation of open and trusting relations between key stakeholders. Here, we go beyond procedural ethics, where the trust built on relational ethics within the project team becomes vital to facilitate such communication and participative ways of working (Cornish et al., 2023).

Further Conceptual Reflections on Rights and Ethics

We return to the importance of immersive iterative engagements and reciprocal gifting that respects the rights of all involved in our disciplinary engagements, in a way that does not repeat the exploitative or extractive mistakes of our past. Our approach to relational ethics encompasses relationality alongside an ethics and duty of care for the communities with whom we work. When we work as a scribe, our role in the community context is not to be a researcher. Rather, we were contributors, with the community leading the initiative. Therein, an aspect of the work of a scribe is to be an accomplice. It is imperative that this working relationship is centred around reciprocity and inclusion, where each party actively gifts and contributes something to the initiative or project at hand.

Working in service to community groups means that accountabilities are central, where our discipline has often prioritized the interests of the scholars or researchers, often at the expense of that of the community. Here, mutual and dialogical accountability is key, such as meeting deadlines, commitments, following the brief of the project, and being accessible and willing to accommodate feedback. In writing the final report for the project, the document was one that was collectively produced by all members of the team (scholars and community members), where we worked together towards a mutual outcome. Co-design was involved in all phases and involved continuous genuine partnerships. Additionally drawing on Islamic worldviews, it was important for us to keep to our word to the community, so trust was vital. Through this process, our engagements with this community ultimately moved towards continuous corporation beyond Project Salaam to include other initiatives. Our engagement with Project Salaam highlights the importance of achieving and maintaining a balance, where while we are accountable to the community, and the interests of the community is the key driving force, it is also possible for the psychologist to benefit. This relational, reciprocal relationship allows us to achieve a win–win orientation, where the community's interests and aims can be achieved (e.g. through supporting, publicizing, and upscaling Project Salaam, and seeking funding for flow-on initiatives), alongside those of the psychologist (e.g. through writing up discipline-defining publications based on the project). An engagement between psychologists and communities where relationships come first, and research agendas comes later allows for such a flexible and mutually beneficial dialogue to occur, where everyone contributes and supports each other.

This stance to relational ethics also means that it does not matter what cultural or faith-based background we identify with. The members of our team who are not Muslims or from a refugee background are more than allies in this research and engagement. Here, we go beyond notions of allyship and reflexive practice. Our engagements with this community are stripped down to basic humanistic values of respect and of working together to achieve a common goal, bringing our diverse backgrounds and skill sets with us. Rather than considering it a weakness, barrier, or leaving it at the door, our diversity is considered a strength, where we value the different worldviews and skillsets that we bring to the table. Our efforts echo that of contemporary approaches to Participatory Action Research, where our engagements are built on a foundation of trust and reciprocity (Cornish et al., 2023). Working with diversity is a necessary reality of working within migrant and forced migrant contexts. More often than not, we find ourselves working alongside peoples from various national/ethnic/faith-based backgrounds.

Relational ethics is also reflective of Islamic perspectives to social solidarity and mutual responsibility in the protection and advancement of community welfare, where we are all seen as brothers and sisters in humanity, regardless of differences in faith or culture (Islamic Relief, 2014). Reciprocity and respect are key values in Islam, and can be linked with the Arabic concepts of *adab* and *akhlaq* (Cassim, Khan-Janif & Martiarini, 2023). *Adab* and *akhlaq* both convey the notion of moral conduct, where *adab* also extends to mean a basic sense of humanity, alongside the notion of hospitality and collectively achieving something good. Both these concepts speak to a Muslim's obligation to be kind, honest, and respectful of others. These values are compatible with contemporary views on human rights. Islam acknowledges that diversity is a reality, and Muslims are encouraged to respect others as a pathway to a safe and peaceful life, and peace of mind (Cassim et al., 2023). Reflecting on core Islamic values of inclusion, some participants of Project Salaam were also Orthodox Christians. Thus, such values constitute an enactment of relational ethics that requires openness and the establishment of dialogue and enduring partnerships with people, that were central to, and informed our engagements within Project Salaam (cf. Hodgetts et al., 2021).

Key Reflective Questions

- What ethical considerations relate to who sets the agenda and designs and leads a community project?
- Why is it important to consider different understandings of human rights in community praxis?
- What are the overlaps and differences between universal and Islamic notions of human rights?

- Given the diversity of your discipline, how does the scope of justice apply in the area you work in?

Acknowledgments

We would like to acknowledge the members of the broader Project Salaam team as key contributors to this work. They are, Shireen Shah Drew, Jamila Slaimankhel, Nazreen Shaban and Mariam Ali.

Further Reading

Bagasra, A. (2021). Socially engaged Islam: Applying social psychological principles to social justice, faith-based activism and altruism in Muslim communities. In N. Pasha-Zaidi (Ed.), *Toward a Positive Psychology of Islam and Muslims* (pp. 29–49). Springer. DOI:10.1007/978-3-030-72606-5_2

Cornish, F., Breton, N., Moreno-Tabarez, U., Delgado, J., Rua, M., de-Graft Aikins, A., & Hodgetts, D. (2023). Participative action research. *Nature Reviews Methods Primers, 3,* Article 34. https://doi.org/10.1038/s43586-023-00214-1

Hodgetts, D., Rua, M., Groot, S., Hopner, V., Drew, N., King, P., & Blake, D. (2021). Relational ethics meets principled practice in community research engagements to understand and address homelessness. *Journal of Community Psychology, 50,* 1980–1992. https://doi.org/10.1002/jcop.22586

Opotow, S. (2012). The scope of justice, intergroup conflict, and peace. In L. Tropp (Ed.), *The Oxford Handbook of Intergroup Conflict* (pp. 72–86). Oxford University Press. https://doi.org/10.1093/oxfordhb/9780199747672.013.0005

References

Bagasra, A. (2021). Socially engaged Islam: Applying social psychological principles to social justice, faith-based activism and altruism in Muslim communities. In N. Pasha-Zaidi. (Ed.), *Toward a positive psychology of Islam and Muslims* (pp. 29–49). Springer. DOI:10.1007/978-3-030-72606-5_2

Beauchamp, T. (2019). The principle of beneficence in applied ethics. In E. N. Zalta (Ed.), *The Stanford Encyclopedia of Philosophy.* https://plato.stanford.edu/archives/spr2019/entries/principle-beneficence/

Cassim, S., Khan-Janif, J., Ali, M., Ali, N., Drew, S. S., Slaimankhel, J., Shaban, N., Hodgetts, D., & Hopner, V. (2023). *Project Salaam: Evaluation Report.* Auckland, New Zealand: Massey University. https://mro.massey.ac.nz/items/40ef9019-d7c6-4928-98cf-bee5eaca59fd

Cassim, S., Khan-Janif, J., & Martiarini, N. (2023). Building enduring relationships for a shared sense of belonging: Culturally derived solidarities between Muslim migrants and Māori. In J. Terruhn & S. Cassim (Ed.), *Transforming the politics of mobility and migration in Aotearoa New Zealand* (pp. 157–172). Anthem Press.

Collins, S. (2001). *Kiwi Muslims under siege. The New Zealand Herald.* https://www.nzherald.co.nz/nz/kiwi-muslims-under-siege/5WR2HNL6LKU3SYPV7AEQLT4T7Q/

Cornish, F., Breton, N. N., Moreno-Tabarez, U., Delgado, J., Rua, M., de-Graft Aikins, A., & Hodgetts, D. (2023). Participative action research. *Nature Reviews Methods Primers, 3*, Article 34. https://doi.org/10.1038/s43586-023-00214-1

Decolonial Psychology Editorial Collective. (2021). General psychology otherwise: A decolonial articulation. *Review of General Psychology, 25*(4), 339–353.

Derickson, K. D., & Routledge, P. (2015). Resourcing scholar-activism: Collaboration, transformation, and the production of knowledge. *The Professional Geographer, 67*, 1–7.

Dewey, J. (1916). *Democracy and education*, The Free Press.

Dewey, J. (1969/1991). *The collected works of John Dewey: The later works* (J. A. Boydston ed.), Southern Illinois University Press.

Education Review Office. (2023). *Education For All Our Children: Embracing Diverse Ethnicities.* https://ero.govt.nz/our-research/education-for-all-our-children-embracing-diverse-ethnicities

Erskine, S. E., & Bilimoria, D. (2019). White allyship of Afro-Diasporic women in the workplace: A transformative strategy for organizational change. *Journal of Leadership & Organizational Studies, 26*, 319–338.

Fine, M., & Asch, A. (1988). Disability beyond stigma: Social interaction, discrimination, and activism. *Journal of Social Issues, 44*(1), 3–21.

Flyvbjerg, B. (2001). *Making social science matter: Why social inquiry fails and how it can succeed again* (S. Sampson, Trans.). Cambridge: Cambridge University Press.

Forber-Pratt, A. J., Mueller, C. O., & Andrews, E. E. (2019). Disability identity and allyship in rehabilitation psychology: Sit, stand, sign, and show up. *Rehabilitation Psychology, 64*, 119–129.

Guimarães, D. S. (2020). *Dialogical multiplication: Principles for an indigenous psychology.* Nature Springer.

Guthrie, R. (2004). *Even the rat was white: A historical view of psychology* (2nd ed.). Pearson.

Hegarty, P. (2017). *A recent history of lesbian and gay psychology: From homophobia to LGBT.* Routledge.

Hodgetts, D., Stolte, O., Sonn, C., Drew, N., Nikora, L. W., & Carr, S. (2020). *Social psychology and everyday life* (2nd ed.). Palgrave Macmillan.

Hodgetts, D., Hopner, V., Carr, S., Bar-Tal, D., Liu, J., Saner, R., Yiu, L., Horgan, J., Searle, R., Massola, G., Hakim, H., Marai, L., King, P., Moghaddam, F. (2023). Human security psychology: A linking construct for an eclectic discipline. *Review of General Psychology, 27*, 177–193.

Hodgetts, D., Rua, M., Groot, S., Hopner, V., Drew, N., King, P., & Blake, D. (2021). Relational ethics meets principled practice in community research engagements to understand and address homelessness. *Journal of Community Psychology, 50*(4), 1980–1992. doi:10.1002/jcop.22586

Islamic Relief (2014). *An Islamic perspective on human development.* https://jliflc.com/wp-content/uploads/2014/07/Human-Development-v3.pdf

Jahoda, M. (1992). Reflections on Marienthal and after. *Journal of Occupational and Organizational Psychology, 65*, 355–358.

Johnson, L. (1991). The trope of the scribe and the question of literary authority in the works of Julian of Norwich and Margery Kempe. *Speculum, 66*(4), 820–838.

Li, W. W., Hung, M. L., & Hodgetts, D. (2021). From a stranger to a 'one-of-us' ally: A new Confucian approach to community allyship. *Qualitative Research in Psychology, 18*(4), 550–570. https://doi.org/10.1080/14780887.2020.1769237

Luukko, M. (2007). The administrative roles of the 'Chief Scribe' and the 'Place Scribe' in the Neo-Assyrian Period. *State Archives of Assyria Bulletin, XVI*, 227–256.

O'Doherty, K., & Hodgetts, D. (2019*). The SAGE handbook of applied social psychology.* SAGE Publications Ltd. https://doi.org/10.4135/9781526417091

Office of Ethnic Communities. (2019). *Conversations with Aotearoa New Zealand's Muslim communities: growing understanding after the Christchurch terror attacks on March 15, 2019.* https://www.ethniccommunities.govt.nz/__data/assets/pdf_file/0019/64711/conversationswithaotearoanewzealandsmuslimcommunities.pdf

Opotow, S. (2012). The scope of justice, intergroup conflict, and peace. In L. Tropp (Ed.), *The Oxford handbook of intergroup conflict* (pp. 72–86). Oxford University Press. https://doi.org/10.1093/oxfordhb/9780199747672.013.0005

Organization of the Islamic Conference. (1990). *Cairo Declaration on Human Rights in Islam.* https://www.refworld.org/docid/3ae6b3822c.html

Peiris-John, R., Kang, K., Bavin, L., Dizon, L., Singh, G., Clark, T., Fleming, T., & Ameratunga, S. (2021). *East Asian, South Asian, Chinese and Indian students in Aotearoa: A Youth19 Report.* Auckland: The University of Auckland. https://static1.squarespace.com/static/5bdbb75ccef37259122e59aa/t/60d3a4202b2d4a2ddd6b7708/1624482883718Youth19+Report+on+South+Asian%2C+East+Asian%2C+Chinese+and+Indian+student.pdf

Pioske, D. (2013). The Scribe of David: A portrait of a life. *Maarav, 20,* 163–188.

Rua, M., Hodgetts, D., Groot, S., Blake, D., Karapu, R., & Neha, E. (2022). A Kaupapa Māori conceptualization and efforts to address the needs of the growing precariat in Aotearoa New Zealand: A situated focus on Māori. *British Journal of Social Psychology, 62*(S1), 39–55. doi:10.1111/bjso.12598

Said, E. (1994). *Representations of the intellectual: The 1993 Reith Lectures.* Vantage.

Vergani, M., Johns, A., Lobo, M., & Monsouri, F., (2015). Examining Islamic religiosity and civic engagement in Melbourne, *Journal of Sociology, 53*(1), 63–78. https://doi.org/10.1177/1440783315621167

Ward, C., Stuart, J., & Adam, Z. M. (2019). A critical narrative review of research about the experiences of being Muslim in New Zealand. *New Zealand Journal of Psychology, 48*(1), 36–746. http://hdl.handle.net/10072/386768

Yogeeswaran, K. M., Afzali, U., Andrews, N. P., Chivers, E. A., Wang, M., Devos, T., & Sibley, C. G. (2019). Exploring New Zealand National Identity and its importance for attitudes toward Muslims and support for diversity. *New Zealand Journal of Psychology, 48*(1), 29–35.

22

Rights-based Leadership and Governance in Health and Social Care Services[*]

Malcolm MacLachlan, Cathal Morgan, Patrick Bracken, Anastasia Campbell, Finbarr Colfer, Priscille Geiser, Caoimhe Gleeson, Chapal Khasnabis, Hasheem Mannan, Satish Mishra, Rosalyn Tamming, and Michael Walsh

Background and context

The rights of persons with disabilities are protected and promoted by the 2006 United Nations Convention on the Rights of Persons with Disabilities (CRPD), the most widely ratified human rights treaty by Member States to the United Nations. It follows decades of work to change attitudes and practices relating to persons with disabilities. The convention asserts the need for seismic change away from viewing persons with disabilities as 'objects of charity, medical treatment and social protection, towards viewing persons with disabilities as subjects with rights, who are capable of claiming those rights and making decisions for their lives based on their free and informed consent as well as being active members of society' (CRPD, 2006). Rights-based changes are required at programmatic, organizational, system, and policy levels in order to ensure that policies, programmes, and services uphold the human rights of all persons with disabilities and are developed in close consultation with organizations of persons with disabilities (CRPD Article 4). The health sector bears a unique responsibility in this regard and especially services for persons with disabilities, mental health conditions, or difficulties associated with ageing. It should also be noted that according to the CRPD all mental health conditions also fall under its remit.

Persons with disabilities have greater healthcare requirements, on average, compared to the broader population (WHO & World Bank, World Disability Report, 2011). Whilst they require access to the same range of general health services as the rest of the population (such as vaccinations and sexual and reproductive health

[*] The first and second authors of this chapter were co-chairs of the Ireland/WHO Working Group, the report of which, parts of this chapter are based on; most of the other authors were also members of this group and they are listed in alphabetical order following the co-chairs.

services), persons with disabilities may need access to specialist services and goods related to their disability (such as specific types of surgery or assistive products). And despite their greater health requirements, persons with disabilities face barriers in accessing healthcare and, consequently, they have less access than others. These barriers include financial barriers; physical barriers related to infrastructure, equipment, and transportation not being accessible; communication barriers, such as health information not being provided in accessible formats; and attitudinal barriers, including discrimination and lack of knowledge on disability issues amongst health workers (OHCHR, 2023).

The WHO Global Report on Health Equity for Persons with Disabilities (WHO, 2022a) demonstrates that while some progress has been made in recent years, we are still far from realizing this right for many persons with disabilities who continue to die earlier, have poorer health, and experience more limitations in everyday functioning than others. These poor health outcomes, it is argued, are due to unfair conditions faced by persons with disabilities in all facets of life, including in the health system itself. The report sheds light on the critical role of health leadership and governance and entails ten targeted actions, which include prioritizing health equity for persons with disabilities; establishing a human rights-based approach to health; assuming a stewardship role for disability inclusion in the health sector; and integrating disability inclusion in the accountability mechanisms of the health sector. Reforming leadership and governance is therefore an essential part of transforming the health and social care sectors and ensuring accountability so that all persons with disabilities can enjoy their right to the highest attainable standards of health.

This chapter is based on a background paper which contributed to the World Health Organization's 'European framework for action to achieve the highest attainable standard of health for persons with disabilities 2022–2030' (WHO, 2022b). The framework aspires to persons with disabilities, through their representative organizations, being fully included and considered in all health planning, delivery, and leadership across the WHO European Region. In this context, Ireland as a Member State agreed to lead on the development of the rights-based leadership and governance component of the framework. This chapter is one of the outputs of the working group established to undertake that task. Within the World Health Organization's building blocks for health systems strengthening, the functions of governance and leadership are charged with ensuring that 'strategic policy frameworks exist and are combined with effective oversight, coalition-building, regulation, attention to system-design, and accountability' (WHO, 2007).

Nothing About Us Without Us

Dainius Pūras, former UN Special Rapporteur on the right of everyone to the enjoyment of the highest attainable standard of physical and mental health, has stated: 'Obstacles for implementation of the rights of persons with disabilities are no longer in bodies or physical or mental health conditions of individuals. Obstacles, which need to be removed, are now in the *physical, social, or other environment, or they may be in attitudes of those who make decisions'* (Pūras, 2022).

The fundamental idea behind the CRPD is equality; access to rights for persons with disabilities on an equal basis to persons without disabilities (Quinn, 2010). Whilst the CRPD articles are interlocking, some are especially relevant to the health service context: Article 5 on Equality and non-discrimination, Article 9 on Accessibility, Article 17 on Protecting the integrity of the person, Article 19 on Living Independently and being included in the community, and Articles 24–26 on Education, Health, and Habilitation and rehabilitation, and Article 28 on Adequate standard of living and social protection. A discussion of each of these is beyond our scope here, but it is important within the ethos of the 'Nothing About Us Without Us' motto of the disability movement, to consider Article 12 Equal recognition before the law, as this relates directly to ideas of leadership and governance in terms of the inclusion of people with disability in decision-making.

Article 12 recognizes that 'persons with disabilities have the right to recognition everywhere as persons before the law', that State parties must 'recognize that persons with disabilities enjoy legal capacity on an equal basis with others in all aspects of life', and that they shall 'take appropriate measures to provide access by persons with disabilities to the support they may require in exercising their legal capacity'. Furthermore, 'measures relating to the exercise of legal capacity respect the rights, will and preferences of the person'.

It is clear from the CRPD that persons with disabilities have the right to be involved in all decisions regarding their health, welfare, and disability services and support. This includes having a voice through shared leadership and governance of services that they use. Article 4.3 requires service providers to 'closely consult with and actively involve persons with disabilities, including children with disabilities, through their representative organizations' regarding the development and implementation of legislation and policies, and Article 33 emphasizes the importance of people with disabilities being actively involved in such monitoring. Thus if people with disabilities are to be involved in the development, implementation, and monitoring of national-level policies, we should also expect this ethos to prevail in the design and leadership of services that directly affect them.

Leadership

Hughes (2009) stated that 'Leadership has a range of definitions, but at its simplest it is concerned with the ability to influence others to achieve goals.' While individuals can be leaders, so too can groups of individuals be leaders. A significant body of research produced by the Centre for Creative Leadership and the King's Fund, demonstrates that, 'where leaders and leadership relationships are well developed, organisations benefit from *direction, alignment* and *commitment*' (see Eckert et al., 2014, p. 2). And they emphasize that 'A collective leadership culture requires new mind-sets, not just new skills' (p. 1). In the context of disability, this requires a significant shift to prevent negative assumptions about persons with disabilities' capacity to contribute.

A collective approach to leadership has been found to promote more effective team working, to enhance the quality of care/service, to improve patient/service user safety, and also to improve staff and service user satisfaction (De Brún & McAuliffe, 2020; De Brún et al., 2019,). Collective leadership is part of the shift away from seeing leaders in terms of individual's attributes, to seeing leadership as being a shared process between a group or team members (Battilana & Casciaro, 2021; Nelson & Daniels, 2012).

The cooperative approach to leadership recognizes and draws on differences in knowledge, experience, and practice according to what will best benefit the service user. This is increasingly common in co-design approaches to health and social services for people with disability; incorporating direct service users themselves (Tucker et al., 2022), family carers (Rathnayake et al., 2021), and requiring new ways of working for staff (Harrison et al., 2021). The idea of service users co-leading the design of their own assistive technologies is also a core principle of the maker-movement (Holloway, 2019).

Part of a cooperative approach therefore also requires a much more inclusive approach to leadership. Randel et al. (2018) describes 'inclusive leadership as a set of leader behaviours that are focused on facilitating group members feeling part of the group (belongingness) and retaining their sense of individuality (uniqueness) while contributing to group processes and outcomes' (p. 191). They also propose that those with stronger pro-diversity beliefs, with a greater sense of humility, and who accept higher levels of cognitive complexity (recognizing and working with contradictions within individuals and groups) will be better inclusive leaders. Inclusive leadership requires being 'able to create environments in which differences are valued and can be incorporated into the main work of an organization to enhance strategies, processes and overall effectiveness' (Chrobot-Mason & Roberson, 2021, p. 32).

Governance

Brennan and Flynn (2013) reviewed 29 extant definitions of clinical governance and found that these incorporated a mixture of activities relating to governance, management, and practice, which they argued, was confusing for those expected to execute such roles. Brennan and Flynn distinguished between three functions that are often conflated within governance in health settings—clinical governance, clinical management, and clinical practice. Lim and Lin (2021) argue that 'governance refers not only to the *processes* through which responsibilities are distributed amongst different actors, but also the *relationships and connections* within a complex web of interlinked stakeholders wishing to influence the processes of governance' (p. 6, italics in the original). Lim and Lin also highlight the importance of 'Stewardship against vested interests through institutional and regulatory reform where necessary' (p. 6).

Disability and Health

Many people with a disability do also have an associated health problem, for instance, a wheelchair user may develop pressure sores, or a person with cerebral palsy may have painful contractures; in such situation's health interventions can be lifesaving and pain relieving. For some persons with disabilities healthcare has a very important function (Shakespeare, 2013). However, it is not the case that everybody with a disability necessarily also has a disease, a disorder, or a deficit of some type, and so it is not appropriate, or rights-based, to construct disability as though it is a health problem (MacLachlan, 2022; MacLachlan & Mannan, 2013), This makes the effective integration of health services and disability services both complex and of paramount importance. As the Missing Billion report (Kuper & Heydt, 2019) highlights 'People with disabilities face higher healthcare needs, more barriers to accessing services, and less health coverage, resulting in worse health outcomes ...' and a corresponding need to 'Ensure that all health services, programming, and trainings consider the needs of people with disabilities' (p. 2).

There is no single profession for whom their skills are required for all people with disability, and for most people with disability they require one, or several, but very rarely all the professions that work in the disability sector. So how should we organize health and social care practitioners—where no single profession is always essential, but several different professions may be beneficial for some individuals, at least sometimes? Traditionally the approach to disability services has been to organize on the basis that the person with a disability is diseased, disordered, or in deficit; and therefore a so-called 'medical model' of service delivery has been used. Giving one profession authority, privilege, and power has created many of the problems associated with the medical model—such as institutionalization and the over-prescription of medication (WHO, 2021). However, 'While abandoning the medical model of disability does not mean rejecting the practice of medicine, medicine cannot be the gatekeeper for people with disabilities' rights' (UNICEF, 2021). In other words, the discipline of medicine should not be determining the right of persons with disabilities; this requires a much broader range of considerations, such as the social and rights models of disability.

Making Teams Work Optimally

While many people with less complex disabilities may be effectively supported by single professions working in a primary care context, those with more complex disabilities will often benefit from availing of a team comprised of different professions. In a multi-disciplinary team, practitioners often work independently, in parallel, with a service user, and team members come together to discuss their experiences. In an interdisciplinary team, practitioners work together—recognizing that there are often overlaps and intersections between their disciplines and that these should constitute part of integrated services and supports. In both cases, the service users should also be centrally involved in discussions about them—'nothing about us without us'.

If team-based interventions are an important mechanism for providing services and supports, then such teams must work as effectively and efficiently as possible. In essence this requires us to consider—independent of specific services or supports— what is the best way for teams to operate? If teams are the central mechanism to deliver services and supports, then teams that do not work well jeopardize both the benefit to an individual service user and represent an inefficient and wasteful use of resources for service providers.

Wei's (2022) synthesis of the results of 36 systematic reviews of interprofessional collaboration found that successful collaborative teamwork arises through a process of first, personal relationship building between individual workers, next working together and then identifying how to actively collaborate through their work. Wei (2022) emphasizes that effective collaborations benefits all stakeholders—service users ('patients'), service providers ('professionals'), and provider organizations—all benefit, each in turn.

Zajac et al.'s (2021) review of the literature noted the benefits of teamwork in relation to a greater diversity of views and expertise, but that 'there are a number of challenges inherent to healthcare that can also hinder performance, including psychological barriers (e.g. professional silos, hierarchies, power differentials) and organizational barriers (e.g. distributed teams, hybrid working models)' (p. 2). According to Weller et al. (2014) 'Recent evidence suggests that improvement in teamwork in healthcare can lead to significant gains in patient safety, measured against efficiency of care, complication rate and mortality', and furthermore they hoped that improvements in teamwork in 'healthcare may be the next major advance in patient outcomes' (p. 149).

Power Asymmetries

Team members are more likely to speak up, voice contrary views, and question orthodoxies in teams where there is a greater sense of psychological safety (O'Donovan & McAuliffe, 2020). Psychological safety is about feeling secure in taking interpersonal risks in, for instance, in a workplace; such safety enhances willingness to contribute ideas and share concerns; it entails feeling comfortable to exchange information and knowledge (Edmondson & Lei, 2014). This contrasts with Fink-Samnick's (2016) concerns: 'The hierarchal culture often allowed to fester in health care organizations continues to be rampant—one fuelling a passive atmosphere that enables bullying, as opposed to one empowering the needed change to combat it' (p 114).

Kearns et al. (2021) systematic evidence review of the impact of power dynamics and hierarchies in healthcare teams incorporated 20 papers relating to power dynamics and team effectiveness and 19 papers concerned power dynamics and service user/patient safety. They concluded that power dynamics inhibits team communication, and in turn this inhibits team members from questioning senior colleagues, impacting the overall effectiveness of the team and service-user/patient safety. Some of the barriers to speaking up Kearns et al. identified included deference to seniors, feelings of intimidation and powerlessness, concerns about reprisals and more general repercussions of speaking up. They also noted perceived poor self-efficacy, a lack of self-confidence, and poor role clarity as deterring some team members from speaking up. Similarly Schmutz et al. (2019) review found that overall—regardless of professional composition, team familiarity, average team size, task type, and type of performance measure—teamwork has a significant effect on performance.

Following the response to Covid-19, the Irish National Clinical Programmes held an event to reflect on learning from the experience of responding to Covid-19 and how that might contribute to a more resilient health service. Philip Crowley, the National Director of Strategy and Research, argued that 'the flattening of the hierarchy promoted better decision making' and that it was important to hold on to this 'more democratic approach' to create a more resilient system. Stephen Mulvany, Acting CEO, also stressed the importance of 'distributed leadership' for resilience.

In line with CRPD Article 4.3, a more democratic approach to health governance requires active consultation with organizations of persons with disabilities, who have a unique role to act as intermediaries and representatives of the diversity of persons with disabilities. Unlike individuals with disabilities consulted as services users, these organizations have a unique mandate to consult and aggregate the collective voice and priorities of their constituencies. Meaningfully engaging organizations of persons with disabilities and building their capacity to provide meaningful contributions is an investment in restoring agency to groups that have been historically discriminated against and necessary to address the power dynamics that are historically weighted heavily towards health professionals.

Dainius Pūras, a psychiatrist and former UN Special Rapporteur for health, states that 'National policies and guidance represent the important principles of the CRPD quite well whereby they guide the design and provision of health and health-related services for persons with disabilities. *However, when implementation starts, often these principles are not properly observed, and most often this happens because of power asymmetries (imbalances) and dominance of the biomedical model.* This is why it is of utmost importance to highlight the existing tensions when the tradition of decision-making (driven by hierarchies) interacts with principles of the CRPD, and to continue to search for creative solutions, with the strong involvement of experts by lived experience' (Pūras, 2022).

Case Study

This case study is based on an actual case with some identifying elements changed. Peter had a history of admission to mental health institutions since being a teenager, when he became depressed and withdrawn following an abusive family situation which lasted for several years prior to admission. He frequently displayed what staff considered to be challenging behaviour and his case notes suggest that the staff did not have the knowledge to manage this behaviour. He was prescribed neuroleptic (anti-psychotic) medication, even though he did not display psychotic behaviour, in the hope of supressing his challenging behaviour. His early case notes suggest that he probably found the response to his problems to be trauma-inducing in itself, thus compounding his earlier trauma.

In his early 20s, Peter continued on a combination of various anti-depressant/anxiety and anti-psychotic medication despite stating a number of times that he would prefer to try living without medication. Unfortunately after increasing doses of medication Peter developed neuroleptic malignant syndrome (NMS)—a severe negative response to his medication—with short term fever, muscle rigidity, and confusion. However, longer-term Peter's behaviour also changed and he was referred to a clinical neuropsychologist who attributed this to frontal lobe syndrome (brain damage), which in Peter's case was associated with a significant reduction in cognitive functioning and with the onset of frequent sexual disinhibition.

Peter was placed in a campus facility where adults with intellectual disability lived in group homes, located beside each other, but where they could visit each other during the daytime. Over a couple of decades Peter lived there and enacted sexual disinhibition in a number of ways, with residents and staff, and people became concerned for each other and their own privacy and safety at times. Following increasing difficulties, the clinical lead for national disability services (Dave) visited the campus facility.

Dave found that 33 out of 35 residents were on some form of psychotropic medication, with the majority being on medication for over a decade. Dave met with a number of staff members and residents. He met with Mary, a care assistant, who was the staff member that spent most time with Peter. To her knowledge Peter had continuously been on medication for the 15 years she had worked at the centre. Mary was asked what was the name of the person who had prescribed Peter's medication:

Mary: 'Well Dr Murphy of course, she is the only psychiatrist who visits us here and she has worked here for as long as I have been here.'
Dave: 'What is Dr Murphy's name?'
Mary: 'What do you mean – its Dr Murphy!', smiles.
Dave: 'Sorry, I mean what is her first name?'
Mary 'Oh, I've no idea, I've never been told, we all just call her Dr Murphy.'
Dave: 'If you thought that Peter was maybe having a problem with his medication, what would you say to Pamela—by the way, that's Dr Murphy's first name.'
Mary: 'God, I don't know; like it wouldn't be for me to say, like anything, sure she's the doctor.'
Dave: 'True, but are you not the person who spends most time with Peter and who most likely knows him best?'
Mary: 'Well yes, but Dr Murphy doesn't really ask me much about him.'

Dave: 'Do you feel you need to be asked, or could you just offer your opinion?'
Mary: 'Oh Christ, no, I mean, like, I wouldn't.'
Dave: 'Well I think we should try and support Pamela by finding ways to let her know when things are going well and when they are not, after all she visits the campus for, what around an hour, every two weeks? So, it's hard for her to know what is going on, isn't it?'
Mary: 'Yes, but she's the doctor.'
Dave: 'Mmmm. Is there anyone else who works as part of the team here who you also call doctor?'
Mary: 'No, everyone is on first-name terms.'
Dave: 'Do you know that Sonya (a speech and language therapist), also has the Dr title—she has a PhD?'
Mary: [Putting her hand over here mouth] 'Oh my God – I'm so sorry, I didn't know! I'll call her doctor too!'
Dave: Laughing. 'No, no, no need, personally I think it's much better just to use everyone's first name. Then it easier to talk to people—staff and residents— in a normal way, what do you think?'
Mary: 'Oh God, I don't know, I need this job'.
Dave: 'Of course, and what about Peter, how does he let people know if he is OK with his medication or with other aspects of his life here?'
Mary: 'Well, when he doesn't like things, he can be very challenging indeed . . . '

Reflection

While this case study is based on real events some aspects have been changed. Peter has a history of receiving services, initially for a mental health condition and then for an acquired disability, in institutional (including campus) settings which are not accepted under the CRPD as they do not allow individuals to live lives in the community. Peter also appears to have had little decision-making power in these settings, having not had his wish to 'try living without medication' accepted. From a service provider perspective it is clear that Mary—the person who spends most time with Peter (the resident)—does not feel that she can or should contribute her ideas. This may partly be because other practitioners do not implicitly or explicitly give her permission to do so, and interact with her as someone who has an equal right to express her views. But it may also be because she is working in a system where she perceives a clear hierarchy, where some people are 'titled' and entitled to dominate and make decisions, whilst others are less entitled to contribute to or make decisions. It is possible that discussions about medication when Peter was in mental health services were similarly off-bounds for others to comment on. If so, then Peter's response to neuroleptics may have been avoided. It is also likely that the prescribing psychiatrist did not have many alternatives to medication, for instance, that other types of health and social care practitioners were not available to work with Peter. This illustrates the importance—especially when teams are understaffed—of ensuring all relevant views are heard, that people participate in decision-making, and they feel secure to do this as a legitimate part of their job. Peter's experience of family abuse may also have been confounded by his subsequent experience of mental health and disability services, which he may have found to be continually traumatizing. If this is the case then it is tragic that the services that sought to ameliorate Peter's original problems actually reproduced them in another form.

Ways Forward

The WHO Task Group which has contributed to the World Health Organization's 'European framework for action to achieve the highest attainable standard of health for persons with disabilities 2022–2030' made recommendations which have been expressed as a series of questions that countries can use to establish the extent to which their health systems are promoting a rights-based approach to leadership and governance. These are provided in Appendix 22.1. Review these questions and consider how the service Peter received would likely score. If you work in—or have worked in—some sort of service environment, how would the teams you have worked in score on these criteria?

At the level of small clinical teams, issues of participation, empowerment, and improved decision-making (for service providers and service users) can best be strengthened by a national structure which reflects some of the values of participation, mutual respect, co-decision-making, and non-hierarchical team working (see Appendix 22.1). If the governance structure for a national clinical programme reflects the dominance of a single profession, then it is also likely that such dominance, disempowerment, and sub-optimal decision-making will play out at the local team level. Thus national structures should reflect the ethos which we want to see practiced locally; and if they don't then we must ask and address why this is.

A key feature of the governance of the National Clinical Programme for People with Disability (NCPPD) in Ireland is through a Disability Advisory Committee (DAC), which has been structured to be inclusive of service users, different types of service providers, and a broad range of involved professions, as well as various aspects of the government provided national service. The Disability Advisory Group (DAG) also has lived experience representatives and is chaired by a person with lived experience of disability.

Figure 22.1 illustrates stakeholder involvement in the DAG. The approach to governance illustrated in Figure 22.1 (see https://www.hse.ie/eng/about/who/cspd/ncps/disability/ for more details) aligns with WHO's work on Effective Health System Governance for Universal Health Coverage (UHC) (see: https://www.who.int/health-topics/universal-health-coverage/health-systems-governance). While this is only one example and other participative structures will be appropriate in different

Appendix 22.1 Rights elements, problem statements and possible solution principles which could contribute to development of a tool for assessing rights-based leadership and governance

#	Rights Element	Problem statement	Solution principle (Possible questions for country assessment tools)
		Engagement in services for persons with disability	
1.	**Accessible information**—are persons with disability provided with information about services in a variety of accessible format?	Information that can be assimilated is the gateway to accessing services, but it may not be provided in a way that persons with hearing, vision, intellectual, or other difficulties may be able to understand.	Is information provided in a variety of formats accessible to the range of difficulties which service users experience? When, where, and by whom? What formats are available? Does your organization provide a list for checking these off?
2.	**Responsiveness**— where services are failing the health needs of persons with disability, what is being done about them?	Service provision occurs in a competitive context, with other demands on resources. Unless data is collected regarding unmet needs, how are these are being communicated, and how can people better physically access services, such unmet needs will not be addressed.	Are the unmet needs of persons with disability recorded? Are people given an explanation if a service cannot be provided to them? Are travel routes and expenses to health facilities identified and facilitated as part of the health service provision?
3.	**Consultation**— are persons with disability involved in all formal discussions concerning the services and supports they personally receive?	Services for persons with disability may be delivered in a paternalistic or charity manner, or where experts or powerful others assume that they know what is best for the person with disability.	Are service users (or their nominated representatives) engaged to participate in all meetings concerning their services? Are they provided with choices aligned to their will and preference, with reasonable accommodations, access, and other commitments taken into account in scheduling discussions?
4.	**Person centred**—are services and supports person-centred, relevant to the context the person lives in, is the person involved in planning them, are services co-produced by the person and actually of service to them?	Service provision may be service-centric where people are expected to fit in with the priorities of service programmes, or of professions.	Is the determination of a person's services based on their own strengths and support needs, their context, their preferences and direction, where provision is then configured around these and fulfils obligations under the UNCRPD (especially re Article 19—Living independently and being included in the community)?

(continued)

Appendix 22.1 Continued

5.	**Decision-making—** some persons with disability are denied representation of their views and opportunities to indicate their decisions.	In many contexts decisions have been made by others— such as courts, parents, or institutional authorities—rather than by persons with disabilities themselves; resulting in disempowerment, infantilizing, and undermining of the right to self-determination.	Is there enacted legislation and established protocols on Supported Decision-Making which staff have been trained in and use; including the option for independent third parties to support decision-making, and is this available on a daily basis, if required? Are involuntary treatment and institutionalization clearly prohibited?
6.	**Needs identification—**Is the provision of services and supports based on identified need and adequately resourced?	The allocation of scarce resources may be determined by the strength of advocacy groups, political pressures, or professional interests, rather than on the basis of greatest need.	Are resources allocated throughout the disability system in a manner that supports the identification of greatest need, including consultations with organizations representing the diversity of persons with disabilities and other disadvantaged groups?
7.	**Procurement—**Are decisions about types of services and products to be procured made with input from people disability representative organizations?	Products and services may be procured at local or national levels without input from those who will use the services.	Are the views of the diversity of persons with disability represented in decision about the procurement of services, supports, or products? Are accessibility standards and universal design mandatory requirements in health procurements?

Effectiveness of service teams for persons disability

8.	**Competency-based leadership—**where people are in leadership positions due to their abilities and established skills, rather than due to their profession or position.	Where formal leaders are appointed to teams these appointments are sometime based on a person's professional training, rather than their competency to complete the necessary leadership tasks.	Where formal leaders are appointed is this based on a match between identified necessary leadership skill sets and competency, irrespective of disciplinary background?
9.	**Effective co-operation** within teams.	Teams are sometimes hierarchically based, with some people being referred to by titles and others by their first name; some people may also seek to dominate discussions, including regularly chairing discussions.	Are all members in a team referred to similarly (either all using first names or all using titles; Ms, Mr, Dr, Prof), is the team chairperson rotated between those who wish to take the role, is there a culture of co-decision-making and is the person with a disability considered to be part of their own team and having the final responsibility?

Appendix 22.1 Continued

10.	**Services provided by persons with disabilities**	There is an underrepresentation of persons with disability in service provision and leadership positions in services. This lack of diversity reflects both barriers to these positions and lost opportunities for improved decision-making in teams. The provision of disability services may benefit especially from people who have lived experience of disability.	What proportion of the workforce are persons with disabilities and are they employed to the same extent across different roles?
11.	**Dominance**—the role of professional bodies, privilege, and power dynamics; and structures.	Some professional bodies have more influence or power than others, and this may deter them from engaging in compromise for the collective good; they may seek to exercise disciplinary capture or dominance.	Are there fora in which all professional bodies involved in services meet with parity of esteem and engage in collective problem solving?
12.	**Governance**—are effective and fair governance arrangements in place?	Governance arrangement may not be clearly demarcated, and/or they may give disproportionate power to some professions or practitioners and fail to include the full network of stakeholders.	Are governance responsibilities clearly identified, and do they include input from all stakeholders, including persons with a disability? Are conditions ensured to guarantee the meaningful participation of OPDs* in decision-making (including capacity building of OPDs, accessible and inclusive governance processes)?
13.	**Diversity**—is representation in governance appropriately diverse and is this the case on decision-making committees?	In hospitals, in general community services, and in disability services there may be some degree of participation or persons with disability, but not always at the levels where decisions are made. There may also be barriers to representative OPDs influencing governance processes.	Is there diversity of persons with disabilities and other marginalized groups on the governing boards and sub-committees of hospitals, general community services and disability service organizations?

(continued)

Appendix 22.1 Continued

Rights of service providers for persons with disability

14.	**Worker training—** are workers trained in a rights-based approach to services?	Workers who are unaware of the rationale, elements of, or examples of good practices in a rights-based approach to services are unlikely to be able to identify situations where rights are lacking, or to implement a truly right-based approach themselves.	What proportion of the workforce has undertaken formal training in a rights-based approach, and at what levels of seniority? What spaces and structures are in place to ensure that they can learn from OPDs and partners to recommend rights-based transformation of services?
15.	**Worker security—** do workers have security of employment?	Some workers in disability and health services are on precarious contracts where they have unreliable hours of employment, short-term contracts and low levels of pay. This may result in even well-motivated workers feeling they must seek employment in other sectors.	What proportion of the workforce is in secure employment? Workers should have contracts that offer the opportunity to be confident of ongoing employment, and at levels of pay that reflect the demands of their jobs and the needs of their clients to have a dependable and skilled workforce.
16.	**Worker advocacy**	Sometimes workers experience moral injury through having to be part of something they fundamentally disagree with; this may result in dissatisfaction, distress, and disengagement from service colleagues and service users.	Do workers have a secure mechanism to voice concerns about leadership, teamwork, or governance; without fear of victimization and retribution, and do they feel heard so that they can advocate for the rights of persons with disability?
17.	**Worker career and skills development**	People working with few skills development or promotion opportunities, may feel less committed to their roles and career, and seek other work, resulting in high workforce turnover, which diminishes the opportunity for quality services.	Do workers, including workers with disabilities, have career pathways and skills development opportunities and does this apply to all levels of work?

* OPD: Organizations for persons with disabilities.

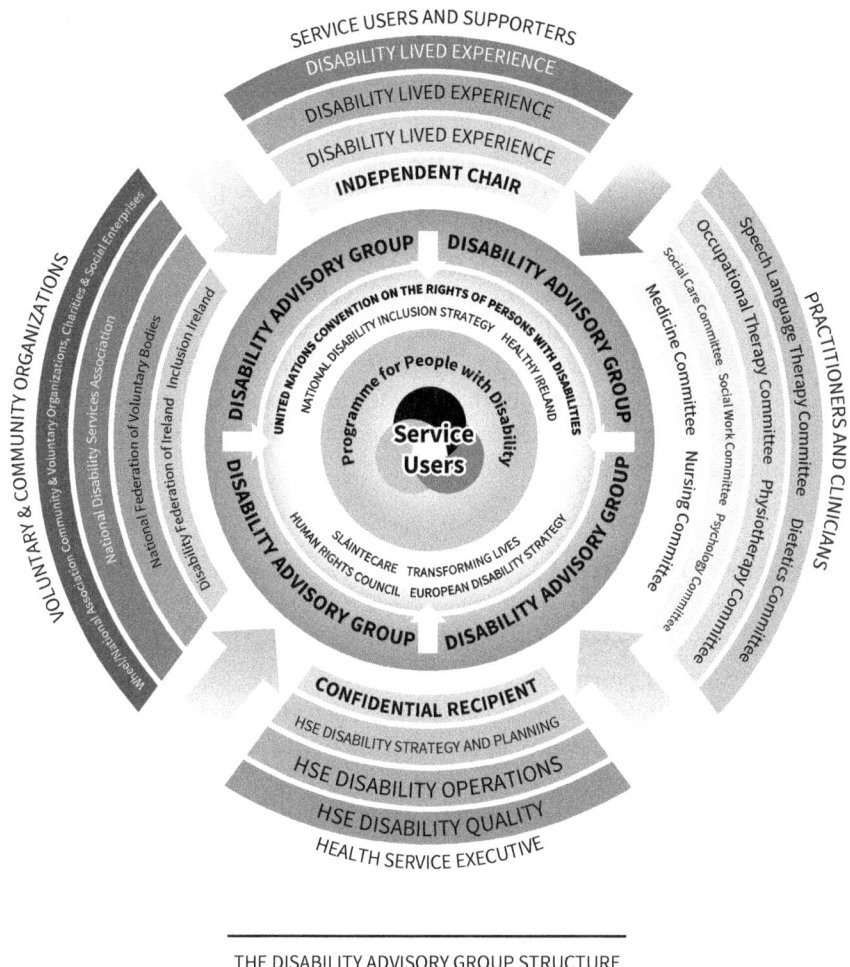

THE DISABILITY ADVISORY GROUP STRUCTURE
with relevant groups of stakeholders and polices informing the
work of the National Clinical Programme for People with
Disability (NCPPD).

Figure 22.1 Representation of stakeholders and guiding national and international policy documents for the Disability Advisory Group of the National Clinical Programme for People with Disability (in Ireland). (see also MacLachlan, 2022).

contexts, it does highlight the symbolic significance of the service user/'patient' being central—allowing service providers to recognize and promote the importance of person-centeredness.

Conclusion

The WHO European Framework for action to achieve the highest attainable standard of health for persons with disabilities 2022–2030 made four recommendations: (1) persons with disabilities must have accessible information about and access to the services they need; (2) persons with disabilities must be central to decisions about the services they receive and involved in the leadership, governance and evaluation of health services; (3) persons with disabilities have the right to have their health services provided through the most effective mechanisms of service delivery, including access to different disciplines working collaboratively through the most effective means of teamworking; and (4) people providing services within health and social care settings also have a right to work in safe working environments, where they feel valued, have secure employment, and feel empowered to question each other and to advocate for the rights of service users. These recommendations contribute to enacting the recommendations of the WHO Global report on health equity for persons with disabilities (2022a), the WHO Health Systems framework (2007), and to realizing a number of articles in the United Nations CRPD.

Reflective Questions

1. Are you aware of power hierarchies in your workplace? If so, how might they affect the services provided?
2. What do you think are the effects of some staff being referred to by a title while others are not—on the services users and the service providers?
3. From the different questions in Appendix 22.1, in practice, which three do you think would be the easiest to address and which three would be the most difficult to address?
4. Which questions in Appendix 22.1 do you feel would be problematic for Peter's case study presented above?
5. Moral stress or injury may occur where a person takes part in or witnesses things that go against their own values or moral beliefs. Do you feel that you have been subject to moral stress or injury in any of your work settings?
6. Have you ever been part of providing a service to others which you feel may have been traumatizing for them? If yes, then how might you do things differently in future?

Further Reading

Battilana, J., & Casciaro, T. (2021). *Power, for all: How it really works and why it's everyone's business*. Simon and Schuster.
World Health Organization & United Nations Human Rights Office of the High Commissioner. (2023). *Mental health, human rights and legislation: guidance and practice*.
MacLachlan, M., Morgan, C., Bracken, P., Campbell, A., Colfer, F., Geiser, P., Gleeson, C., Khasnabis, C., Mannan, H., Mishra, S., Naughton, C., Tamming, R. E., Shakespeare, T.,

& Walsh, M. (2024). *Towards a Rights-based Approach to Strengthening Leadership and Governance in Health Services.* Maynooth University: ALL Institute.

References

Battilana, J., & Casciaro, T. (2021). *Power, for all: How it really works and why it's everyone's business.* Simon and Schuster.

Brennan, N. M., & Flynn, M. A. (2013). Differentiating clinical governance, clinical management, and clinical practice. *Clinical Governance, 18*(2), 114–131. https://doi.org/10.1108/14777271311317909

Chrobot-Mason, D., & Roberson, Q. (2021). Inclusive leadership. In P. G. Northouse (Ed.), *Leadership: Theory and practice* (9th ed., p. 32) Sage Publications.

De Brún, A., & McAuliffe, E. (2020). Identifying the context, mechanisms and outcomes underlying collective leadership in teams: building a realist programme theory. *BMC Health Services Research, 20*, Article 261. https://doi.org/10.1186/s12913-020-05129-1

De Brún, A., O'Donovan, R., & McAuliffe, E. (2019). Interventions to develop collectivistic leadership in healthcare settings: a systematic review. *BMC Health Service Research, 19*, Article 72. https://doi.org/10.1186/s12913-019-3883-x

Eckert, R., West, M., Altman, D., Steward, K., & Pasmore, W. A. (2014). *Delivering a collective leadership strategy for health care.* King's Fund.

Edmondson, A. C., & Lei, Z. (2014). Psychological safety: The history, renaissance, and future of an interpersonal construct. *Annual Review of Organizational Psychology and Organizational Behavior, 1*(1), 23–43.

Fink-Samnick, E. (2016). The new age of bullying and violence in health care: Part 2: Advancing professional education, practice culture, and advocacy. *Professional Case Management, 21*(3), 114–26. doi: 10.1097/NCM.0000000000000146

Harrison, R., Chin, M., & She, E. N. (2021). What does co-design mean for Australia's diverse clinical workforce? *Australian Health Review, 46*(1), 60–61.

Holloway, C. (2019). Disability interaction (dix) a manifesto. *Interactions, 26*(2), 44–49.

Hughes, R. (2009). Editorial: Time for leadership development interventions in the public health nutrition workforce. *Public Health Nutrition, 12*(8), 1029–1029. doi:10.1017/S1368980009990395

Kearns, E., Khurshid, Z., Anjara, S., De Brún, A., Rowan, R., & McAuliffe, E. (2021). P92 Power dynamics in healthcare teams – a barrier to team effectiveness and patient safety: A systematic review. *BJS Open, 5*(1), 92. doi: 10.1093/bjsopen/zrab032.091

Kuper, H., & Heydt, P. (2019). *The missing billion: Access to health service for 1 billion people with disabilities.* London School of Hygiene and Tropical Medicine.

Lim, M. Y. H., & Lin V. (2021). Governance in health workforce: how do we improve on the concept? A network-based, stakeholder-driven approach. *Human Resources for Health, 19*(1), 1. doi: 10.1186/s12960-020-00545-0

MacLachlan, M. (2022). Structure, power and practice: Designing a new rights-based national clinical programme for people with disability in Ireland. *Clinical Psychology Forum, 353*, 43–48.

MacLachlan, M., & Mannan, H. (2013). Is disability a health problem? *Social Inclusion, 1*(2), 139–141.

Nielsen, K., & Daniels, K., (2012). Does shared and differentiated transformational leadership predict followers' working conditions and well-being? *Leadership. Quarterly, 23*(3), 383–397. https://doi.org/10.1016/j.leaqua.2011.09.001

O'Donovan, R., & McAuliffe, E. (2020). A systematic review of factors that enable psychological safety in healthcare teams. *International Journal for Quality in Health Care, 32*(4), 240–250. https://doi.org/10.1093/intqhc/mzaa025

Office of the High Commissioner for Human Rights. (2023). *CRPD Article 25: Illustrative indicators on health.* Geneva: OHCHR. https://www.ohchr.org/sites/default/files/article-25-indicators-en.pdf

Pūras, D. (2022). Personal Communication: commenting on an earlier draft of this paper.

Quinn, G. (2010). The UN Convention on the Rights of Persons with Disabilities—Implications for persons with Intellectual Disabilities. *Jo Mills Memorial Lecture, 10th World Down Syndrome Congress.*

Randel, A. E., Galvin, B. M., Shore, L. M., Ehrhart, K. H., Chung, B. G., Dean, M. A., & Kedharnath, U. (2018). Inclusive leadership: Realizing positive outcomes through belongingness and being valued for uniqueness. *Human Resource Management Review, 28*(2), 190–203.

Rathnayake, S., Moyle, W., Jones, C., & Calleja, P. (2021). Co-design of an mHealth application for family caregivers of people with dementia to address functional disability care needs. *Informatics for Health and Social Care, 46*(1), 1–17.

Shakespeare, T. (2013). *Disability rights and wrongs revisited.* Routledge.

Schmutz, J. B., Meier, L. L., & Manser, T. (2019). How effective is teamwork really? The relationship between teamwork and performance in healthcare teams: a systematic review and meta-analysis. *British Medical Journal Open, 9*(9), 1–16. doi:10.1136/ bmjopen-2018-028280

Tucker, R., Frawley, P., Lozanovska, M., & Prain, M. (2022). Co-designing in Australia housing for people with intellectual disability: an integrative literature review. *Journal of Housing and the Built Environment, 37,* 2215–2235. https://doi.org/10.1007/s10901-022-09948-y

UNCRPD. (2006). *United Nations Convention on the Rights of Persons with Disabilities.* New York: United Nations.

UNICEF. (2021). *A Rights-Based Approach to Disability in the Context of Mental Health.* United Nations Children's Fund (UNICEF), New York.

Wei, H. (2022). The development of an evidence-informed Convergent Care Theory: Working together to achieve optimal health outcomes. *International Journal of Nursing Science, 9*(1), 11–25. doi: 10.1016/j.ijnss.2021.12.009

Weller, J., Boyd, M., & Cumin, D. (2014). Teams, tribes, and patient safety: overcoming barriers to effective teamwork in healthcare. *Postgrad Medical Journal, 90*(1061), 149–154. doi: 10.1136/postgradmedj-2012-131168

World Health Organization. (2007). *Everybody's business: strengthening health systems to improve health outcomes. WHO's framework for action.* Geneva: World Health Organization. https://apps.who.int/iris/handle/10665/43918

World Health Organization. (2011). World Report on Disability. Retrieved September 13, 2022, https://www.who.int/teams/noncommunicable-diseases/sensory-functions-disability-and-rehabilitation/world-report-on-disability

World Health Organization. (2021). *Guidance on Community Mental Health Services. promoting person-centred and rights-based approaches.* Geneva: WHO. https://www.who.int/publications/i/item/guidance-and-technical-packages-on-community-mental-health-services

World Health Organization. (2022a). *Global report on health equity for persons with disabilities.* Geneva: WHO. https://www.who.int/publications/i/item/9789240063600

World Health Organization. (2022b). *European framework for action to achieve the highest attainable standard of health for persons with disabilities 2022–2030.* Copenhagen: WHO Regional Office for Europe.

World Health Organization & United Nations Human Rights Office of the High Commissioner. (2023). *Mental health, human rights and legislation: guidance and practice*. Geneva.

Zajac, S., Woods, A., Tannenbaum, S., Salas, E., & Holladay C. L. (2021). Overcoming Challenges to Teamwork in Healthcare: A Team Effectiveness Framework and Evidence-Based Guidance. *Frontiers in Communication*, 6(606445), 1–20. https://doi.org/10.3389/fcomm.2021.606445

Index

For the benefit of digital users, indexed terms that span two pages (e.g., 52–53) may, on occasion, appear on only one of those pages.

Tables and figures are indicated by an italic *t* and *f* following the page number.